281
Current Topics in Microbiology and Immunology

Editors

R.W. Compans, Atlanta/Georgia
M.D. Cooper, Birmingham/Alabama
H. Koprowski, Philadelphia/Pennsylvania
F. Melchers, Basel · M.B.A. Oldstone, La Jolla/California
S. Olsnes, Oslo · M. Potter, Bethesda/Maryland
P.K. Vogt, La Jolla/California · H. Wagner, Munich

Springer
Berlin
Heidelberg
New York
Hong Kong
London
Milan
Paris
Tokyo

J.A.T. Young (Ed.)

Cellular Factors Involved in Early Steps of Retroviral Replication

With 21 Figures and 1 Table

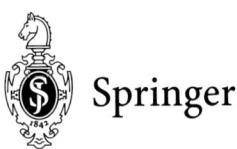 Springer

John A.T. Young
The Howard M. Temin, Professor in Cancer Research
University Wisconsin, Madison, Department of Oncology
McArdle Laboratory for Cancer Research, 1400 University Avenue
Madison, WI 53706, USA
e-mail: johnyoung@wisc.edu

***Cover Illustration (part) by Jeffrey D. Dvorin and Michael H. Malim
(see complete figure this volume)
Model for early steps in HIV-1 life cycle***

Following binding and membrane fusion, the viral core is released into the cytoplasm. A series of uncoating steps follow, preparing the intracellular viral nucleoprotein complex (NPC) for reverse transcription. During or after this step, the viral reverse transcription complex (RTC) is transported along microtubules toward the nucleus. The RTC, together with cellular proteins interacts with the nuclear pore promoting active nuclear import followed by additional uncoating steps that lead to the formation of the preintegration complex (PIC). The PIC directs the integration of viral DNA into a host cell chromosome leading to the formation of the provirus.

ISSN 0070-217X
ISBN 3-540-00844-6
Springer-Verlag Berlin Heidelberg New York

Library of Congress Catalog Card Number 72-152360

This work is subject to copyright. All rights are reserved, whether the whole or part of the material is concerned, specifically the rights of translation, reprinting, reuse of illustrations, recitation, broadcasting, reproduction on microfilm or in any other way, and storage in data banks. Duplication of this publication or parts thereof is permitted only under the provisions of the German Copyright Law of September 9, 1965, in its current version, and permission for use must always be obtained from Springer-Verlag. Violations are liable for prosecution under the German Copyright Law.

Springer-Verlag Berlin Heidelberg New York
a member of BertelsmannSpringer Science+Business Media GmbH

http://www.springer.de

© Springer-Verlag Berlin Heidelberg 2003
Library of Congress Catalog Card Number 15-12910
Printed in Germany. Not for Sale.

The use of general descriptive names, registered names, trademarks, etc. in this publication does not imply, even in the absence of a specific statement, that such names are exempt from the relevant protective laws and regulations and therefore free for general use.

Cover Design: Design & Production GmbH, Heidelberg
Typesetting: Stürtz AG, Würzburg
Production Editor: Angélique Gcouta, Berlin
Printed on acid-free paper   SPIN: 10915059   27/3020   5 4 3 2 1 0

Preface

The early steps of retroviral replication involve virus-cell membrane fusion, reverse transcription, and integration of the double-stranded viral DNA genome into a host cell chromosome. To facilitate these events, retroviruses exploit a number of diverse cellular factors including specific cell surface receptors, components of the cellular cytoskeleton, and factors involved in nucleocytoplasmic transport.

The first step of retroviral entry involves virion adsorption to the target cell surface followed by viral envelope (Env) glycoprotein interactions with specific cell surface receptors and coreceptors. Many retroviral receptors and coreceptors have been identified over the course of the last 15 years. The vast majority of these proteins have multiple membrane-spanning domains and include G-protein-coupled chemokine receptors and amino acid, or ion, transporters. However, other retroviral receptors are simple type-1 membrane proteins such as CD4 for human and simian immunodeficiency viruses and the low-density lipoprotein receptor-related and tumor necrosis factor receptor-related receptors for alpharetroviruses.

It is widely accepted that entry begins with receptor/coreceptor-induced conformational changes in Env. For most retroviruses, these changes are thought to be sufficient to induce virus-cell membrane fusion at the cell surface. However, in the case of the alpharetroviruses, there is a strong body of evidence indicating that receptor-induced changes render Env competent for mediating fusion only in response to the low-pH environment of an acidic endosomal compartment. Knowledge gained from studying these basic mechanisms of retroviral entry is being applied to the design of novel approaches for selectively targeting retroviral vectors to specific cell types for gene therapy applications.

After fusion, the viral nucleoprotein complex containing two copies of viral genomic RNA is released into the target cell cytoplasm where "uncoating" occurs before reverse transcription. This uncoating step is one of the most poorly defined of all retroviral replication steps, and consequently it is now becoming the subject of intense scientific interest. The viral reverse transcription complex (RTC) is trafficked to the nucleus by a mechanism that is also not at all well understood. However, in the case of HIV-1, this transport is predicted to involve microtubules and components of the cellular nucleocytoplasmic transport machinery. Once in the nucleus, the viral preintegration complex (PIC) mediates the integration of viral DNA into a host cell chromosome by a mechanism influenced by cellular factors including HMGA1 proteins and barrier-to-autointegration factor (BAF).

The chapters in this volume provide a comprehensive overview of our current understanding of the roles played by cellular factors in facilitation of retroviral replication. A better understanding of these functions will provide critical new insights into retrovirus-host cell interactions and is likely to prove useful for the future development of effective antiretroviral therapies.

May 2003   John A.T. Young

List of Contents

HIV-1 Entry and Its Inhibition
T.C. Pierson and R.W. Doms   1

Cell Surface Receptors for Gammaretroviruses
C.S. Tailor, D. Lavillette, M. Marin, and D. Kabat 29

Alpharetrovirus Envelope-Receptor Interactions
R.J.O. Barnard and J.A.T. Young 107

Targeting Retroviral and Lentiviral Vectors
V. Sandrin, S.J. Russell, and F.-L. Cosset 137

Intracellular Trafficking of HIV-1 Cores: Journey to the Center
of the Cell
J.D. Dvorin and M.H. Malim 179

The Roles of Cellular Factors in Retroviral Integration
A. Engelman 209

Subject Index 239

List of Contributors

(Their addresses can be found at the beginning of their respective chapters.)

BARNARD, R.J.O.   107

COSSET, F.-L.   137

DOMS, R.W.   1

DVORIN, J.D.   179

ENGELMAN, A.   209

KABAT, D.   29

LAVILLETTE, D.   29

MALIM, M.H.   179

MARIN, M.   29

PIERSON, T.C.   1

RUSSELL, S.J.   137

SANDRIN, V.   137

TAILOR, C.S.   29

YOUNG, J.A.T.   107

HIV-1 Entry and Its Inhibition

T. C. Pierson · R. W. Doms

Department of Microbiology, University of Pennsylvania,
301C Johnson Pavilion, 3610 Hamilton Walk, Philadelphia, PA 19104, USA
E-mail: tpierson@mail.med.upenn.edu
E-mail: doms@mail.med.upenn.edu

1	Introduction	2
2	HIV-1 Entry	3
2.1	Attachment to the Cell Surface	3
2.2	CD4 Binding	5
2.3	Chemokine Receptors	7
2.4	CD4-Independent HIV-1 Infection: A Special Case	8
2.5	The Fusion Machinery: gp41	9
3	Targeting the Entry Process	10
3.1	Inhibitors of CD4 Binding	10
3.2	Inhibitors of the CCR5-gp120 Interaction	10
3.3	Inhibitors of the CXCR4-gp120 Interaction	11
3.4	Peptides Derived from gp41 Inhibit HIV-1 Infection	12
3.4.1	T20 and T1249	12
3.4.2	Small-Molecule Inhibitors of Six-Helix Bundle Formation	14
4	Bringing it Together: A Model of Membrane Fusion	14
4.1	A Requirement for Cooperativity	16
	References	17

Abstract Entry of HIV-1 virions into cells is a complex and dynamic process carried out by envelope (Env) glycoproteins on the surface of the virion that promote the thermodynamically unfavorable fusion of highly stable viral and target cell membranes. Insight gained from studies of the mechanism of viral entry allowed insight into the design of novel inhibitors of HIV-1 entry, several of which are now in clinical trials. This review highlights the mechanism by which viral and cellular proteins mediate entry of HIV-1 into permissive cells, with an emphasis on targeting this process in the design of novel therapies that target distinct steps of the entry process, including antagonizing receptor binding events and blocking conformational changes intimately involved in membrane fusion.

1
Introduction

Current antiviral regimens for treatment of HIV-1 infection employ combinations of three classes of drugs that target two different points in the retroviral lifecycle (reviewed in Richman 2001). Widespread use of these drugs has resulted in a dramatic decrease in mortality associated with the onset of HIV-1-related disease (AIDS) (Gulick et al. 1997; Hammer et al. 1997). The development of class resistance, transmission of resistant viruses (Boden et al. 1999; Brenner et al. 2002; Little et al. 1999; Yerly et al. 1999), and treatment fatigue due to the development of serious drug-associated pathology (Carr and Cooper 2000; Carr et al. 1999; Safrin and Grunfeld 1999) highlight the challenges of managing HIV-1 chemotherapy and the importance of continued development of novel therapies. This review discusses the mechanism by which viral and cellular proteins mediate entry of HIV-1 into permissive cells with an emphasis on targeting this process in the design of novel therapies.

Entry of HIV-1 virions into cells is a complex and dynamic process carried out by envelope (Env) glycoprotein on the surface of the virion that promotes the thermodynamically unfavorable fusion of highly stable viral and target cell membranes. The Env protein is initially synthesized as a homotrimeric polyprotein that is cleaved in the Golgi by the cellular protease furin into two functionally distinct subunits, gp120 and gp41. After cleavage, gp120 remains noncovalently associated with the membrane-spanning gp41. The role of gp120 during virus entry involves the sequential binding of host cell attachment factors, the CD4 receptor, and a coreceptor resulting in conformational changes in the gp41 subunit that ultimately lead to fusion between the viral and cellular membranes. HIV-1 tropism is largely controlled at the level of virus entry. Most HIV-1 strains use the chemokine receptors CCR5 (referred to as R5 strains) or CXCR4 (X4 strains) as coreceptors to effect cellular entry (Berger et al. 1998; reviewed in Berger et al. 1999), and it is the differential use of these coreceptors by different HIV-1 strains coupled with their patterns of expression on CD4-positive cells that largely governs viral tropism.

2
HIV-1 Entry

2.1
Attachment to the Cell Surface

The first step in HIV-1 infection involves attachment of the virion to the surface of the host cell. Although CD4 is the primary receptor for HIV (Dalgleish et al. 1984; Klatzmann et al. 1984; Maddon et al. 1986; McDougal et al. 1986) and is required for efficient viral infection, gp120 has the capacity to bind to several different molecules on the cell surface, such as DC-SIGN and heparan sulfate proteoglycans. In addition, HIV-1 virions have been shown to selectively incorporate host cell proteins, such as ICAM-1, which have the capacity to bind to their cognate receptors and facilitate attachment independent of the viral envelope proteins (reviewed in Tremblay et al. 1998). Together, attachment factors may serve to anchor virus on the surface of the cell, increasing the likelihood that it may subsequently encounter the receptors needed for virus entry and thereby increase the efficiency of virus infection.

DC-SIGN is a type II integral membrane protein with an extracellular calcium dependent (C type) lectin-binding domain that exhibits a specificity for oligosaccharides containing high-mannose structures (Feinberg et al. 2001; Mitchell et al. 2001), such as those found on the heavily glycosylated Env protein (Mizuochi et al. 1990; reviewed in Pohlmann et al. 2001a). DC-SIGN is highly expressed on dendritic cells (DCs) and binds to ICAM-3 to promote the interaction of DCs and naïve T cells (Geijtenbeek et al. 2000b). Importantly, DC-SIGN has been shown to bind HIV-1, HIV-2, and SIV to enhance infection *in cis* and *in trans* (Geijtenbeek et al. 2000a; Lee et al. 2001; Pohlmann et al. 2001b) (Fig. 1). The capacity of DC-SIGN to facilitate virus transmission and entry is not simply a function of concentrating HIV-1 virions on the cell surface. For example, murine DC-SIGN binds but does not transmit HIV-1 (Baribaud et al. 2001), and some chimeras constructed between DC-SIGN and its closely related homolog, DC-SIGNR (Bashirova et al. 2001; Pohlmann et al. 2001d), also fail to transmit bound virus (Pohlmann et al. 2001c). Thus the requirements for binding and transmission are distinct. A possible explanation for these findings is that on binding DC-SIGN, HIV-1 virions appear to be endocytosed into a low-pH compartment distinct from the late endosome, a process that was shown to be

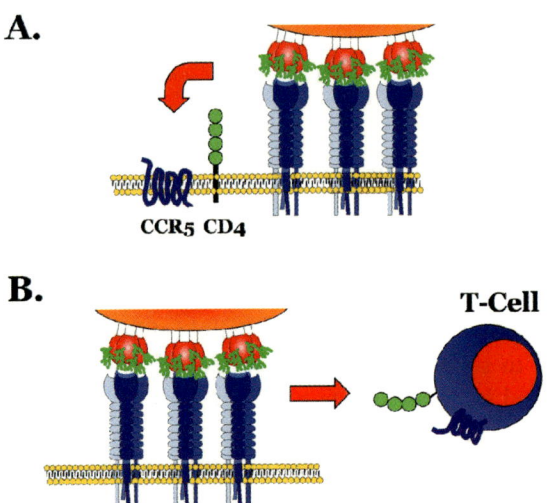

Fig. 1A, B Role of DC-SIGN in HIV-1 attachment and enhancement of infection. DC-SIGN is a C-type lectin expressed on dendritic cells capable of binding high-mannose oligosaccharides such as those on the surface of gp120. Binding of gp120 leads to attachment of the virus to the cell and can result in enhanced transmission of virus either *in cis* (**A**) or *in trans* (**B**). This interaction may have important significance for the trafficking of virions from peripheral mucosal tissues to secondary lymphoid organs where widespread infection of T lymphocytes may occur. (Modified from Pohlmann et. al. 2001)

required for enhanced transmission in the cell type studied (Kwon et al. 2002). This result is generally consistent with electron micrographs demonstrating the presence of intact viral particles inside DCs exposed to HIV-1 (Frank et al. 2002; Hladik et al. 1999).

Because DC-SIGN is expressed on mucosal DCs, it may play a role in sexual transmission of HIV-1 as these are among the first cells that HIV-1 encounters. By taking advantage of the adhesive and migratory properties of DCs, HIV-1 may be efficiently ferried to secondary lymphoid organs, the major site of virus replication in vivo (Steinman, 2000). If this model is true, then virus interactions with DC-SIGN may represent a new therapeutic target, particularly in the context of microbicides. However, other as yet unidentified molecules on DCs can also mediate virus binding and transmission (Baribaud et al. 2002; Turville et al. 2001; Wu et al. 2002). More generally, these results call for enhanced study of virus attachment factors in general, including those on other primary cell types.

2.2
CD4 Binding

A hallmark advance in our understanding of the interaction of gp120 with cellular receptors came with the crystal structure of a large fragment of the gp120 subunit complexed with a soluble fragment of CD4 and a Fab binding to an epitope exposed only after CD4 binding (Kwong et al. 1998). The structure revealed that gp120 is composed of two major domains (inner and outer) linked by a region referred to as the bridging sheet (Fig. 2A, B). The interaction of gp120 and CD4 occurs at the interface of the inner and outer domains (Kwong et al. 1998). Consistent with early biochemical and genetic evidence, the CD4 residues involved in gp120 binding are restricted to the second complementary determining region (CDR2) at the amino terminus of CD4 (Arthos et al. 1989; Clayton et al. 1988; Mizukami et al. 1988; Peterson and Seed 1988). In contrast, several discontinuous regions of gp120 are involved in CD4 binding (Kwong et al. 1998). A striking structural feature of the gp120-CD4 interface is the presence of two rather large cavities resulting from poor complementarity between the CD4 and gp120 surfaces (Kwong et al. 1998) (Fig. 2C, D). The larger of the two cavities contains variable gp120 residues that do not contact CD4 directly and is filled with water molecules. The smaller cavity, located at the junction of the bridging sheet and both inner and outer domains, appears to have a more central role in binding CD4. This 152-Å^3 cavity is lined entirely by hydrophobic residues of gp120 that form a small pocket into which Phe43 of CD4 inserts. Mutational analysis of Phe43 demonstrates that it is essential for gp120 binding (Arthos et al. 1989).

The gp120-CD4 interaction results in a complex series of structural changes in Env that result in the exposure of envelope surfaces previously masked by variable loops and formation or stabilization of the bridging sheet (Kwong et al. 1998; Sattentau and Moore, 1991; Sattentau and Moore 1995). Although structural information describing unbound native gp120 is not yet available, thermodynamic measurements reveal that the changes in Env structure resulting from CD4 binding are extensive, and involve not only the peripheral loops but the inner and outer domains of the core as well (Myszka et al. 2000). Therefore, binding CD4

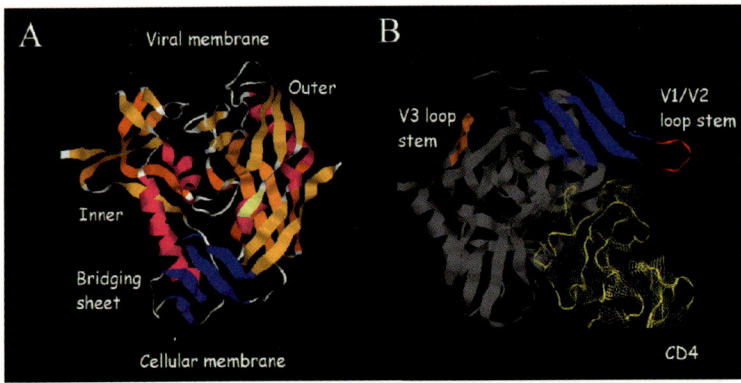
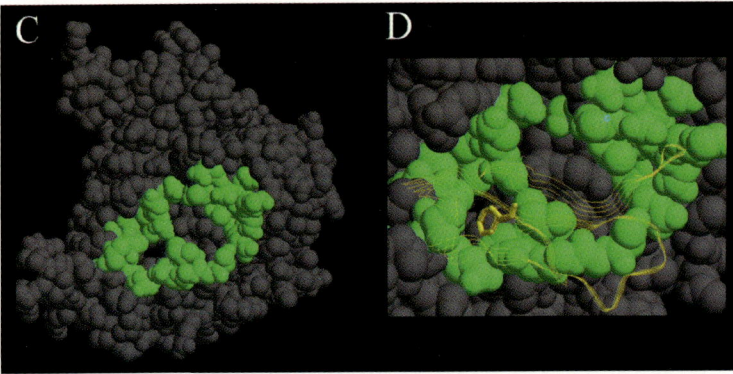

Fig. 2A–D Structural details of the gp120 core. **A** The crystal structure of a partially deglycosylated core domain of gp120 that was genetically modified such that the V1/V2 and V3 loops are absent reveals a structure composed of inner and outer domains connected by a region referred to as the bridging sheet (shown in *blue*). The bridging sheet is located on the surface of gp120 proximal to the cellular membrane, and the inner domain is adjacent to the axis of the gp120 trimer. **B** When viewed from the perspective of the cellular membrane, the location of the bridging sheet proximal to the variable loops can be appreciated. In this image CD4 is shown in *yellow*, position of the V3 loop stem in *orange*, V1/V2 stem in *red*, and the bridging sheet in *blue*. **C** The CD4 binding site on gp120 (shown in *green*) is found at the junction of the inner and outer domains of gp120. Although a considerable amount of surface area is involved, the gp120-CD4 interface demonstrates poor complementarity. Two large pockets are present, the smaller of which serves as a pocket into which inserts the highly conserved Phe43 of CD4 (**D**). (Images prepared by Mark Biscone, University of Pennsylvania)

appears to allow for the formation of a more stable form of gp120 which is capable of binding coreceptors and initiating fusion.

Primary HIV-1 strains cannot bind chemokine receptors efficiently in the absence of CD4. Therefore, it is likely that a major consequence of CD4 binding is the exposure of a coreceptor-binding site on gp120. Binding and mutagenesis studies suggest that the chemokine receptor binding site on gp120 is composed of highly conserved residues localized in or around the bridging sheet (Basmaciogullari et al. 2002; Rizzuto et al. 1998). This region of envelope, located between the bases of the V1/2 and V3 loops, faces the target cell membrane after CD4 binding, and so is in a position to interact with a chemokine receptor on the target cell surface (Kwong et al. 1998).

The structure of gp120 also sheds light on the mechanism by which HIV-1 evades the humoral immune response. Much of the surface of gp120 is masked by the presence of carbohydrate or is buried in the interface between adjoining subunits of the trimer (reviewed in Poignard et al. 2001). Regions of Env that are highly conserved because of their role in fusion, such as the CD4 binding pocket and coreceptor binding site, are protected by highly variable loops (V1/V2 and V2/V3, respectively) (Kwong et al. 1998). Current challenges involve employing new insights into the structure of Env in the generation of broadly neutralizing antibodies capable of recognizing these conserved structures, perhaps through immunization strategies aimed at targeting intermediates in the fusion process.

2.3
Chemokine Receptors

Although the role of CD4 as a receptor for HIV-1 was appreciated soon after the discovery of the virus, several lines of evidence suggested the role of additional receptors during HIV-1 infection (reviewed in Berger et al. 1999). The identification of the first HIV-1 coreceptor was accomplished by an elegant genetic approach in which a human cDNA library was screened for members capable of rendering a CD4-expressing murine cell line permissive for HIV-1 entry. This approach identified a member of the seven-transmembrane G protein-coupled superfamily of proteins, named CXCR4, capable of mediating entry of T cell line-adapted strains of HIV-1 into cells (Feng et al. 1996). Interestingly, CXCR4 was shown to play no role in the entry of macrophage tropic viruses, establishing a link between viral tropism and chemokine receptor utilization. Insight gained from this work, and the observation that a group of CC-chemokines blocked replication of some HIV-1 strains (Cocchi et al. 1995), allowed for the rapid identification of the chemokine receptor CCR5 as the coreceptor used by most primary HIV-1 strains (Alkhatib et al. 1996; Choe et al. 1996; Deng et al. 1996; Doranz et al. 1996; Dragic et al. 1996) (reviewed in Doms and Peiper, 1997 and references within).

The strongest evidence for the importance of CCR5 in HIV-1 pathogenesis is the profound resistance to HIV-1 infection of individuals homozygous for a 32-base pair inactivating deletion in CCR5 (Liu et al. 1996; Samson et al. 1996). Although individuals who have only one copy of the mutant allele exhibit only a modest degree of protection from virus infection, once infected heterozygotes typically exhibit a 2- to 4-year survival advantage, most likely caused by a modest reduction in CCR5 expression levels. The resistance of individuals who lack CCR5 to virus infection coupled with the fact that there are no significant deficits associated with the absence of this receptor make CCR5 an attractive drug target.

2.4
CD4-Independent HIV-1 Infection: A Special Case

Although the majority of HIV-1 strains utilize CD4 during entry, some SIV, HIV-2, and HIV-1 strains can bind coreceptors in the absence of CD4 (Dumonceaux et al. 1998; Edinger et al. 1997; Endres et al. 1996; Reeves et al. 1997; Reeves and Schulz 1997). This feature may confer on these viruses a more expanded tropism in vivo in situations in which CD4 is absent or limiting (Edinger et al. 1997; Reeves et al. 1999). A consequence of CD4 independence appears to be an increased sensitivity to neutralization that may be a result of stable exposure of the coreceptor-binding site (Edwards et al. 2001; Hoffman et al. 1999). Interestingly, the sera of naturally infected individuals frequently have the potential to neutralize CD4-independent viruses (Edwards et al. 2001), although the mechanisms for this are not clear. Whether such genetically "triggered" Envs will prove to be more effective immunogens remains to be determined.

2.5
The Fusion Machinery: gp41

Structural and biochemical studies of the transmembrane fusion protein of HIV-1 (gp41) provided great insight into the mechanism of virus entry and the design of novel fusion inhibitors. Analysis of the primary sequence of the ectodomain of gp41 reveals two helical regions containing conserved hydrophobic residues arranged in a 4–3 heptad repeat (Chambers et al. 1990; Delwart et al. 1990; Gallaher et al. 1989). The first helical region (HR1) is found adjacent to the glycine-rich amino-terminal fusion peptide, and the second (HR2) is located adjacent to the membrane-spanning portion of the gp41 ectodomain. During membrane fusion, it is thought that the HR1 domain forms a triple-stranded coiled coil with the adjoining HR1 domains in the Env trimer, projecting the fusion peptide in the direction of the cellular membrane. Then, after coreceptor binding, the molecule folds back on itself, forming a hairpin structure in which each HR2 domain in the trimer packs into grooves on the exterior surface of the triple-stranded coiled coil (Chan et al. 1997; Weissenhorn et al. 1997). A striking feature of the central coiled coil of gp41 is the presence of three large hydrophobic pockets found in the grooves that accommodate the HR2 helices. The residues forming the cavity are highly conserved among both HIV-1s and SIVs, making this cavity an attractive target for the design of low-molecular-weight antiviral compounds (Chan et al. 1997; Eckert et al. 1999). Interestingly, the structure of the gp41 six-helix bundle is similar not only to that of other retroviral fusion proteins (Fass and Kim, 1995) but also to that of several evolutionarily unrelated enveloped viruses including influenza (Bullough et al. 1994), simian parainfluenza virus 5 (Baker et al. 1999), and Ebola (Weissenhorn et al. 1998), suggesting a common mechanism of fusion. The role of the formation of the six-helix bundle in driving fusion is discussed below (reviewed in Weissenhorn et al. 1999).

3
Targeting the Entry Process

3.1
Inhibitors of CD4 Binding

The interaction of gp120 with CD4 was identified as a potential therapeutic target soon after the role of CD4 in HIV-1 infection became clear. Initial attempts involved the use of soluble versions of CD4 (sCD4) to block infection (Deen et al. 1988; Fisher et al. 1988; Hussey et al. 1988; Smith et al. 1987; Traunecker et al. 1988). Although sCD4 was shown to be efficacious against common laboratory strains of HIV-1, further studies demonstrated that primary isolates were relatively resistant to inhibition with sCD4 (Ashkenazi et al. 1991; Daar et al. 1990; Moore et al. 1993). A more promising approach involves the use of Pro5452, a recombinant fusion protein of both the heavy and light chains of an IgG2a antibody and the two amino-terminal Ig domains of CD4 (Allaway et al. 1995). An advantage of Pro5452 over sCD4 is that the interaction is tetravalent and thus binds Env with a higher avidity (Zhu et al. 2001). This chimeric molecule has been shown to neutralize many strains of HIV-1 ex vivo and can protect hu-PBL-SCID mice from virus challenge (Gauduin et al. 1996; Gauduin et al. 1998; Trkola et al. 1995). Clinical trials in both adults and children have been reported and demonstrate that Pro5452 is effective at reducing viral burden in vivo (Jacobson et al. 2000; Shearer et al. 2000).

3.2
Inhibitors of the CCR5-gp120 Interaction

The profound resistance of healthy individuals who do not express functional CCR5 to HIV-1 infection highlights its utility as a potential drug target (Liu et al. 1996; Samson et al. 1996). Several approaches toward antagonizing the gp120-CCR5 interaction have been pursued. Although the natural chemokine ligands for CCR5 as well as several of their synthetic derivatives have some capacity to inhibit the replication of R5 strains of HIV-1 (Cocchi et al. 1995), their utility as antiviral agents in vivo is limited.

In contrast, small-molecule CCR5 inhibitors have the advantage of oral bioavailability, improved pharmacokinetics, and most likely, reduced cost. Several nonpeptide small-molecule inhibitors of CCR5 binding are under development (Baba et al. 1999; Dragic et al. 2000; Maeda et al. 2001; Strizki et al. 2001). TAK-779 is a small organic molecule (531.13 Da) that inhibits replication of R5 strains when present at nanomolar concentrations (Baba et al. 1999; Dragic et al. 2000). Interestingly, TAK-779 binds in a cavity formed among several of the transmembrane helices of CCR5 but does not result in CCR5 signaling or internalization (Baba et al. 1999). Although TAK-779 does not block replication of HIV-1 utilizing CXCR4, it has some activity against viruses utilizing CCR2b such as SIVrcm (Zhang et al. 2000). SCH-C is a low-molecular-weight oxime-piperdine compound that binds CCR5 and blocks replication of a large number of primary R5 viruses at nanomolar concentrations in vitro and in the SCID-hu Thy/Liv mouse model (Strizki et al. 2001). SCH-C is now in clinical trials, and early results from a Phase 1b study show that it reduces virus load in vivo.

3.3
Inhibitors of the CXCR4-gp120 Interaction

The interaction of CXCR4 and gp120 is also a potentially viable target for therapy. Unlike the situation for CCR5, long-term blockade of CXCR4 may have negative consequences, as evidenced by the requirement of CXCR4 and its ligand SDF-1a for murine development (Nagasawa et al. 1996; Tachibana et al. 1998; Zou et al. 1998). The best-studied low-molecular-weight compound that targets the gp120-CXCR4 interaction is the bicyclam AMD3100 (De Clercq et al. 1994). AMD3100 blocks entry of viruses through a blockade of CXCR4, with no detectable inhibition of R5 strains (Donzella et al. 1998; Schols et al. 1997). Although AMD3100 has been shown to be effective in murine models of infection (Datema et al. 1996), human clinical trials were halted because of a failure to meet efficacy goals and undesirable cardiac effects (Hendrix C., 2002). As a proof of principle, AMD3100 was shown to significantly reduce viral load in the one patient in the trial with documented X4 virus and to eliminate X4 viruses from those volunteers with a mixture of R5 and X4 variants (Schols, 2002). Several other CXCR4 inhibitors are in development including the polyphemusin analogs T22 (Murakami et al. 1997; Nakashima et al. 1992), T134 (Arakaki et al. 1999), and T140 (Tamamura et al. 1998) (derived from defensin peptides in the blood of the horseshoe crab), as well as the d-Arg peptide ALX40-4 (Doranz et al.

1997). Importantly, ALX40-4C was well tolerated in a Phase I clinical trial, indicating that CXCR4 inhibition may be tolerated in adults (Doranz et al. 2001).

Strategies directed at blocking gp120-chemokine receptor interactions have the potential to drive the selection of viral variants utilizing different receptors during entry. This may be particularly problematic when antagonizing CCR5 as the evolution of viruses that utilize CXCR4 has been associated with progression to AIDS. Mosier et al. demonstrated the selection of virus utilizing CXCR4 after the use of NNY-RANTES in the hu-PBL-SCID system (Mosier et al. 1999). Similar studies demonstrate that escape from coreceptor blockade ex vivo involves adaptation at the level of coreceptor choice (Este et al. 1999). However, other mechanisms of adaptation are possible. A recent study demonstrated that adaptation of an R5 strain to growth in the presence of a CCR5 antagonist (AD101) involved an alteration in the manner in which the virus interacted with CCR5 rather than a switch in coreceptor usage (Trkola et al. 2002). The implications of this for viral pathogenesis are not known. However, the use of coreceptor antagonists will have practical implications for clinical management. The use of a CXCR4 antagonist in a patient who harbors R5 virus strains would not be expected to have a significant impact on virus load, nor would a CCR5 antagonist be expected to reduce virus load in a patient who harbors mostly X4 virus strains. Thus virus phenotype as well as virus load may have to be measured in order to develop an appropriate treatment strategy for any given patient.

3.4
Peptides Derived from gp41 Inhibit HIV-1 Infection

3.4.1
T20 and T1249

T20 is a synthetic peptide composed of a 36-amino acid sequence that mimics the HR2 region of gp41. In vitro studies demonstrate that this peptide inhibitor binds to the triple-stranded coiled coil formed by the HR1 domain and is potent at nanomolar concentrations against diverse laboratory and primary virus isolates of HIV-1 (Derdeyn et al. 2000; Derdeyn et al. 2001; Rimsky et al. 1998; Wild et al. 1993; Wild et al. 1992). A Phase I/IIB trial of T20 safety and efficacy has been conducted and demonstrated a substantial 1.9 log reduction in plasma viral load in four patients receiving 100 mg/ml of peptide twice daily (Kilby et al. 1998). Continued assessment of the clinical utility of T20, as part of a salvage HAART regimen, is underway (reviewed in LaBranche et al. 2001). T1249 is a second-generation peptide inhibitor derived from the HR2 sequence of HIV-1, HIV-2, and SIV. T1249 binds in a region that overlaps much of the T20 binding site but is positioned to cover the highly conserved deep hydrophobic pocket described above. In agreement with the highly conserved structure of many viral fusion proteins, similar peptide inhibitors have been designed for other viruses including paramyxovirus (Lambert et al. 1996), Ebola (Watanabe et al. 2000), and RSV (Netter and Bates, submitted).

Although T20 and T1249 exhibit broad antiviral activity, there is considerable variation in the sensitivity of HIV-1 to T20 and other peptide inhibitors. In vitro selection of an X4 virus resistant to T20 inhibition identified three highly conserved amino acids in HR1 that are involved in T20 resistance (Rimsky, 1998). Additionally, resistant virus was found in treated volunteers receiving T20 monotherapy (LaBranche et al. 2001). To date, the genotype of these resistant viruses has not been reported. In addition, Derdeyn and colleagues (Derdeyn et al. 2000, 2001) found that sensitivity to T20 could be determined in part by determinants outside of gp41. With proviruses that differed only in the V3 region, a larger amount of T20 (0.6–0.8 logs) was required to block infection of viruses utilizing CCR5 compared with those binding to CXCR4 during entry (Derdeyn et al. 2000). The difference in sensitivity of viruses to T20 was recently shown to be a function of the affinity for coreceptor (Reeves et al. 2002).

Current peptide inhibitors like T20 and T1249 are derived from HR2 and are referred to as C-peptides. C-peptides bind to the central coiled coil of HR1 to block fusion. N-peptide inhibitors, derived from sequence in HR1, have been studied with respect to their capacity to block HIV-1 infection. These N-peptides are less potent than those derived from HR2, and they tend to form aggregates in solution (micromolar affinity) (Lu et al. 1995; Wild et al. 1992). However, use of five covalently linked N-peptides that mimic the arrangement of the HR1 helices in the six-helix bundle was shown to block HIV-1 entry at nanomolar concentrations, confirming HR2 as a viable therapeutic target (Root et al. 2001).

3.4.2
Small-Molecule Inhibitors of Six-Helix Bundle Formation

The significant challenges that exist for the delivery of therapeutic concentrations of large (4,000 Da) peptide inhibitors such as T20 has driven the development of a small -molecule inhibitor of HIV-1 entry (Eckert et al. 1999). As a proof of principle, Eckert and colleagues used mirror-image phage display technology to identify a small cyclic D peptide that bound solely in the hydrophobic pocket and was capable of blocking entry at micromolar concentrations. Further development in this area may result in the development of antiviral compounds with fewer pharmacological challenges than the current generation of peptide-based therapies that target formation of the six-helix bundle.

4
Bringing it Together: A Model of Membrane Fusion

The development of inhibitors targeting HIV-1 entry has allowed several key advances in our understanding of the mechanism of how HIV-1 Env orchestrates fusion. Fusion mediated by HIV-1 Env is temperature dependent (Frey et al. 1995). Incubation of cells expressing HIV-1 Env with receptor-bearing cells at lower temperatures allows for some, but not all, of the events leading up to fusion to occur. Experiments using this temperature-arrested state (TAS) in conjunction with a myriad of different entry inhibitors have allowed the entry process to be separated and ordered into several discrete steps (Gallo et al. 2001; Melikyan et al. 2000). When these studies were coupled with other biochemical, immunological, and structural studies, a general model of the entry of HIV-1 emerged.

After attachment to the cell surface, gp120 trimers bind CD4 with high affinity. Recent evidence suggests that interaction with three different CD4 molecules is required for efficient activation of Env (R.W. Doms, unpublished data; Layne et al. 1990). Fusion does not occur immediately after gp120-CD4 interaction. Instead, a lag phase of 15–20 min in which fusion is not detected is characteristic (Frey et al. 1995; Weiss et al. 1996). To understand the significance of the lag phase, the fusion kinetics of a CD4-independent virus was compared to the parental CD4 dependent clone and revealed a more rapid fusion rate with a significantly reduced lag time (Gallo et al. 2001). This result identifies the con-

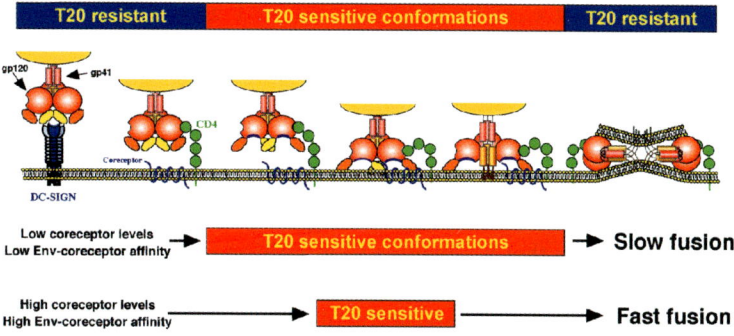

Fig. 3 Model for HIV-1 Env-mediated membrane fusion. After attachment to the cell surface, gp120 binds with high affinity to CD4 (shown in *green*). It is thought that three such binding events are required for efficient activation of a HIV-1 Env trimer. CD4 binding results in a dramatic conformational rearrangement of gp120 that results in exposure of both the coreceptor binding site and the helical repeat regions (HR1 and HR2) of gp41. Exposure of the HR1 domain makes Env sensitive to the fusion inhibitor T20 that binds to this domain. Binding to coreceptor (shown in *blue*) then occurs and is required for membrane fusion. Fusion also involves the insertion of the hydrophobic amino terminal fusion peptide of gp41 in the host cell membrane, followed by formation of the six-helix bundle and membrane fusion. As Envs that have already formed the bundle are no longer sensitive to T20, a finite window of opportunity for blockade by T20 exists between CD4 binding and membrane fusion. Factors that affect the rate with which Env promotes fusion after CD4 binding, such as affinity for coreceptor and coreceptor expression levels, may modulate sensitivity to T20 inhibition

formational changes associated with CD4 binding as rate limiting for fusion, a result consistent with the slow rate reported for the reorganization of the envelope core upon receptor binding (Myszka et al. 2000). Additional factors contributing to the lag occurring before fusion may reflect the requirement for multiple gp120 trimers to engage receptors on the target cell, as discussed in more detail below.

The ability of peptide inhibitors such as T20 or T1249 to block fusion is dependent on exposure of HR1 during the fusion process. For example, treatment of intact virions with T20, followed by removal of unbound T20, does not block entry (Furuta et al. 1998). Thus T20 does not bind to the native Env protein. Conversely, T20 is effective even when added up to 15 min after incubation of envelope and receptor (Munoz-Barroso et al. 1998). Together, these results define a kinetic window in which peptide inhibitors are efficacious (Fig. 3). Analysis of fusion at a

TAS demonstrates that CD4 binding exposes HR1 and is sufficient to render Env sensitive to T20 in the absence of detectable fusion (Gallo et al. 2001; Melikyan et al. 2000). This observation defines an intermediate of fusion, referred to as the pre-hairpin intermediate, which serves as the target of peptide inhibitors such as T20 and T1249. Taken together, the "triggering" of Env by CD4 involves both functional changes in gp120 (formation of the coreceptor binding site) and repositioning of gp41 in a conformation that is sensitive to inhibition by peptide.

Interaction of gp120 with chemokine receptors is required for HIV-1 entry. The precise function of coreceptor binding is not yet clear. Binding coreceptor may improve the efficiency and kinetics of subsequent steps in the fusion process, such as formation of the six-helix bundle (Doms 2000). In contrast to CD4, which extends well above the glycocalyx, chemokine receptors do not protrude far off the surface of the cell. This feature may facilitate insertion of the fusion peptide into the target cell membrane on chemokine receptor binding.

After CD4 and coreceptor engagement, the fusion peptide of gp41 inserts into the membrane of the target cell and a dramatic conformational change ensues that results in the formation of the six-helix bundle in which the amino terminus (inserted in the target membrane) and the carboxy terminus (inserted in the viral membrane) are pulled into close opposition. A recent study by Melikyan and colleagues provided new insight into the relationship between formation of the six-helix structure and membrane fusion (Melikyan et al. 2000). They demonstrate that addition of stearoyl-lysophosphatidylcholine (LPC), a lipid that induces positive curvature in membranes, to the outer leaflet of membranes abolishes fusion. Using LPC in conjunction with T20, they were unable to separate formation of the six-helix bundle from lipid mixing, suggesting that the formation of the six-helix bundle occurs coincident with membrane fusion. The large amount of free energy released during the transition to the highly stable six-helix bundle may serve to drive the otherwise energetically unfavorable process of fusion pore formation.

4.1
A Requirement for Cooperativity

Penetrating the membrane of a permissive host cell is an energetically formidable task mediated by the glycoproteins of enveloped viruses. The fusion of many viruses, such as influenza, is dependent on exposure to low pH. A consequence of this mechanism is that on exposure to low pH, the fusion potential of all the surface envelope is activated simultaneously, allowing for the formation of a fusion pore in a cooperative fashion involving several envelopes. In contrast, HIV-1 Env trimers are activated by receptor binding rather than protonation. This has important consequences for the kinetics and efficiency of HIV-1 entry. First, the density of receptor on the cell surface impacts the efficiency and rate of fusion. Efficient activation of gp120 requires engagement by three CD4 molecules (R.W. Doms, unpublished data). Several recent studies demonstrate that four to six CCR5 receptors are required for formation of a fusion pore (Kuhmann et al. 2000; Platt et al. 2001). Although the amount of CD4 is not limiting in most instances in vivo (Lee et al. 1999), susceptibility to HIV-1 infection is often a function of coreceptor expression, which differs among cell types and state of activation (Lee et al. 1999; Rabin et al. 1999). As discussed above, engagement of CD4 activates Env for both coreceptor binding and fusion peptide insertion. Because engagement of coreceptor is an obligate step, the proximity of a cluster of coreceptors to virus bound to CD4 may affect fusion kinetics and contribute to the lag phase discussed above. This could be especially true if CD4 and coreceptor are not found in the same membrane microdomains on the cell surface, as has been reported for CD4 and CXCR4 (Kozak et al. 2002; Manes et al. 2000). The affinity of the Env-coreceptor interaction also plays an important role as it regulates the probability that a given Env will be fully engaged by the required number of coreceptors at any given time (reviewed in Doms, 2000). Therefore, the requirement that multiple sequential envelope-receptor interactions occur before efficient fusion governs the efficiency, selectivity, and kinetics of HIV-1 entry. Our increased understanding of this dynamic process has allowed the development of some novel opportunities for intervention.

References

Alkhatib, G, Combadiere, C, Broder, CC, Feng, Y, Kennedy, PE, Murphy, PM, and Berger, EA (1996) CC CKR5: a RANTES, MIP-1alpha, MIP-1beta receptor as a fusion cofactor for macrophage-tropic HIV-1, Science 272: 1955–1958

Allaway, GP, Davis-Bruno, KL, Beaudry, GA, Garcia, EB, Wong, EL, Ryder, AM, Hasel, KW, Gauduin, MC, Koup, RA, McDougal, JS, and et al. (1995) Expression and characterization of CD4-IgG2, a novel heterotetramer that neutralizes primary HIV type 1 isolates, AIDS Res Hum Retroviruses 11: 533–9

Arakaki, R, Tamamura, H, Premanathan, M, Kanbara, K, Ramanan, S, Mochizuki, K, Baba, M, Fujii, N, and Nakashima, H (1999) T134, a small-molecule CXCR4 inhibitor, has no cross-drug resistance with AMD3100, a CXCR4 antagonist with a different structure, J Virol 73: 1719–1723

Arthos, J, Deen, KC, Chaikin, MA, Fornwald, JA, Sathe, G, Sattentau, QJ, Clapham, PR, Weiss, RA, McDougal, JS, Pietropaolo, C, et al.(1989) Identification of the residues in human CD4 critical for the binding of HIV, Cell 57: 469–481

Ashkenazi, A, Smith, DH, Marsters, SA, Riddle, L, Gregory, TJ, Ho, DD, and Capon, DJ (1991) Resistance of primary isolates of human immunodeficiency virus type 1 to soluble CD4 is independent of CD4-gp120 binding affinity, Proc Natl Acad Sci USA 88: 7056–7060

Baba, M, Nishimura, O, Kanzaki, N, Okamoto, M, Sawada, H, Iizawa, Y, Shiraishi, M, Aramaki, Y, Okonogi, K, Ogawa, Y, et al. (1999) A small-molecule, nonpeptide CCR5 antagonist with highly potent and selective anti-HIV-1 activity, Proc Natl Acad Sci USA 96: 5698–5703

Baker, KA, Dutch, RE, Lamb, RA, and Jardetzky, TS (1999) Structural basis for paramyxovirus-mediated membrane fusion, Mol Cell 3: 309–19

Baribaud, F, Pohlmann, S, Leslie, G, Mortari, F, and Doms, RW (2002) Quantitative expression and virus transmission analysis of DC-SIGN on monocyte-derived dendritic cells, J Virol 76: 9135–42

Baribaud, F, Pohlmann, S, Sparwasser, T, Kimata, MT, Choi, YK, Haggarty, BS, Ahmad, N, Macfarlan, T, Edwards, TG, Leslie, GJ, et al. (2001) Functional and antigenic characterization of human, rhesus macaque, pigtailed macaque, and murine DC-SIGN, J Virol 75: 10281–10299

Bashirova, AA, Geijtenbeek, TB, van Duijnhoven, GC, van Vliet, SJ, Eilering, JB, Martin, MP, Wu, L, Martin, TD, Viebig, N, Knolle, PA, et al. (2001) A dendritic cell-specific intercellular adhesion molecule 3-grabbing nonintegrin (DC-SIGN)-related protein is highly expressed on human liver sinusoidal endothelial cells and promotes HIV-1 infection, J Exp Med 193: 671–8

Basmaciogullari, S, Babcock, GJ, Van Ryk, D, Wojtowicz, W, and Sodroski, J (2002) Identification of conserved and variable structures in the human immunodeficiency virus gp120 glycoprotein of importance for CXCR4 binding, J Virol 76: 10791–800

Berger, EA, Doms, RW, Fenyo, EM, Korber, BT, Littman, DR, Moore, JP, Sattentau, QJ, Schuitemaker, H, Sodroski, J, and Weiss, RA (1998) A new classification for HIV-1, Nature 391: 240

Berger, EA, Murphy, PM, and Farber, JM (1999) Chemokine receptors as HIV-1 coreceptors: roles in viral entry, tropism, and disease, Annu Rev Immunol 17: 657–700

Boden, D, Hurley, A, Zhang, L, Cao, Y, Guo, Y, Jones, E, Tsay, J, Ip, J, Farthing, C, Limoli, K, et al. (1999) HIV-1 drug resistance in newly infected individuals, JAMA 282: 1135–41

Brenner, BG, Routy, JP, Petrella, M, Moisi, D, Oliveira, M, Detorio, M, Spira, B, Essabag, V, Conway, B, Lalonde, R, et al. (2002) Persistence and fitness of multidrug-resistant human immunodeficiency virus type 1 acquired in primary infection, J Virol 76: 1753-61

Bullough, PA, Hughson, FM, Skehel, JJ, and Wiley, DC (1994) Structure of influenza haemagglutinin at the pH of membrane fusion, Nature 371: 37-43

Carr, A, and Cooper, DA (2000) Adverse effects of antiretroviral therapy, Lancet 356: 1423-30

Carr, A, Samaras, K, Thorisdottir, A, Kaufmann, GR, Chisholm, DJ, and Cooper, DA (1999) Diagnosis, prediction, and natural course of HIV-1 protease-inhibitor- associated lipodystrophy, hyperlipidaemia, and diabetes mellitus: a cohort study, Lancet 353: 2093-9

Chambers, P, Pringle, CR, and Easton, AJ (1990) Heptad repeat sequences are located adjacent to hydrophobic regions in several types of virus fusion glycoproteins, J Gen Virol 71: 3075-80

Chan, DC, Fass, D, Berger, JM, and Kim, PS (1997) Core structure of gp41 from the HIV envelope glycoprotein, Cell 89: 263-273

Choe, H, Farzan, M, Sun, Y, Sullivan, N, Rollins, B, Ponath, PD, Wu, L, Mackay, CR, LaRosa, G, Newman, W, et al. (1996) The beta-chemokine receptors CCR3 and CCR5 facilitate infection by primary HIV-1 isolates, Cell 85: 1135-1148

Clayton, LK, Hussey, RE, Steinbrich, R, Ramachandran, H, Husain, Y, and Reinherz, EL (1988) Substitution of murine for human CD4 residues identifies amino acids critical for HIV-gp120 binding, Nature 335: 363-6

Cocchi, F, DeVico, AL, Garzino-Demo, A, Arya, SK, Gallo, RC, and Lusso, P (1995) Identification of RANTES, MIP-1 alpha, and MIP-1 beta as the major HIV- suppressive factors produced by CD8+ T cells, Science 270: 1811-1815

Daar, ES, Li, XL, Moudgil, T, and Ho, DD (1990) High concentrations of recombinant soluble CD4 are required to neutralize primary human immunodeficiency virus type 1 isolates, Proc Natl Acad Sci USA 87: 6574-6578

Dalgleish, AG, Beverley, PC, Clapham, PR, Crawford, DH, Greaves, MF, and Weiss, RA (1984) The CD4 (T4) antigen is an essential component of the receptor for the AIDS retrovirus, Nature 312: 763-767

Datema, R, Rabin, L, Hincenbergs, M, Moreno, MB, Warren, S, Linquist, V, Rosenwirth, B, Seifert, J, and McCune, JM (1996) Antiviral efficacy in vivo of the anti-human immunodeficiency virus bicyclam SDZ SID 791 (JM 3100), an inhibitor of infectious cell entry, Antimicrob Agents Chemother 40: 750-4

De Clercq, E, Yamamoto, N, Pauwels, R, Balzarini, J, Witvrouw, M, De Vreese, K, Debyser, Z, Rosenwirth, B, Peichl, P, Datema, R, et al. (1994) Highly potent and selective inhibition of human immunodeficiency virus by the bicyclam derivative JM3100, Antimicrob Agents Chemother 38: 668-674

Deen, KC, McDougal, JS, Inacker, R, Folena-Wasserman, G, Arthos, J, Rosenberg, J, Maddon, PJ, Axel, R, and Sweet, RW (1988) A soluble form of CD4 (T4) protein inhibits AIDS virus infection, Nature 331: 82-84

Delwart, EL, Mosialos, G, and Gilmore, T (1990) Retroviral envelope glycoproteins contain a "leucine zipper"-like repeat, AIDS Res Hum Retroviruses 6: 703-6

Deng, H, Liu, R, Ellmeier, W, Choe, S, Unutmaz, D, Burkhart, M, Di Marzio, P, Marmon, S, Sutton, RE, Hill, CM, et al. (1996) Identification of a major co-receptor for primary isolates of HIV-1, Nature 381: 661-666

Derdeyn, CA, Decker, JM, Sfakianos, JN, Wu, X, O'Brien, WA, Ratner, L, Kappes, JC, Shaw, GM, and Hunter, E (2000) Sensitivity of human immunodeficiency virus type 1 to the fusion inhibitor T-20 is modulated by coreceptor specificity defined by the V3 loop of gp120, J Virol 74: 8358–67

Derdeyn, CA, Decker, JM, Sfakianos, JN, Zhang, Z, O'Brien, WA, Ratner, L, Shaw, GM, and Hunter, E (2001) Sensitivity of human immunodeficiency virus type 1 to fusion inhibitors targeted to the gp41 first heptad repeat involves distinct regions of gp41 and is consistently modulated by gp120 interactions with the coreceptor, J Virol 75: 8605–14

Doms, RW (2000) Beyond receptor expression: the influence of receptor conformation, density, and affinity in HIV-1 infection, Virology 276: 229–237

Doms, RW, and Peiper, SC (1997) Unwelcomed guests with master keys: how HIV uses chemokine receptors for cellular entry, Virology 235: 179–90

Donzella, GA, Schols, D, Lin, SW, Este, JA, Nagashima, KA, Maddon, PJ, Allaway, GP, Sakmar, TP, Henson, G, De Clercq, E, and Moore, JP (1998) AMD3100, a small molecule inhibitor of HIV-1 entry via the CXCR4 co-receptor, Nat Med 4: 72–77

Doranz, BJ, Filion, LG, Diaz-Mitoma, F, Sitar, DS, Sahai, J, Baribaud, F, Orsini, MJ, Benovic, JL, Cameron, W, and Doms, RW (2001) Safe use of the CXCR4 inhibitor ALX40-4C in humans, AIDS Res Hum Retroviruses 17: 475–486

Doranz, BJ, Grovit-Ferbas, K, Sharron, MP, Mao, SH, Goetz, MB, Daar, ES, Doms, RW, and O'Brien, WA (1997) A small-molecule inhibitor directed against the chemokine receptor CXCR4 prevents its use as an HIV-1 coreceptor, J Exp Med 186: 1395–1400

Doranz, BJ, Rucker, J, Yi, Y, Smyth, RJ, Samson, M, Peiper, SC, Parmentier, M, Collman, RG, and Doms, RW (1996) A dual-tropic primary HIV-1 isolate that uses fusin and the beta-chemokine receptors CKR-5, CKR-3, and CKR-2b as fusion cofactors, Cell 85: 1149–1158

Dragic, T, Litwin, V, Allaway, GP, Martin, SR, Huang, Y, Nagashima, KA, Cayanan, C, Maddon, PJ, Koup, RA, Moore, JP, and Paxton, WA (1996) HIV-1 entry into CD4+ cells is mediated by the chemokine receptor CC-CKR-5, Nature 381: 667–673

Dragic, T, Trkola, A, Thompson, DA, Cormier, EG, Kajumo, FA, Maxwell, E, Lin, SW, Ying, W, Smith, SO, Sakmar, TP, and Moore, JP (2000) A binding pocket for a small molecule inhibitor of HIV-1 entry within the transmembrane helices of CCR5, Proc Natl Acad Sci U S A 97: 5639–5644

Dumonceaux, J, Nisole, S, Chanel, C, Quivet, L, Amara, A, Baleux, F, Briand, P, and Hazan, U (1998) Spontaneous mutations in the env gene of the human immunodeficiency virus type 1 NDK isolate are associated with a CD4-independent entry phenotype, J Virol 72: 512–519

Eckert, DM, Malashkevich, VN, Hong, LH, Carr, PA, and Kim, PS (1999) Inhibiting HIV-1 entry: discovery of D-peptide inhibitors that target the gp41 coiled-coil pocket, Cell 99: 103–15

Edinger, AL, Mankowski, JL, Doranz, BJ, Margulies, BJ, Lee, B, Rucker, J, Sharron, M, Hoffman, TL, Berson, JF, Zink, MC, et al. (1997) CD4-independent, CCR5-dependent infection of brain capillary endothelial cells by a neurovirulent simian immunodeficiency virus strain, Proc Natl Acad Sci USA 94: 14742–14747

Edwards, TG, Hoffman, TL, Baribaud, F, Wyss, S, LaBranche, CC, Romano, J, Adkinson, J, Sharron, M, Hoxie, JA, and Doms, RW (2001) Relationships between

CD4 independence, neutralization sensitivity, and exposure of a CD4-induced epitope in a human immunodeficiency virus type 1 envelope protein, J Virol 75: 5230–5239

Endres, MJ, Clapham, PR, Marsh, M, Ahuja, M, Turner, JD, McKnight, A, Thomas, JF, Stoebenau-Haggarty, B, Choe, S, Vance, PJ, et al. (1996) CD4-independent infection by HIV-2 is mediated by fusin/CXCR4, Cell 87: 745–756

Este, JA, Cabrera, C, Blanco, J, Gutierrez, A, Bridger, G, Henson, G, Clotet, B, Schols, D, and De Clercq, E (1999) Shift of clinical human immunodeficiency virus type 1 isolates from X4 to R5 and prevention of emergence of the syncytium-inducing phenotype by blockade of CXCR4, J Virol 73: 5577–85

Fass, D, and Kim, PS (1995) Dissection of a retrovirus envelope protein reveals structural similarity to influenza hemagglutinin, Curr Biol 5: 1377–83

Feinberg, H, Mitchell, DA, Drickamer, K, and Weis, WI (2001) Structural basis for selective recognition of oligosaccharides by DC-SIGN and DC-SIGNR, Science 294: 2163–6

Feng, Y, Broder, CC, Kennedy, PE, and Berger, EA (1996) HIV-1 entry cofactor: functional cDNA cloning of a seven-transmembrane, G protein-coupled receptor, Science 272: 872–877

Fisher, RA, Bertonis, JM, Meier, W, Johnson, VA, Costopoulos, DS, Liu, T, Tizard, R, Walker, BD, Hirsch, MS, Schooley, RT, and Flavell, RA (1988) HIV infection is blocked in vitro by recombinant soluble CD4, Nature 331: 76–78

Frank, I, Piatak, M, Jr., Stoessel, H, Romani, N, Bonnyay, D, Lifson, JD, and Pope, M (2002) Infectious and whole inactivated simian immunodeficiency viruses interact similarly with primate dendritic cells (DCs): differential intracellular fate of virions in mature and immature DCs, J Virol 76: 2936–51

Frey, S, Marsh, M, Gunther, S, Pelchen-Matthews, A, Stephens, P, Ortlepp, S, and Stegmann, T (1995) Temperature dependence of cell-cell fusion induced by the envelope glycoprotein of human immunodeficiency virus type I, J Virol 69: 1462–1472

Furuta, RA, Wild, CT, Weng, Y, and Weiss, CD (1998) Capture of an early fusion-active conformation of HIV-1 gp41, Nat Struct Biol 5: 276–9

Gallaher, WR, Ball, JM, Garry, RF, Griffin, MC, and Montelaro, RC (1989) A general model for the transmembrane proteins of HIV and other retroviruses, AIDS Res Hum Retroviruses 5: 431–440

Gallo, SA, Puri, A, and Blumenthal, R (2001) HIV-1 gp41 six-helix bundle formation occurs rapidly after the engagement of gp120 by CXCR4 in the HIV-1 Env-mediated fusion process, Biochemistry (Mosc) 40: 12231–6

Gauduin, MC, Allaway, GP, Maddon, PJ, Barbas, CF 3rd, Burton, DR, and Koup, RA (1996) Effective ex vivo neutralization of human immunodeficiency virus type 1 in plasma by recombinant immunoglobulin molecules, J Virol 70: 2586–92

Gauduin, MC, Allaway, GP, Olson, WC, Weir, R, Maddon, PJ, and Koup, RA (1998) CD4-immunoglobulin G2 protects Hu-PBL-SCID mice against challenge by primary human immunodeficiency virus type 1 isolates, J Virol 72: 3475–8

Geijtenbeek, TB, Kwon, DS, Torensma, R, van Vliet, SJ, van Duijnhoven, GC, Middel, J, Cornelissen, IL, Nottet, HS, KewalRamani, VN, Littman, DR, et al. (2000a) DC-SIGN, a dendritic cell-specific HIV-1-binding protein that enhances trans-infection of T cells, Cell 100: 587–597

Geijtenbeek, TB, Torensma, R, van Vliet, SJ, van Duijnhoven, GC, Adema, GJ, van Kooyk, Y, and Figdor, CG (2000b) Identification of DC-SIGN, a novel dendritic cell-specific ICAM-3 receptor that supports primary immune responses, Cell 100: 575–585

Gulick, RM, Mellors, JW, Havlir, D, Eron, JJ, Gonzalez, C, McMahon, D, Richman, DD, Valentine, FT, Jonas, L, Meibohm, A, et al. (1997) Treatment with indinavir, zidovudine, and lamivudine in adults with human immunodeficiency virus infection and prior antiretroviral therapy, N Engl J Med 337: 734–9

Hammer, SM, Squires, KE, Hughes, MD, Grimes, JM, Demeter, LM, Currier, JS, Eron, JJ, Jr., Feinberg, JE, Balfour, HH, Jr., Deyton, LR, et al. (1997) A controlled trial of two nucleoside analogues plus indinavir in persons with human immunodeficiency virus infection and CD4 cell counts of 200 per cubic millimeter or less. AIDS Clinical Trials Group 320 Study Team, N Engl J Med 337: 725–33

Hendrix C., AC, M. Lederman, R. Pollard, S. Brown, M. Glesby, C. Flexner, G. Bridger, K. Badel, R. MacFarland, G. Henson, and G. Calandra, the AMD-3100 HIV Study Group (2002) AMD-3100 CXXCR4 Receptor Blocker Fails to Reduce HIV Viral Load by >1 Log following 10-Day Continuous Infusion. Paper presented at: 9th Conference on Retroviruses and Opportunistic Infections

Hladik, F, Lentz, G, Akridge, RE, Peterson, G, Kelley, H, McElroy, A, and McElrath, MJ (1999) Dendritic cell-T-cell interactions support coreceptor-independent human immunodeficiency virus type 1 transmission in the human genital tract, J Virol 73: 5833–42

Hoffman, TL, LaBranche, CC, Zhang, W, Canziani, G, Robinson, J, Chaiken, I, Hoxie, JA, and Doms, RW (1999) Stable exposure of the coreceptor-binding site in a CD4-independent HIV-1 envelope protein, Proc Natl Acad Sci USA 96: 6359–6364

Hussey, RE, Richardson, NE, Kowalski, M, Brown, NR, Chang, HC, Siliciano, RF, Dorfman, T, Walker, B, Sodroski, J, and Reinherz, EL (1988) A soluble CD4 protein selectively inhibits HIV replication and syncytium formation, Nature 331: 78–81

Jacobson, JM, Lowy, I, Fletcher, CV, O'Neill, TJ, Tran, DN, Ketas, TJ, Trkola, A, Klotman, ME, Maddon, PJ, Olson, WC, and Israel, RJ (2000) Single-dose safety, pharmacology, and antiviral activity of the human immunodeficiency virus (HIV) type 1 entry inhibitor PRO 542 in HIV-infected adults, J Infect Dis 182: 326–9

Kilby, JM, Hopkins, S, Venetta, TM, DiMassimo, B, Cloud, GA, Lee, JY, Alldredge, L, Hunter, E, Lambert, D, Bolognesi, D, et al. (1998) Potent suppression of HIV-1 replication in humans by T-20, a peptide inhibitor of gp41-mediated virus entry, Nat Med 4: 1302–1307

Klatzmann, D, Champagne, E, Chamaret, S, Gruest, J, Guetard, D, Hercend, T, Gluckman, JC, and Montagnier, L (1984) T-lymphocyte T4 molecule behaves as the receptor for human retrovirus LAV, Nature 312: 767–768

Kozak, SL, Heard, JM, and Kabat, D (2002) Segregation of CD4 and CXCR4 into distinct lipid microdomains in T lymphocytes suggests a mechanism for membrane destabilization by human immunodeficiency virus, J Virol 76: 1802–15

Kuhmann, SE, Platt, EJ, Kozak, SL, and Kabat, D (2000) Cooperation of multiple CCR5 coreceptors is required for infections by human immunodeficiency virus type 1, J Virol 74: 7005–15

Kwon, DS, Gregorio, G, Bitton, N, Hendrickson, WA, and Littman, DR (2002) DC-SIGN-mediated internalization of HIV is required for trans-enhancement of T cell infection, Immunity 16: 135–44

Kwong, PD, Wyatt, R, Robinson, J, Sweet, RW, Sodroski, J, and Hendrickson, WA (1998) Structure of an HIV gp120 envelope glycoprotein in complex with the CD4 receptor and a neutralizing human antibody, Nature 393: 648–659

LaBranche, CC, Galasso, G, Moore, JP, Bolognesi, DP, Hirsch, MS, and Hammer, SM (2001) HIV fusion and its inhibition, Antiviral Res 50: 95–115

Lambert, DM, Barney, S, Lambert, AL, Guthrie, K, Medinas, R, Davis, DE, Bucy, T, Erickson, J, Merutka, G, and Petteway, SR Jr. (1996) Peptides from conserved regions of paramyxovirus fusion (F) proteins are potent inhibitors of viral fusion, Proc Natl Acad Sci U S A 93: 2186–91

Layne, SP, Merges, MJ, Dembo, M, Spouge, JL, and Nara, PL (1990) HIV requires multiple gp120 molecules for CD4-mediated infection, Nature 346: 277–279

Lee, B, Leslie, G, Soilleux, E, O'Doherty, U, Baik, S, Levroney, E, Flummerfelt, K, Swiggard, W, Coleman, N, Malim, M, and Doms, RW (2001) cis Expression of DC-SIGN allows for more efficient entry of human and simian immunodeficiency viruses via CD4 and a coreceptor, J Virol 75: 12028–38

Lee, B, Sharron, M, Montaner, LJ, Weissman, D, and Doms, RW (1999) Quantification of CD4, CCR5, and CXCR4 levels on lymphocyte subsets, dendritic cells, and differentially conditioned monocyte-derived macrophages, Proc Natl Acad Sci USA 96: 5215–5220

Little, SJ, Daar, ES, D'Aquila, RT, Keiser, PH, Connick, E, Whitcomb, JM, Hellmann, NS, Petropoulos, CJ, Sutton, L, Pitt, JA, et al. (1999) Reduced antiretroviral drug susceptibility among patients with primary HIV infection, JAMA 282: 1142–9

Liu, R, Paxton, WA, Choe, S, Ceradini, D, Martin, SR, Horuk, R, MacDonald, ME, Stuhlmann, H, Koup, RA, and Landau, NR (1996) Homozygous defect in HIV-1 coreceptor accounts for resistance of some multiply-exposed individuals to HIV-1 infection, Cell 86: 367–377

Lu, M, Blacklow, SC, and Kim, PS (1995) A trimeric structural domain of the HIV-1 transmembrane glycoprotein, Nat Struct Biol 2: 1075–1082

Maddon, PJ, Dalgleish, AG, McDougal, JS, Clapham, PR, Weiss, RA, and Axel, R (1986) The T4 gene encodes the AIDS virus receptor and is expressed in the immune system and the brain, Cell 47: 333–348

Maeda, K, Yoshimura, K, Shibayama, S, Habashita, H, Tada, H, Sagawa, K, Miyakawa, T, Aoki, M, Fukushima, D, and Mitsuya, H (2001) Novel low molecular weight spirodiketopiperazine derivatives potently inhibit R5 HIV-1 infection through their antagonistic effects on CCR5, J Biol Chem 276: 35194–200

Manes, S, del Real, G, Lacalle, RA, Lucas, P, Gomez-Mouton, C, Sanchez-Palomino, S, Delgado, R, Alcami, J, Mira, E, and Martinez, AC (2000) Membrane raft microdomains mediate lateral assemblies required for HIV-1 infection, EMBO Rep 1: 190–6

McDougal, JS, Kennedy, MS, Sligh, JM, Cort, SP, Mawle, A, and Nicholson, JK (1986) Binding of HTLV-III/LAV to T4+ T cells by a complex of the 110 K viral protein and the T4 molecule, Science 231: 382–385

Melikyan, GB, Markosyan, RM, Hemmati, H, Delmedico, MK, Lambert, DM, and Cohen, FS (2000) Evidence that the transition of HIV-1 gp41 into a six-helix bundle, not the bundle configuration, induces membrane fusion, J Cell Biol 151: 413–423

Mitchell, DA, Fadden, AJ, and Drickamer, K (2001) A novel mechanism of carbohydrate recognition by the C-type lectins DC-SIGN and DC-SIGNR. Subunit organization and binding to multivalent ligands, J Biol Chem 276: 28939-45

Mizukami, T, Fuerst, TR, Berger, EA, and Moss, B (1988) Binding region for human immunodeficiency virus (HIV) and epitopes for HIV-blocking monoclonal antibodies of the CD4 molecule defined by site-directed mutagenesis, Proc Natl Acad Sci U S A 85: 9273–7

Mizuochi, T, Matthews, TJ, Kato, M, Hamako, J, Titani, K, Solomon, J, and Feizi, T (1990) Diversity of oligosaccharide structures on the envelope glycoprotein gp120 of human immunodeficiency virus 1 from the lymphoblastoid cell line H9. Presence of complex-type oligosaccharides with bisecting N-acetylglucosamine residues, J Biol Chem 265: 8519–24

Moore, JP, Burkly, LC, Connor, RI, Cao, Y, Tizard, R, Ho, DD, and Fisher, RA (1993) Adaptation of two primary human immunodeficiency virus type 1 isolates to growth in transformed T cell lines correlates with alterations in the responses of their envelope glycoproteins to soluble CD4, AIDS Res Hum Retroviruses 9: 529–539

Mosier, DE, Picchio, GR, Gulizia, RJ, Sabbe, R, Poignard, P, Picard, L, Offord, RE, Thompson, DA, and Wilken, J (1999) Highly potent RANTES analogues either prevent CCR5-using human immunodeficiency virus type 1 infection in vivo or rapidly select for CXCR4-using variants, J Virol 73: 3544–50

Munoz-Barroso, I, Durell, S, Sakaguchi, K, Appella, E, and Blumenthal, R (1998) Dilation of the human immunodeficiency virus-1 envelope glycoprotein fusion pore revealed by the inhibitory action of a synthetic peptide from gp41, J Cell Biol 140: 315–323

Murakami, T, Nakajima, T, Koyanagi, Y, Tachibana, K, Fujii, N, Tamamura, H, Yoshida, N, Waki, M, Matsumoto, A, Yoshie, O, et al. (1997) A small molecule CXCR4 inhibitor that blocks T cell line-tropic HIV-1 infection, J Exp Med 186: 1389–1393

Myszka, DG, Sweet, RW, Hensley, P, Brigham-Burke, M, Kwong, PD, Hendrickson, WA, Wyatt, R, Sodroski, J, and Doyle, ML (2000) Energetics of the HIV gp120-CD4 binding reaction, Proc Natl Acad Sci U S A 97: 9026–31

Nagasawa, T, Hirota, S, Tachibana, K, Takakura, N, Nishikawa, S, Kitamura, Y, Yoshida, N, Kikutani, H, and Kishimoto, T (1996) Defects of B-cell lymphopoiesis and bone-marrow myelopoiesis in mice lacking the CXC chemokine PBSF/SDF-1, Nature 382: 635–638

Nakashima, H, Masuda, M, Murakami, T, Koyanagi, Y, Matsumoto, A, Fujii, N, and Yamamoto, N (1992) Anti-human immunodeficiency virus activity of a novel synthetic peptide, T22 ([Tyr-5,12, Lys-7]polyphemusin II): a possible inhibitor of virus-cell fusion, Antimicrob Agents Chemother 36: 1249–55

Peterson, A, and Seed, B (1988) Genetic analysis of monoclonal antibody and HIV binding sites on the human lymphocyte antigen CD4, Cell 54: 65–72

Platt, EJ, Kuhmann, SE, Rose, PP, and Kabat, D (2001) Adaptive mutations in the V3 loop of gp120 enhance fusogenicity of human immunodeficiency virus type 1 and enable use of a CCR5 coreceptor that lacks the amino-terminal sulfated region, J Virol 75: 12266–78

Pohlmann, S, Baribaud, F, and Doms, RW (2001a) DC-SIGN and DC-SIGNR: helping hands for HIV, Trends Immunol 22: 643–646

Pohlmann, S, Baribaud, F, Lee, B, Leslie, GJ, Sanchez, MD, Hiebenthal-Millow, K, Munch, J, Kirchhoff, F, and Doms, RW (2001b) DC-SIGN interactions with human immunodeficiency virus type 1 and 2 and simian immunodeficiency virus, J Virol 75: 4664–4672

Pohlmann, S, Leslie, GJ, Edwards, TG, Macfarlan, T, Reeves, JD, Hiebenthal-Millow, K, Kirchhoff, F, Baribaud, F, and Doms, RW (2001c) DC-SIGN interactions with human immunodeficiency virus: virus binding and transfer are dissociable functions, J Virol 75: 10523–10526

Pohlmann, S, Soilleux, EJ, Baribaud, F, Leslie, GJ, Morris, LS, Trowsdale, J, Lee, B, Coleman, N, and Doms, RW (2001d) DC-SIGNR, a DC-SIGN homologue expressed in endothelial cells, binds to human and simian immunodeficiency viruses and activates infection in trans, Proc Natl Acad Sci U S A 98: 2670–2675

Poignard, P, Saphire, EO, Parren, PW, and Burton, DR (2001) gp120: Biologic aspects of structural features, Annu Rev Immunol 19: 253–74

Rabin, RL, Park, MK, Liao, F, Swofford, R, Stephany, D, and Farber, JM (1999) Chemokine receptor responses on T cells are achieved through regulation of both receptor expression and signaling, J Immunol 162: 3840–50

Reeves, JD, Gallo, SA, Ahmad, N, Miamidian, JL, Harvey, PE, Sharron, M, Pohlmann, S, Sfakianos, JN, Derdeyn, CA, Blumenthal, R, et al. (2002) Sensitivity of HIV-1 to entry inhibitors correlates with envelope/coreceptor affinity, receptor density, and fusion kinetics, Proc Natl Acad Sci U S A 99: 16249–16254

Reeves, JD, Hibbitts, S, Simmons, G, McKnight, Azevedo-Pereira, JM, Moniz-Pereira, J, and Clapham, PR (1999) Primary human immunodeficiency virus type 2 (HIV-2) isolates infect CD4-negative cells via CCR5 and CXCR4: Comparison with HIV-1 and simian immunodeficiency virus and relevance to cell tropism in vivo, J Virol 73: 7795–7804

Reeves, JD, McKnight, A, Potempa, S, Simmons, G, Gray, PW, Power, CA, Wells, T, Weiss, RA, and Talbot, SJ (1997) CD4-independent infection by HIV-2 (ROD/B): use of the 7-transmembrane receptors CXCR-4, CCR-3, and V28 for entry, Virology 231: 130–134

Reeves, JD, and Schulz, TF (1997) The CD4-independent tropism of human immunodeficiency virus type 2 involves several regions of the envelope protein and correlates with a reduced activation threshold for envelope-mediated fusion, J Virol 71: 1453–1465

Richman, DD (2001) HIV chemotherapy, Nature 410: 995–1001

Rimsky, LT, Shugars, DC, and Matthews, TJ (1998) Determinants of human immunodeficiency virus type 1 resistance to gp41-derived inhibitory peptides, J Virol 72: 986–993

Rizzuto, CD, Wyatt, R, Hernandez-Ramos, N, Sun, Y, Kwong, PD, Hendrickson, WA, and Sodroski, J (1998) A conserved HIV gp120 glycoprotein structure involved in chemokine receptor binding, Science 280: 1949–1953

Root, MJ, Kay, MS, and Kim, PS (2001) Protein design of an HIV-1 entry inhibitor, Science 291: 884–8

Safrin, S, and Grunfeld, C (1999) Fat distribution and metabolic changes in patients with HIV infection, AIDS 13: 2493–505

Samson, M, Libert, F, Doranz, BJ, Rucker, J, Liesnard, C, Farber, CM, Saragosti, S, Lapoumeroulie, C, Cognaux, J, Forceille, C, et al. (1996) Resistance to HIV-1 infection in caucasian individuals bearing mutant alleles of the CCR-5 chemokine receptor gene, Nature 382: 722–725

Sattentau, QJ, and Moore, JP (1991) Conformational changes induced in the human immunodeficiency virus envelope glycoprotein by soluble CD4 binding, J Exp Med 174: 407–415

Sattentau, QJ, and Moore, JP (1995) Human immunodeficiency virus type 1 neutralization is determined by epitope exposure on the gp120 oligomer, J Exp Med 182: 185–196

Schols, D, S. Claes, E. De Clercq, C. Hendrix, G. Bridger, G. Calandra, G.W. Henson, S. Fransen, W. Huang, J.M. Whitcomb, C.J. Petropoulos, and AMD-3100 HIV Study Group (2002) AMD-3100, a CXCR4 Antagonist, Reduced HIV VIral Load and X4 Levels in Humans. Paper presented at: 9th Conference on Retroviruses and Opportunistic Infections

Schols, D, Struyf, S, Van Damme, J, Este, JA, Henson, G, and De Clercq, E (1997) Inhibition of T-tropic HIV strains by selective antagonization of the chemokine receptor CXCR4, J Exp Med 186: 1383–1388

Shearer, WT, Israel, RJ, Starr, S, Fletcher, CV, Wara, D, Rathore, M, Church, J, DeVille, J, Fenton, T, Graham, B, et al. (2000) Recombinant CD4-IgG2 in human immunodeficiency virus type 1-infected children: phase 1/2 study. The Pediatric AIDS Clinical Trials Group Protocol 351 Study Team, J Infect Dis 182: 1774–9

Smith, DH, Byrn, RA, Marsters, SA, Gregory, T, Groopman, JE, and Capon, DJ (1987) Blocking of HIV-1 infectivity by a soluble, secreted form of the CD4 antigen, Science 238: 1704–1707

Steinman, RM (2000) DC-SIGN: a guide to some mysteries of dendritic cells, Cell 100: 491–4

Strizki, JM, Xu, S, Wagner, NE, Wojcik, L, Liu, J, Hou, Y, Endres, M, Palani, A, Shapiro, S, Clader, JW, et al. (2001) SCH-C (SCH 351125), an orally bioavailable, small molecule antagonist of the chemokine receptor CCR5, is a potent inhibitor of HIV-1 infection in vitro and in vivo, Proc Natl Acad Sci U S A 98: 12718–23

Tachibana, K, Hirota, S, Iizasa, H, Yoshida, H, Kawabata, K, Kataoka, Y, Kitamura, Y, Matsushima, K, Yoshida, N, Nishikawa, S, et al. (1998) The chemokine receptor CXCR4 is essential for vascularization of the gastrointestinal tract, Nature 393: 591–594

Tamamura, H, Xu, Y, Hattori, T, Zhang, X, Arakaki, R, Kanbara, K, Omagari, A, Otaka, A, Ibuka, T, Yamamoto, N, et al. (1998) A low-molecular-weight inhibitor against the chemokine receptor CXCR4: a strong anti-HIV peptide T140, Biochem Biophys Res Commun 253: 877–82

Traunecker, A, Luke, W, and Karjalainen, K (1988) Soluble CD4 molecules neutralize human immunodeficiency virus type 1, Nature 331: 84–86

Tremblay, MJ, Fortin, JF, and Cantin, R (1998) The acquisition of host-encoded proteins by nascent HIV-1, Immunol Today 19: 346–51

Trkola, A, Kuhmann, SE, Strizki, JM, Maxwell, E, Ketas, T, Morgan, T, Pugach, P, Xu, S, Wojcik, L, Tagat, J, et al. (2002) HIV-1 escape from a small molecule, CCR5-specific entry inhibitor does not involve CXCR4 use, Proc Natl Acad Sci USA 99: 395–400

Trkola, A, Pomales, AB, Yuan, H, Korber, B, Maddon, PJ, Allaway, GP, Katinger, H, Barbas, CF, 3rd, Burton, DR, Ho, DD, et al. (1995) Cross-clade neutralization of primary isolates of human immunodeficiency virus type 1 by human monoclonal antibodies and tetrameric CD4-IgG, J Virol 69: 6609–17

Turville, SG, Arthos, J, Donald, KM, Lynch, G, Naif, H, Clark, G, Hart, D, and Cunningham, AL (2001) HIV gp120 receptors on human dendritic cells, Blood 98: 2482–8

Watanabe, S, Takada, A, Watanabe, T, Ito, H, Kida, H, and Kawaoka, Y (2000) Functional importance of the coiled-coil of the Ebola virus glycoprotein, J Virol 74: 10194–201

Weiss, CD, Barnett, SW, Cacalano, N, Killeen, N, Littman, DR, and White, JM (1996) Studies of HIV-1 envelope glycoprotein-mediated fusion using a simple fluorescence assay, AIDS 10: 241–6

Weissenhorn, W, Calder, LJ, Wharton, SA, Skehel, JJ, and Wiley, DC (1998) The central structural feature of the membrane fusion protein subunit from the Ebola virus glycoprotein is a long triple-stranded coiled coil, Proc Natl Acad Sci USA 95: 6032–6

Weissenhorn, W, Dessen, A, Calder, LJ, Harrison, SC, Skehel, JJ, and Wiley, DC (1999) Structural basis for membrane fusion by enveloped viruses, Mol Membr Biol 16: 3–9

Weissenhorn, W, Dessen, A, Harrison, SC, Skehel, JJ, and Wiley, DC (1997) Atomic structure of the ectodomain from HIV-1 gp41, Nature 387: 426–430

Wild, C, Greenwell, T, and Matthews, T (1993) A synthetic peptide from HIV-1 gp41 is a potent inhibitor of virus-mediated cell-cell fusion, AIDS Res Hum Retroviruses 9: 1051–1053

Wild, C, Oas, T, McDanal, C, Bolognesi, D, and Matthews, T (1992) A synthetic peptide inhibitor of human immunodeficiency virus replication: correlation between solution structure and viral inhibition, Proc Natl Acad Sci USA 89: 10537–10541

Wu, L, Bashirova, AA, Martin, TD, Villamide, L, Mehlhop, E, Chertov, AO, Unutmaz, D, Pope, M, Carrington, M, and KewalRamani, VN (2002) Rhesus macaque dendritic cells efficiently transmit primate lentiviruses independently of DC-SIGN, Proc Natl Acad Sci USA 99: 1568–73

Yerly, S, Kaiser, L, Race, E, Bru, JP, Clavel, F, and Perrin, L (1999) Transmission of antiretroviral-drug-resistant HIV-1 variants, Lancet 354: 729–33

Zhang, Y, Lou, B, Lal, RB, Gettie, A, Marx, PA, and Moore, JP (2000) Use of inhibitors to evaluate coreceptor usage by simian and simian/human immunodeficiency viruses and human immunodeficiency virus type 2 in primary cells, J Virol 74: 6893–6910

Zhu, P, Olson, WC, and Roux, KH (2001) Structural flexibility and functional valence of CD4-IgG2 (PRO 542): potential for cross-linking human immunodeficiency virus type 1 envelope spikes, J Virol 75: 6682–6

Zou, YR, Kottmann, AH, Kuroda, M, Taniuchi, I, and Littman, DR (1998) Function of the chemokine receptor CXCR4 in haematopoiesis and in cerebellar development, Nature 393: 595–599

Cell Surface Receptors for Gammaretroviruses

C. S. Tailor[1] · D. Lavillette[2] · M. Marin[2] · D. Kabat[2]

[1] Infection, Immunity Injury and Repair Program, Hospital for Sick Children,
Toronto, ON M5G 1 XB, Canada

[2] Department of Biochemistry and Molecular Biology,
Oregon Health and Science University, 3181 SW Sam Jackson Park Road,
Mailcode L-224, Portland, OR 97201-3098, USA
E-mail: kabat@ohsu.edu

1	Introduction	31
2	Historical Perspectives Concerning Interference.	33
3	The γ-Retrovirus Receptors Are Few in Number, and They All Contain Multiple Transmembrane Sequences.	37
4	Despite the Rarity of Receptor Repertoire Expansions Throughout Millions of Years of Retrovirus Evolution, Limited Switches Can Occur Within Single Infected Animals	45
4.1	Evolution of Coreceptor Usage in HIV-1/AIDS	45
4.2	In Vivo Adaptations of Ecotropic MuLVs and Formation of Polytropic MuLVs	46
4.3	Evolution of Altered Receptor Usages in Domestic Cats Infected with FeLV-A.	48
5	Threshold Effects of Receptor Concentrations on γ-Retroviral Infections.	50
6	Receptor Transport Activities Are Not Required for γ-Retrovirus Infections	52
7	Host Range Control of γ-Retrovirus Entry into Cells	56
7.1	Previous Hypotheses and Recent Alternative Interpretations.	56
7.2	Mouse CAT1, the Receptor for Ecotropic MuLVs	59
7.3	Pit 1 and Pit 2 Receptors.	63
7.4	Xenotropic and Polytropic MuLVs	66
7.5	The RD114 Superfamily of Retroviruses	69
7.6	The FeLV-C Receptor.	73
7.7	A Pair of PERV-A Receptors.	74
8	The Role(s) of Receptors in γ-Retrovirus Infections.	75
8.1	General Issues	75
8.2	Adsorption onto Cell Surfaces.	75
8.3	Binding to Receptors Initiates a Pathway of Cooperative Interactions Between Env Glycoproteins	77
9	Summary	81
References.		83

Abstract Evidence obtained during the last few years has greatly extended our understanding of the cell surface receptors that mediate infections of retroviruses and has provided many surprising insights. In contrast to other cell surface components such as lectins or proteoglycans that influence infections indirectly by enhancing virus adsorption onto specific cells, the true receptors induce conformational changes in the viral envelope glycoproteins that are essential for infection. One surprise is that all of the cell surface receptors for γ-retroviruses are proteins that have multiple transmembrane (TM) sequences, compatible with their identification in known instances as transporters for important solutes. In striking contrast, almost all other animal viruses use receptors that exclusively have single TM sequences, with the sole proven exception we know of being the coreceptors used by lentiviruses. This evidence strongly suggests that virus genera have been prevented because of their previous evolutionary adaptations from switching their specificities between single-TM and multi-TM receptors. This evidence also implies that γ-retroviruses formed by divergent evolution from a common origin millions of years ago and that individual viruses have occasionally jumped between species (zoonoses) while retaining their commitment to using the orthologous receptor of the new host. Another surprise is that many γ-retroviruses use not just one receptor but pairs of closely related receptors as alternatives. This appears to have enhanced viral survival by severely limiting the likelihood of host escape mutations. All of the receptors used by γ-retroviruses contain hypervariable regions that are often heavily glycosylated and that control the viral host range properties, consistent with the idea that these sequences are battlegrounds of virus-host coevolution. However, in contrast to previous assumptions, we propose that γ-retroviruses have become adapted to recognize conserved sites that are important for the receptor's natural function and that the hypervariable sequences have been elaborated by the hosts as defense bulwarks that surround the conserved viral attachment sites. Previously, it was believed that binding to receptors directly triggers a series of conformational changes in the viral envelope glycoproteins that culminate in fusion of the viral and cellular membranes. However, new evidence suggests that γ-retroviral association with receptors triggers an obligatory interaction or cross-talk between envelope glycoproteins on the viral surface. If this intermediate step is prevented, infection fails. Conversely, in several circumstances this cross-talk can be induced in the absence of a cell surface receptor for the virus, in which case infection can proceed efficiently. This new evidence strongly implies that the role of cell surface receptors in infections of γ-retroviruses (and perhaps of other enveloped animal viruses) is more complex and interesting than was previously imagined.

Recently, another gammaretroviral receptor with multiple transmembrane sequences was cloned. See Prassolov, Y., Zhang, D., Ivanov, D., Lohler, J., Ross, S.R., and Stocking, C. Sodium-dependent myo-inositol transporter 1 is a receptor for Mus cervicolor M813 murine leukemia virus.

1
Introduction

Research during the last few years has greatly advanced our understanding of the cell surface receptors for retroviruses and their roles in controlling viral host ranges and in mediating interference, a process whereby infection of a cell with a retrovirus that encodes an envelope glycoprotein (Env) usually prevents superinfection by viruses that use the same receptor as the primary virus. These advances were achieved largely by identification and molecular cloning of the cell surface proteins that have been subverted for use as retroviral receptors and by parallel advances in studies of the viral Env glycoproteins that bind to the receptors. Another key area of new insights concerns the physical chemical process of viral adsorption and of pulling the virus closely onto the cellular membrane. Indeed, adsorption is a severely limiting step in retroviral infections of cultured cells, and the initial attachment often does not involve the receptors that ultimately mediate infections (Andreadis et al. 2000; Guibinga et al. 2002; Pizzato et al. 1999, 2001; Sharma et al. 2000; Ugolini et al. 1999). Thus we need to distinguish between cell surface molecules such as heparan sulfate proteoglycans, DC-SIGN, or integrins that can enhance infections by concentrating retroviruses onto cells (Bounou et al. 2002; Geijtenbeek et al. 2000; Jinno-Oue et al. 2001; Lee et al. 2001; Mondor et al. 1998; Pöhlmann et al. 2001a; Saphire et al. 2001) from authentic receptors that induce conformational changes in Env glycoproteins that are prerequisite for fusion of the viral and cellular membranes.

Retroviral membranes are studded with trimeric Env glycoprotein "knobs" that have monomers consisting of two subunits, a surface (SU) glycoprotein that binds to receptors and a transmembrane subunit that participates in the membrane fusion reaction (Hunter 1997; Hunter and Swanstrom 1990; Wilk et al. 2000). In contrast to previous assumptions, recent evidence suggests that γ-retrovirus binding to receptors probably does not directly trigger the membrane fusion process. Rather, it induces a conformational change in SU that enables neighboring SU molecules in the virus to interact in a manner that appears to be necessary and in some instances even sufficient for the membrane fusion step of infection (Anderson et al. 2000; Barnett and Cunningham 2001; Barnett et al. 2001; Lavillette et al. 2000, 2001, 2002b). In specific cases, γ-retrovirus binding to receptors can be bypassed by *trans*-acting SU-related factors (Barnett and Cunningham 2001; Barnett et al. 2001; Lavillette et al. 2002b). We will discuss this evidence because it helps to define the role(s) that receptors perform in the infection pathway. Moreover, it supports other evidence that multiple receptors and SU glycoproteins may be required for membrane fusion (Bachrach et al. 2000; Battini et al. 1995; Blumenthal et al. 1996; Boulay et al. 1988; Chung et al. 1999; Damico and Bates 2000; Danieli et al. 1996; Ellens et al. 1990; Frey et al. 1995; Gunther-Ausborn et al. 2000; Kuhmann et al. 2000; Layne et al. 1990; Platt et al. 1998; Salaün et al. 2002; Siess et al. 1996; Valsesia-Wittmann et al. 1997) and suggests that "cross-talk" and collaboration occurs between Env molecules on retroviral surfaces (Anderson et al. 2000; Lavillette et al. 2000; Rein et al. 1998; Salzwedel and Berger 2000; Zhao et al. 1997).

An important feature of our review derives from our belief that the γ-retrovirus interference groups each formed by divergent evolution from a common origin and that the members of each group have remained faithful to their receptor for millions of years. Consistent with this hypothesis, γ-retroviruses use a surprisingly small number of receptors, which all have the common feature of being proteins with multiple transmembrane (TM) sequences. In contrast, nearly all other groups of animal viruses including the α- and β-retroviruses (Adkins et al. 1997; Ban et al. 1993; Bates et al. 1993; Brojatsch et al. 1996; Golovkina et al. 1998; Rai et al. 2001; Young et al. 1993) exclusively use receptors that have single TM sequences, with the sole proven exception we know of being the coreceptors used by lentiviruses. On the basis of this and other evidence, we propose that a commitment to using receptors with common structural features has been a previously unrecognized general aspect of animal virus evolution. Despite this commitment of viruses to using specific types of cell surface receptors, it is notable that limited switches in receptor specificities are very common in nature and underlie many important aspects of viral diseases, including AIDS, feline leukemia, and the use of animal reservoirs by influenza A viruses. We attempt to explain this apparent paradox between the long-term evolutionary commitment of viruses to their receptors and their often facile ability to shift to somewhat different receptors very quickly.

It has been generally accepted that many membrane enveloped viruses such as influenza A, Semliki Forest virus, and mouse mammary tumor viruses enter cells by receptor-mediated endocytosis and that membrane fusion is triggered by a decrease in pH that occurs within the endosomes (Flint et al. 2000; Kielian and Helenius 1986; Mothes et al. 2000; Redmond et al. 1984; Ross et al. 2002; Skehel et al. 1995; White et al. 1980; White 1995). In contrast, other viruses such as HIV-1 and most γ-retroviruses are believed to fuse at cell surfaces because of receptor-triggered changes in conformations of Env glycoproteins (Damico and Bates 2000; Damico et al. 1998; Flint et al. 2000; Gilbert et al. 1990, 1995; Katen et al. 2001; Kizhatil and Albritton 1997; McClure et al. 1990; Portis et al. 1985; Ragheb and Anderson 1994; Sommerfelt 1999), and these viruses often cause considerable fusion of uninfected with infected cells at neutral pH (Lavillette et al. 2002a; Ragheb and Anderson 1994; Rein et al. 1998; Siess et al. 1996; Zhao et al. 1997). Although there is no clear evidence for acid-induced fusogenic changes in γ-retroviral Env glycoproteins, some evidence concerning these issues has been ambiguous or dependent on the cells used for the assays (Katen et al. 2001; Kizhatil and Albritton 1997; McClure et al. 1990; Mothes et al. 2000; Portis et al. 1985; Sommerfelt 1999).

For different perspectives concerning γ-retrovirus entry pathways and for more details regarding particular topics, we refer the reader to other recent reviews (Boeke and Stoye 1997; Flint et al. 2000a,b; Hernandez et al. 1996; Hunter 1997; Hunter and Swanstrom 1990; Hunter et al. 2000; Overbaugh et al. 2001; Rosenberg and Jolicoeur 1997; Sommerfelt 1999; Weiss 1992) and to the original articles that are cited here and in those other sources.

2
Historical Perspectives Concerning Interference

Retroviruses were historically classified on the basis of multiple criteria including their core morphologies, their species of origin and interference properties, the diseases they induce, the complexities of their genomes, and the evolutionary lineages of their sequences (Coffin 1992; Hunter et al. 2000; Vogt 1997). It should be understood that all of these criteria are ambiguous and that extensive genetic recombination has occurred throughout retroviral evolution (Benit et al. 2001; Jin et al. 1994; Martin et al. 1999; Ott et al. 1990). Indeed, although HIV-1 is a relatively new virus, recombination between evolutionarily distinct HIV-1 lineages (termed clades) has already occurred and recombination also occurs frequently within infected individuals (Jung et al. 2002; Robertson et al. 1995). As a consequence, evolutionary distances and trees can depend dramatically on whether they are based on comparisons of reverse transcriptase or of other sequences (Benit et al. 2001; Martin et al. 1999). For example, the type D primate retroviruses were recently classified as β-retroviruses (Hunter et al. 2000; Overbaugh et al. 2001). However, they are recombinants that have Env glycoproteins closely related to the γ-retroviruses RD114, BaEV, and HERV-W (Boeke and Stoye 1997; Hunter et al. 2000; Kekuda et al. 1997), and these viruses also use a common cell surface receptor (Blond et al. 2000; Lavillette et al. 2002a; Rasko et al. 1999; Tailor et al. 1999). Moreover, the evolutionary lineages of retroviruses do not always correspond to the lineages of their host species because interspecies jumps (termed zoonoses) have occurred (Benit et al. 2001; Martin et al. 1999). Although retroviral zoonoses appear to be most frequent between closely related species, larger jumps have also occurred. For example, the gibbon ape leukemia virus (GALV) occurs in Asia, but its closest known relatives occur in mice and also in marsupial koalas in Australia (Martin et al. 1999). Presumably, there must have been an intermediate host in the transfer involving Australia, but it is unclear how this could have occurred. Thus retroviral lineages cannot be unambiguously rooted by knowledge of host species evolution.

Until recently, the γ-retroviruses were described as the mammalian type C oncoretroviruses. Evidence concerning their cell surface receptors was derived indirectly by determining their host ranges and cross-interference properties (Hunter 1997; Hunter and Swanstrom 1990; Rein and Schultz 1984). For example, murine γ-retroviruses were classified into four principal host range/interference groups termed ecotropic, amphotropic, polytropic (sometimes called dualtropic), and xenotropic (Hunter 1997; Levy 1978; Rein and Schultz 1984), and these groupings were later expanded to include the 10A1 and the *Mus dunni* endogenous viruses (Bonham et al. 1997; Miller and Wolgamot 1997; Miller et al.

1996; Prassolov et al. 2001). Although it was initially believed that each interference group would use a distinct cell surface receptor, it was subsequently found that the interference groupings depended unexpectedly on the cells used for the assays (Chesebro and Wehrly 1985) and were often nonreciprocal (Chesebro and Wehrly 1985; Miller and Wolgamot 1997). Thus, for example, xenotropic MuLVs are endogenously inherited in mice and are naturally produced in some inbred strains such as NZB, but they cannot infect cells of these inbred mice and were therefore termed xenotropic (Lee et al. 1984; Levy 1973, 1978; O'Neill et al. 1986; Tomonaga and Coffin 1998). Similarly, some other endogenous γ-retroviruses such as the baboon endogenous virus and the feline endogenous virus RD114 cannot infect the species in which they are inherited (Boeke and Stoye 1997; Levy 1978). It is likely that mutations in the cell surface receptors accumulated after these viruses had become endogenous, thus protecting the species from additional infections. Because xenotropic MuLVs cannot infect or bind to receptors on NZB cells, it is perhaps not surprising in hindsight that expression of the NZB viral Env glycoprotein in NZB fibroblasts did not cause any interference to infections by polytropic MuLVs (Chesebro and Wehrly 1985; Levy 1978; Rein and Schultz 1984). However, it was later observed that xenotropic MuLVs strongly interfere with polytropic MuLV infections in human or mink cells and even in fibroblasts from Asian wild mice such as *Mus dunni* that are susceptible to both groups of virus, implying that these viruses might use a common receptor in these cells (Bassin et al. 1982; Kozak 1985; Miller and Wolgamot 1997; Ruscetti et al. 1981). However, interference in these cells is nonreciprocal, with polytropic MuLVs causing only weak or negligible interference to superinfections by xenotropic MuLVs (Chesebro and Wehrly 1985; Miller and Wolgamot 1997). Indeed, polytropic MuLVs generally only interfere weakly with superinfections by other polytropic MuLVs, and this results in massive pathogenic superinfections by these viruses in cell cultures and in vivo (Chesebro and Wehrly 1985; Herr and Gilbert 1984; Kozak 1985; Marin et al. 1999; Yoshimura et al. 2001). Similarly, several other highly pathogenic retroviruses such as FeLV-T and SNVs also bind to their receptors only weakly and therefore cause only weak interference to superinfection (Anderson et al. 2000; Delwart and Panganiban 1989; Donahue et al. 1991; Keshet and Temin 1979; Kristal et al. 1993; Moser et al. 1998; Overbaugh et al. 2001; Reinhart et al. 1993; Rohn et al. 1998; Temin 1988; Weller et al. 1980). Such results were very difficult to understand before receptor cDNAs were cloned and analyzed. The basic outcome of the recent cloning studies is that polytropic and xenotropic MuLVs are closely related viruses that use a common receptor termed the X-receptor that is highly polymorphic in different mouse strains (Battini et al. 1999; Marin et al. 1999; Tailor et al. 1999a; Yang et al. 1999). The complexities in the interference results derive from the fact that retroviruses that use a common receptor need not have the same host ranges or binding affinities for the receptor ortholog that occurs in a particular animal. In addition, in some cases retroviruses can use several related cell surface proteins as receptors (see below). Similar complexities occur in other groups of retroviruses including the avian leukosis virus groups B, D, and E, which do not always cross-interfere despite the fact that they use a common polymorphic receptor (Adkins et al. 1997, 2001).

Interference appears to operate by multiple synergistic mechanisms that have different efficiencies. Coexpression of an Env glycoprotein with its receptor generally results in association of the newly synthesized proteins within the rough endoplasmic reticulum, which inhibits processing of both components to the cell surfaces (Chen and Townes 2000; Heard and Danos 1991; Hunter 1997; Jobbagy et al. 2000; Kim and Cunningham 1993; Murakami and Freed 2000). In addition, Env glycoprotein or SU that is shed from cells or added exogenously can bind to the cell surface receptor and in some cases stimulate partial receptor endocytosis (Hunter 1997; Overbaugh et al. 2001). If these processes that remove receptors from cell surfaces were efficient, the normal function of the receptor would be eliminated with attendant pathological consequences. Although such severe downmodulation of receptors may occur in some instances, chronic infections by γ-retroviruses generally do not cause complete removal of receptors from cell surfaces and it appears that the residual receptor is active in performing its normal cellular function, despite the fact that it becomes saturated with SU and therefore unavailable to serve as a receptor for superinfecting viruses (Wang et al. 1992).

Coexpression of Env with its receptor in infected cells can inhibit processing of the Env glycoprotein to cell surfaces. If this is severe, infectious virus production is reduced, especially in cells that synthesize less Env than receptor. In this context, it should be understood that the extent of viral protein expression depends substantially on the site of proviral DNA integration in the host cell chromosomes and can therefore differ by at least 100-fold in different infected cells (see, e.g., Kabat et al. 1994; Kuhmann et al. 2000)). Consequently, the degree of interference and of infectious virus production varies within a chronically infected population of cells. In the case of HIV-1, the virus overcomes this problem by using two viral-encoded accessory proteins, Nef and Vpu, to eliminate the CD4 receptor from infected cells (Chen et al. 1996; Piguet et al. 1998, 1999; Schubert et al. 1998). Because CD4 is not essential for viability of T cells or macrophages, its elimination enhances virus production and release (Bour et al. 1999; Cortex et al. 2002; Lama et al. 1999; Ross et al. 1999).

Despite the enormous number of target cells available to a retrovirus in vivo, it is clear that interference has a major influence on the infection process within animals (Corbin et al. 1994; Gardner et al. 1986; Ikeda and Sugimura 1989). In diseased tissues, large proportions of cells often become infected. Accordingly, replication-defective retroviruses such as the Friend spleen focus-forming virus or the Moloney sarcoma virus are efficiently produced in mice in concert with a replication-competent helper virus (Kabat 1989; Rosenberg and Jolicoeur 1997). In this situation, the defective pseudotyped virus often enters the cell first and it is later rescued into virions after the same cell becomes infected by the helper virus. Similarly, retroviruses that do not cause significant interference such as FeLV-T or polytropic MuLVs have a replicative advantage in chronically infected animals and they often accumulate at high proviral copy numbers per cell late in the process of infection (Herr and Gilbert 1984; Keshet and Temin 1979; Reinhart et al. 1993; Weller et al. 1980; Yoshimura et al. 2001).

3
The γ-Retrovirus Receptors Are Few in Number, and They All Contain Multiple Transmembrane Sequences

Figure 1A summarizes current evidence concerning the cell surface receptors used by γ-retroviruses, including depictions of their presumptive topologies and with their abbreviated names listed below and the virus groups that use them listed above. They are also shown from left to right in the order in which they were molecularly cloned and identified, with the PERV-A receptors being the most recent additions.

It should be understood that all retroviruses likely bind at least weakly to multiple cell surface components not shown in Fig. 1, such as heparan sulfate proteoglycans, DC-SIGN, integrins, or glycolipids (Bounou et al. 2002; Cantin et al. 1997; Fortin et al. 1997; Jinno-Que et al. 2001; Lee

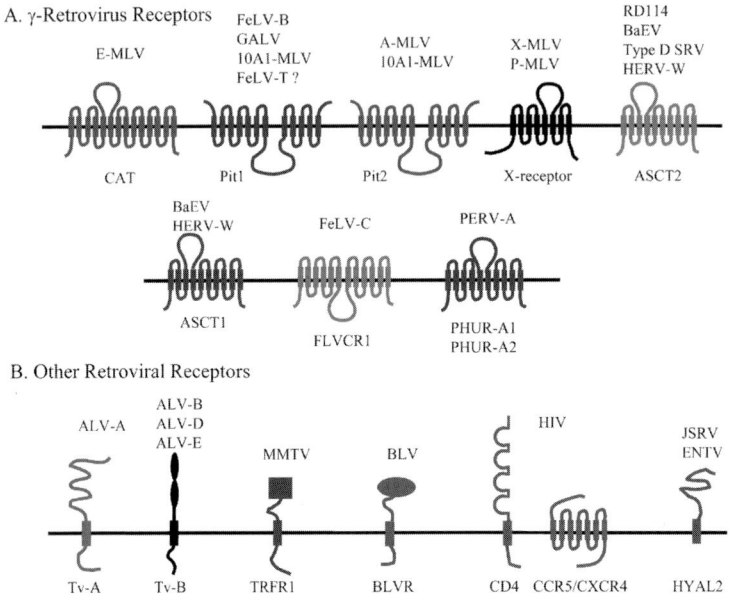

Fig. 1A, B Schematic representation of the cell surface receptors of γ-retroviruses and their comparison to other retroviral receptors. **A** γ-Retrovirus Receptors. All of the known receptors used by γ-retroviruses contain multiple transmembrane (*TM*) segments with short extracellular loops, compatible with their identifications as solute transporters. E-MLV uses a cationic amino acid transporter of mice (*mCAT-1*) as a receptor, whereas FeLV-B, GALV, A-MLV and 10A1-MLV use the sodium-dependent phosphate symporters Pit1 and/or Pit2. The large group of retroviruses that include RD114, BaEV, HERV-W and type D simian retroviruses (*SRVs*) use the neutral amino acid transporter, ASCT2. Recent studies showed that BaEV and HERV-W can also use the related neutral amino acid transporter ASCT1 as a receptor. The normal cellular functions of the receptors for X-MLV/P-MLV (*X-receptor*) and for FeLV-C (*FLVCR1*) are unknown. However, FLVCR1 is a member of the major facilitator superfamily of transporters, suggesting that it is likely to be a transporter of organic anions. The PERV-A receptors have not been functionally characterized, but they occur in many tissues and may also be transporters. **B** Receptors for other retroviruses. This shows the receptors for the avian leukosis virus (*ALV*) subgroups A, B, D, and E, mouse mammary tumor virus (*MMTV*), the complex bovine leukemia virus (*BLV*), the Jagsiekte sheep lung carcinoma virus, and the two different receptors used by human immunodeficiency virus (*HIV*). Interestingly, the receptors for these other retroviruses, are type 1 membrane proteins with only one hydrophobic TM segment, with the exception of the lentiviruses such as HIV-1, which use chemokine receptors with seven TM domains. The Jagsiekte receptor is attached to the cells by a single phosphatidylinositol-linked lipid anchor rather than by a TM peptide (Overbaugh et al. 2001; Rai et al. 2001). The MMTV receptor is transferrin receptor 1 (*TRFR1*) (Ross et al. 2002)

et al. 2001; Mondor et al. 1998; Saphire et al. 1999, 2001). Although such binding substances probably do not induce conformational changes in SU glycoproteins that are necessary for membrane fusion, they can enhance viral adsorption and substantially increase efficiencies of infections, thus contributing to pathogenesis (Alvarez et al. 2002; Bounou et al. 2002; Geijtenbeek et al. 2000; Jinno-Que et al. 2001; Lee et al. 2001; Saphire et al. 2001). Because such binding proteins contribute to infections, it can be difficult to unambiguously distinguish them from receptors that directly mediate the membrane fusion process, especially for retroviruses that bind to their authentic receptors only weakly (e.g., in the cases of FeLV-T or polytropic MuLVs; Anderson et al. 2000; Donahue et al. 1991; Herr and Gilbert 1984; Kristal et al. 1993; Lauring et al. 2001; Marin et al. 1999; Reinhart et al. 1993; Temin 1988; Yoshimura et al. 2001). We emphasize this because pathogenic variants of different animal viruses have often been associated with abilities to bind to apparently novel cell surface components and it has sometimes been inferred that the viruses have switched their receptor specificities. In these instances it has generally not been established that the cell surface binding components are receptors that directly mediate infections.

Because many details concerning the γ-retrovirus receptors are described in following sections, we make only several general conclusions here. First, the receptors all contain multiple TM sequences, consistent with their identification in known instances as transporters of small solutes. Thus CAT1 is a facilitative transporter for cationic amino acids (Kavanaugh et al. 1994b; Kim et al. 1991; Wang et al. 1991); Pit1 and Pit2 are Na^+-dependent phosphate symporters (Kavanaugh et al. 1994a; Olah et al. 1994; Wilson et al. 1995); and ASCT1 and ASCT2 are Na^+-dependent exchangers of neutral amino acids (Marin et al. 1999; Rasko et al. 1999; Tailor et al. 1999b; Torres-Zamorano et al. 1998; Utsunomiya-Tate et al. 1996). In addition, the receptor for FeLV-C (FLVCR1) is a member of the major facilitator superfamily of transporters (Pao et al. 1998; Quigley et al. 2000; Tailor et al. 1999c) although its solute specificity is unknown. Second, the viruses listed in Fig. 1 are broad groupings with numerous members. For example, hundreds of ecotropic MuLVs have been isolated and/or cloned. The GALV group has subgroups including viruses that infect woolly monkeys (Delassus et al. 1989; Martin et al. 1999). Other close relatives occur in mice (MuRRS) and in koalas (Martin et al. 1999), and it is likely that they also use Pit1 as a receptor. The HERV-W family of human endogenous retroviruses contains approximately 646 representative sequences in the human genome (Pavlicek et al. 2002), and it is also closely related to other viruses including the HERV-H and MuERV-U1 families (Benit et al. 2001). Considered from this perspective, the total number of viruses represented by the summary in Fig. 1A is very large and likely includes the majority of γ-retroviruses. Indeed, only a small number of γ-retroviruses that have been analyzed for their infectivities do not use the receptors shown in Fig. 1A. These include the *Mus dunni* endogenous virus (MDEV) and FeLV-A groups, which use unknown receptors. Third, it should also be understood that each member of a virus group differs from other isolates and that they also differ to a degree in their interactions with receptors. Thus, for example, some FeLV-B isolates use human Pit2 in addition to human Pit1, whereas others use only human Pit1 (Sugai et al. 2001). In domestic cats, FeLV-Bs frequently can use both of the feline Pit proteins as receptors (Anderson et al. 2001). Similarly, GALV uses hamster Pit2 (Wilson et al. 1995). Thus the receptor specificities listed in Fig. 1 pertain to particular members of the virus group as assayed with receptors derived from one or a small number of species. Fourth, many γ-retroviruses use receptors that have close relatives (e.g., Pit1 or Pit2, ASCT1 or ASCT2, FLVCR1 or FLVCR2, and PHuR-A1 or PHuR-A2) and these viruses generally have an inherent ability to use both receptors, at least in certain species as illustrated by the above examples of GALV and FeLV-B. Frequently, the inability of a virus to use one member of a related pair of receptors can be changed by a single amino acid substitution in that receptor (see below). Furthermore, it is likely that additional examples of closely related receptor pairs will be identified in the future for reasons discussed below. For example, we have proposed that the FeLV-A receptor is likely to be closely related to FLVCR1 (Tailor and Kabat 1997). In addition, there is evidence that ecotropic MuLVs can weakly use mouse CAT3, a transporter that is related to mouse CAT1 (mCAT1) (Masuda et al. 1999). FeLV-C isolates can use FLVCR1 and, to a lesser extent, FLVCR2 (C. Tailor, unpublished results). Use of closely related pairs of receptors has been advantageous for γ-retroviruses, presumably in part because it makes host escape mutations much less likely (see below).

A corollary of the above conclusions is that the receptors shown in Fig. 1A probably include a substantial proportion of the receptors that have been successfully exploited by γ-retroviruses and that they are certainly at least representative of all the receptors that have been used.

Thus the total number of receptors used by γ-retroviruses is quite small. Furthermore, several of these receptors are closely related pairs (~60% identity), which implies an additional limitation in their overall diversity. This idea is also strongly supported by the fact that γ-retroviral interference groups initially identified within different species were later shown to use a common receptor (e.g., the FeLV-B and GALV groups). Such overlaps would be unexpected if the total number of receptors was very large. Considered together with the fact that these receptors are all structurally similar in having multiple TM sequences, these results strongly imply that expansions in the repertoire of receptors have been severely limited and constrained throughout millions of years of γ-retrovirus evolution.

It was recently suggested that unrelated γ-retroviruses may have independently chosen to use a common receptor by a process of convergent evolution (Overbaugh et al. 2001), presumably because of some advantageous but unknown aspect of the receptor's structure or function. However, we believe that an hypothesis of convergent evolution would be very difficult to reconcile with the fact that more distantly related families of retroviruses use receptors that exclusively have single TM domains (see Fig. 1B; Adkins et al. 1997, 2001; Ban et al. 1993; Bates et al. 1993; Brojatsch et al. 1996; Golovkina et al. 1998; Rai et al. 2001; Ross et al. 2002; Young et al. 1993). These retroviruses include the avian leukosis viruses, MMTV, bovine leukemia virus, and Jaagsiekte sheep lung carcinoma virus groups, which have lifestyles similar to those of the γ-retroviruses. Furthermore, there is very solid evidence for divergent evolution of γ-retroviruses within their specific interference groups. Most strikingly, the only avian retroviruses known to use a receptor with multiple TM domains is the SNV/REV-A group that is closely related to the baboon endogenous virus (BaEV) and probably originated by a rare zoonosis from a primate into a bird followed by adaptive infectious radiation into gallinaceous and anseriform birds (Barbacid et al. 1979; Boeke and Stoye 1997; Hunter 1997; Kewalramani et al. 1992; Koo et al. 1992, 1991; Martin et al. 1999). Similarly, the RD114 feline endogeneous retrovirus and BaEVs appear to have derived from a common ancestor (Mang et al. 1999; van der Kkuyl et al. 1999), as did the xenotropic and polytropic MuLVs (Khan 1984). The Env sequences that can be used to trace evolutionary lineages are also compatible with the hypothesis that the interference groups of γ-retroviruses each derived by divergent evolution from a common ancestor, although it is also clear that genetic recombinations have shuffled these sequences and made it difficult to trace the lineages of the receptor-recognition domains of the SU glycoproteins (Benit et al. 2001). However, the immunosuppressive domain of the transmembrane Env subunit has provided useful lineage information (Benit et al. 2001). Similarly, the amino-terminal PHQ motif in SU that is involved in *trans*-stimulation (Lavillette et al. 2000) is conserved in several γ-retrovirus interference groups but is absent or modified in other interference groups, implying distinct evolutionary lineages (D. Lavillette, unpublished results). Divergent evolution also occurs during retroviral replication *in* vivo, which can involve minor shifts in usage between closely related receptors (e.g., shifts of CCR5 to CXCR4 coreceptor usage for HIV-1) as discussed below and during in vitro selection in cultured cells that express different orthologs of a common receptor for avian leukosis virus subgroups B, D, and E (Holmen et al. 2001; Taplitz and Coffin 1997).

Despite this strong evidence for divergent evolution of the γ-retrovirus interference groups, we emphasize that a limited degree of convergent evolution in receptor choice cannot be fully excluded. This has been proposed mainly with respect to the γ-retroviruses that use Pit1 and Pit2 receptors, in part because it has been difficult to identify close lineage relationships among some of these viruses and because several studies implied that GALV, FeLV-B, and A-MuLV viruses may interact rather differently with distinct regions of the Pit receptors (Overbaugh et al. 2001; Pedersen et al. 1995). In contrast, other evidence suggests that these viruses interact with the same regions of these receptors (Dreyer et al. 2000; Eiden et al. 1996; Johann et al. 1993; Lundoft et al. 1998; Tailor and Kabat 1997; Tailor et al. 1993, 2000b). Indeed, corresponding sites in the FeLV-B and A-MuLV SU glycoproteins interact with homologous sites in Pit1 and Pit2 in a common orientation (Tailor and Kabat 1997; Tailor et al. 2000b). We believe that the simplest interpretation of the available evidence is that these viruses all interact with Pit1 and Pit2 in a common orientation that involves several contact sites in both the receptors and the SU glycoproteins. However, the affinities of interactions at specific contact sites can differ for particular virus isolates. Similarly, R5 and X4 strains of HIV-1 interact somewhat differently with different regions of their coreceptors, as do distinct isolates of SIV (Brelot et al. 1997; Chabot and Broder 2000; Edinger et al. 1997; Lu et al. 1997; Picard et al. 1997; Pontow and Ratner 2001). Nevertheless, all of these immunodeficiency viruses diverged from a common ancestor, and the structures of the SU-coreceptor complexes must also be very similar.

On the basis of the above considerations, we propose that throughout a period of evolution that may have exceeded 100 million years the γ-retroviruses have been only rarely able to expand their repertoire of cell surface receptors. Presumably, an early γ-retrovirus progenitor became adapted to use a receptor with multiple TMs, and its descendants thereby were committed to the constraints imposed by this adaptation. Consequently, the few successful receptor switches that subsequently occurred had this same structural constraint. Thus, as is typical in evolution, an initial accident that is followed by adaptation imposes severe limits on subsequent evolutionary options.

Our conclusion that γ-retroviruses have had difficulty in expanding their repertoire of receptors also may apply to other virus groups. Thus avian leukosis viruses use a small number of receptors that have the common feature of being single-TM proteins (see Fig. 1B). Intriguingly, this is also true of other animal viruses. For example, all proven receptors for coronaviruses, herpesviruses, adenoviruses, and picornaviruses have only single TM domains (Flint et al. 2000a). Indeed, there are only a few receptors for animal viruses other than γ-retroviruses that have been reported to have multiple TM sequences, with CD81, a tetraspanin binding factor for hepatitis C virus (Baranowski et al. 2001; Higginbottom et al. 2000; Pileri et al. 1998), and the lentivirus coreceptors being the most convincing examples. However, a single -TM protein, the low-density lipoprotein receptor, was recently shown to be a specific entry receptor for hepatitis C virus (Agnello et al. 1999; Baranowski et al. 2001), and CD81 is evidently only a binding factor (Meola et al. 2000; Petracca et al. 2000; Pileri et al. 1998). In addition, it was reported that rabies virus may use an acetylcholine receptor with multiple TM sequences (Burrage et al. 1985; Flint et al. 2000a; Thoulouze et al. 1998), but this is not essential for infection and is also believed to be a binding protein rather than a true receptor.

Our proposal that all virus groups have been severely limited throughout evolution in the types of receptors they can employ may initially appear inconsistent with evidence that some viruses can switch their receptor specificities with apparent ease. This has been most dramatically suggested by shifts of influenza A viruses between animal reservoirs, which involve single amino acid changes in the viral hemagglutinin that enable recognition of different sialic acid structures (e.g., *N*-acetyl or

N-glycolyl neuraminic acids in $\alpha 2,6$ or $\alpha 2,3$ linkages to galactose) that predominate in the different host species (Baranowski et al. 2001; Rogers et al. 1985; Skehel and Wiley 2000; Suzuki et al. 1989, 2000). Similarly, slight changes in specificity for receptors accompanied emergence in 1978 of the canine parvovirus (Domingo et al. 1999; Parker et al. 2001). However, these are small shifts in receptor specificities rather than global jumps to dissimilar receptors. Similar slight shifts are involved in the change from CCR5 to CXCR4 coreceptor usage during AIDS progression (Scarlatti et al. 1997). Small shifts in usages of closely similar receptors also have been reported to occur during cell culture selections of subgroup B, D, and E avian leukosis viruses that all use polymorphic variants of the same TVB receptor (Holmen et al. 2001; Taplitz and Coffin 1997) and during cell culture selections of HIV-1 variants (Platt et al. 2001). These issues are discussed further below (see Sect. 4).

Several viruses have been reported to use multiple alternative receptors or even alternative pathways for infection of cells. For example, measles virus isolates appear to be capable of using CD46 or SLAM, which both contain single TM domains (Baranowski et al. 2001; Oldstone et al. 1999; Tatsuo et al. 2000). Complex viruses such as herpesviruses that contain several distinct envelope glycoproteins are also typically able to bind to several cell surface components (Baranowski et al. 2001; Borza and Hutt-Fletcher 2002; Flint et al. 2000a). The foot-and-mouth disease picornavirus (FMDV) may also use multiple receptors including heparan sulfates and integrins and may in addition be able to invade cells via immunoglobulin F_c receptors when the virus is coated with antibodies (Baranowski et al. 2001; Mason et al. 1994). This alternative entry route is also used by the dengue flavivirus, which may explain the extremely strong pathogenesis that occurs when it reinfects previously exposed individuals (Baranowski et al. 2001). In the case of FMDV, it has not been established whether heparan sulfate is a true receptor that directly mediates infection or merely a binding factor that influences infection indirectly by enhancing virus adsorption. HIV-1 infections are also strongly stimulated by accessory cell surface binding components including heparan sulfates, glycolipids, and DC-SIGN (Bounou et al. 2002; Geijtenbeek et al. 2000; Lee et al. 2001; Pöhlmann et al. 2001a,b; Zhang et al. 2002). Similarly, a paralysis-inducing neurotropic variant of Friend MuLV binds more strongly than the parental virus to heparan sulfate, and it thereby becomes more infectious for brain capillary endothelial cells while still remaining dependent on the CAT1 receptor (Jinno-Oue et al. 2001). These examples illustrate how changes in affinities for accessory binding substances can dramatically alter cellular tropisms and pathogenesis of viruses, and why it has often been difficult to distinguish such accessory binding factors from true receptors or coreceptors that are essential for infections. On the basis of these considerations, we believe that the available evidence strongly supports our proposal that all virus groups have been severely constrained in the types of receptors they can employ for infection of cells. However, some viruses have evolved several pathways for infection, and viruses such as HIV-1 have evolved distinct sites in a single SU glycoprotein for recognition of dissimilar receptors and coreceptors. In addition, viruses including γ-retroviruses have become adapted to interact with accessory binding factors on cell surfaces, and these accessory associations often have major effects on viral transmission and pathogenesis.

4
Despite the Rarity of Receptor Repertoire Expansions Throughout Millions of Years of Retrovirus Evolution, Limited Switches Can Occur Within Single Infected Animals

4.1
Evolution of Coreceptor Usage in HIV-1/AIDS

It is well-known that HIV-1 invades cells via a sequential interaction of its gp120 SU glycoprotein with at least two cell surface proteins, the CD4 receptor and a coreceptor (Choe et al. 1996; Deng et al. 1996; Doranz et al. 1996; Dragic et al. 1996; Feng et al. 1996; Flint et al. 2000a,b; Moore et al. 1997; Weiss 1992). CD4 is normally involved in T cell activation, whereas coreceptors are closely related members of a group of heterotrimeric G protein-coupled receptors that are activated by small chemoattractant cytokines termed chemokines (Littman 1998). Like other retroviruses HIV-1 mutates rapidly in vivo, and one consequence is often an expansion in its coreceptor specificity. HIV-1 involved in initial transmission exclusively uses CCR5 as a coreceptor (Liu et al. 1996). However, during viral evolution within approximately 50% of infected individuals, mutations of gp120 in one disulfide-bonded loop called variable loop 3 (V3) expand the coreceptor repertoire to allow additional or eventually even exclusive use of CXCR4 (Connor et al. 1997; Pollakis et al. 2001; Polzer et al. 2001; Scarlatti et al. 1997; Speck et al. 1997). Utilization of CXCR4 enables HIV-1 to more readily infect the immunologically naive, unactivated $CD26^{low}$ $CD45RA^+$ $CD45R0^-$ subset of T lymphocytes, and this expansion in cell tropism coincides with and is likely to be the proximal cause of an accelerated destruction of the host immune system (Blaak et al. 2000; Bleul et al. 1997; Camerini et al. 2000; Kreisberg et al. 2001; Kwa et al. 2001; Lee et al. 1999; Schramm et al. 2000; Unutmaz and Littman 1997).

This cycle of viral variation within infected individuals is poorly understood. However, it recapitulates itself in each infected individual. Thus, even when transmission occurs by a blood transfusion or needle stick that contains X4 strains of HIV-1, the virus reverts to R5 specificity early in the new infection (Beaumont et al. 2001; Cornelissen et al. 1995), suggesting that entry via the mucosal endothelium is not required for selection of the CCR5 specificity. Rather, it is likely that R5 strains of HIV-1 have a selective advantage in the milieu of the newly infected individual, in part because CCR5 is a substantially stronger coreceptor than CXCR4 (Doranz et al. 1996, 1999; Hoffman et al. 2000; Mondor et al. 1998) and in part because at the early phase of infection there are abundant memory T cells that express adequate concentrations of CD4 and CCR5 (Blaak et al. 2000; Bleul et al. 1997; Lee et al. 1999; Unutmaz and Littman 1997). CXCR4 contains an N-linked oligosaccharide in its amino-terminal region that inhibits its utilization by R5 strains of HIV-1 (Chabot et al. 2000). Viral transmission to these memory T cells is also facilitated by antigen-presenting follicular dendritic cells that contain DC-SIGN (Geijtenbeek et al. 2000; Lin et al. 2000). After substantial disruption of the lymph node follicles and depletion of the follicular dendritic cells and memory T cells, the immune system becomes weaker and viral variants that can more efficiently use CXCR4 begin to have improved opportunities.

4.2
In Vivo Adaptations of Ecotropic MuLVs
and Formation of Polytropic MuLVs

Infections with ecotropic MuLVs (E-MuLVs) have also resulted in selection of adapted viral variants. Normally, E-MuLVs can infect cells of mice or rats but cannot infect Chinese hamster ovary cells (CHO-K1 cells) unless the cells are pretreated with tunicamycin, which inhibits N-linked glycosylation of proteins (Masuda et al. 1996; Miller and Miller

1992; Wilson and Eiden 1991). However, passage of the Friend strain of E-MuLV in rats reproducibly causes paralysis with degeneration of the central nervous system, and the virus recovered from these passages also causes the same disease when injected into newborn mice (Masuda et al. 1992, 1996a,b; Park et al. 1994; Takase-Yoden and Watanabe 1999). Compared with the original molecular clone of Friend E-MuLV, the Env SU glycoprotein of the passaged virus PVC-211 is altered in a variable region that contains disulfide-bonded loops and is known to be involved in receptor binding (Battini et al. 1998; Fass et al. 1997; Masuda et al. 1996a,b). In addition, this variant Friend virus is able to efficiently infect CHO-K1 cells in the absence of tunicamycin, and it binds relatively strongly to heparan sulfates (Jinno-Oue et al. 2001; Masuda et al. 1996b). These novel properties of the PVC-211 virus are all caused by mutations in the SU glycoprotein (Masuda et al. 1996b). An implication of these results is that growth of the Friend E-MuLV in rats, which contain a CAT1 protein distinct from the mouse ortholog, selected for SU changes that coincidentally enabled efficient infection of CHO-K1 cells and invasions of brain capillary endothelial cells. Indeed, as described below, the CAT1 orthologs in rats and hamsters have common sequences that distinguish them from mouse CAT1.

When E-MuLVs are injected into mice or when they are expressed endogenously as in newborn AKR strain mice, they often recombine with endogenously inherited polytropic *env* sequences to produce recombinant viruses that encode chimeric Env glycoproteins, with the amino-terminal receptor-binding domains of SU deriving from polytropic endogenous sequences and the remainder corresponding to the E-MuLV parental virus (Fischinger et al. 1975; Kabat 1989; Rosenberg and Jolicoeur 1997; Stoye et al. 1991). In addition, recombinations also often occur in the viral LTRs (Kabat 1989; O'Neill et al. 1986; Stoye et al. 1991). These recombinant viruses have a polytropic host range and use the X-receptor for infection (Battini et al. 1999; Tailor et al. 1999a; Yang et al. 1999). Because they form as recombinants when E-MuLVs replicate in mice, polytropic MuLVs were first discovered as "contaminants" in preparations of E-MuLVs (Fischinger et al. 1975; Hartley et al. 1977; Kabat 1989; Rosenberg and Jolicoeur 1997). In such preparations, the polytropic MuLVs generally are pseudotyped with the E-MuLV envelope, a phenomenon called "genomic masking" (Fischinger et al. 1978). Accordingly, isolation of polytropic MuLVs generally has required infection of mouse cells at low multiplicities by the contaminated E-MuLVs, followed by harvest of the released virions before the E-MuLV can spread into all cells and subsequent infection of cells that are resistant to E-MuLVs such as CCL64 mink cells (Fischinger et al. 1975, 1978; Hartley et al. 1977). Because polytropic MuLVs cause foci in mink cells they have been termed mink cell focus-inducing viruses (MCFs). MCFs cause only weak interference, and they massively superinfect susceptible cells *in* vitro and in vivo (Hartley et al. 1977; Herr and Gilbert 1984; Marin et al. 1999; Yoshimura et al. 2001).

Interestingly, many diseases of mice initially believed to be caused by E-MuLVs were later shown to be substantially accelerated by the MCF contaminants (Chesebro et al. 1984; Cloyd et al. 1980; Hartley et al. 1977; Kabat 1989; Rosenberg and Jolicoeur 1997; Stoye et al. 1991), and they were in several cases inhibited by the R_{mcf} gene that blocks the X-receptor and interferes with MCF infections (Bassin et al. 1982; Jung et al. 2002; Kabat 1989; Kozak 1985; Ruscetti et al. 1981, 1985). These results implied that polytropic MuLVs may be causal agents for many diseases including T cell leukemias, lymphomas, and erythroleukemias (Hartley et al. 1977; Kabat 1989; Ruscetti et al. 1981). This hypothesis has been difficult to test with pure MCFs because there are inhibitory lipoprotein factors in sera of many mice that specifically inactivate polytropic and xenotropic MuLVs by an unknown mechanism (Levy 1978; Wu et al. 2002). In contrast, when MCFs are partially or fully genomically masked by replication in the presence of E-MuLVs, the MCFs resist this inactivation system and contribute to pathogenesis. Consequently, the mixture of an E-MuLV plus an MCF is often much more pathogenic than either virus alone.

4.3
Evolution of Altered Receptor Usages in Domestic Cats Infected with FeLV-A

Although domestic cats initially become infected via saliva only with the FeLV-A subgroup of feline leukemia viruses, which use an unknown cell surface receptor, chronically infected animals often also contain FeLV-B, FeLV-C, and/or FeLV-T viruses (Linenberger and Abkowitz 1995; Moser et al. 1998; Overbaugh et al. 1988, 2001). The FeLV-B viruses form by recombination of the replicating FeLV-A with endogenously inherited FeLV-B *env* gene sequences that occur in high copy numbers in the genome of these animals (Boomer et al. 1994; Overbaugh et al. 1988; Roy-

Burman 1995; Sheets et al. 1993; Stewart et al. 1986). This recombination closely resembles the formation of MCFs in mice initially infected with E-MuLVs (see above). Accordingly, the FeLV-B recombinants encode chimeric SU glycoproteins that have amino-terminal receptor-binding domains corresponding to the endogenous FeLV-B-specific portion (Roy-Burman 1995; Sheets et al. 1992; Stewart et al. 1986). Interestingly, the endogenous FeLV-B envelope sequences are more homologous to the amino termini of the amphotropic and 10A1 MuLV SU sequences than to the corresponding regions of other FeLV Env glycoproteins. This similarity to murine retroviruses suggests that FeLV-B may have formed as a zoonosis of cats by a virus of rodent origin. Accordingly, FeLV-B and 10A1 MuLV both use human Pit proteins as receptors (see Fig. 1A; Miller and Miller 1994; Takeuchi et al. 1992; Wilson et al. 1994). Although it is believed that endogenously inherited FeLV-B SU glycoproteins preferentially employ feline Pit1 as a receptor, many FeLV-B isolates from infected cats also employ feline Pit2, and these probably are adapted variants with a broadened cellular tropism that evolved *in* vivo (Anderson et al. 2001; Boomer et al. 1997). The contributions of FeLV-B to pathogenesis have been difficult to determine unambiguously (Bechtel et al. 1999; Neil et al. 1991). However, FeLV-B Env glycoproteins can in some cases facilitate infections by other viral subgroups (Anderson et al. 2000; Lauring et al. 2001, 2002).

In contrast, formation of FeLV-C viruses occurs sporadically in FeLV-A-infected cats because of accumulation of a small number of mutations in one disulfide-bonded loop of the SU glycoprotein (Brojatsch et al. 1992; Neil et al. 1991; Rigby et al. 1992). These mutations shift the receptor specificity from that of FeLV-A toward use of the FLVCR1 receptor. Interestingly, formation of FeLV-C *in* vivo coincides with onset of aplastic anemia also called fatal red cell aplasia (Abkowitz et al. 1987; Linenberger and Abkowitz 1992, 1995; Onions et al. 1982; Rojko et al. 1996). Accordingly, infections of cats with FeLV-C induce this disease, which can also be mimicked in bone marrow cultures (Abkowitz et al. 1987; Linenberger and Abkowitz 1992, 1995; Onions et al. 1982; Rojko et al. 1986; Testa et al. 1983). FLVCR1 expression occurs in multiple hematopoietic lineages, which also become infected by FeLV-C *in* vivo and *in* vitro, suggesting that erythroblasts or their supporting bone marrow microenvironment may be especially sensitive to the virus rather than uniquely susceptible to infection (Abkowitz et al. 1987; Dean et al. 1992; Linenberger and Abkowitz 1992, 1995). Because SU glycoproteins of

FeLV-C and FeLV-A differ specifically only at a few positions in one disulfide-bonded loop region, and because analogous changes in disulfide-bonded loops cause small shifts in receptor or coreceptor specificities for HIV-1 (Connor et al. 1997; Pollakis et al. 2001; Polzer et al. 2001; Scarlatti et al. 1997; Speck et al. 1997), E-MuLVs (Masuda et al. 1992, 1996a,b; Park et al. 1994), and avian leukosis viruses (Holmen et al. 2001; Taplitz and Coffin 1997), we have proposed that FeLV-A probably uses a receptor that is very similar in structure to FLVCR1 (Tailor et al. 1999c). Thus we anticipate that the FeLV-A receptor may also be a member of the major facilitator superfamily of transporters (Pao et al. 1998).

In addition to FeLV subgroups A, B, and C, several virus isolates from domestic cats have been termed FeLV-T because they selectively destroy T cell cultures and cause a severe feline acquired immunodeficiency syndrome (FAIDS) (Donahue et al. 1991; Overbaugh et al. 1988; Rohn et al. 1998). FeLV-T SU glycoproteins appear to have only minute binding affinities for susceptible cells, and they accordingly cause negligible interferences to superinfections (Donahue et al. 1991; Kristal et al. 1993; Overbaugh et al. 1988, 2001; Reinhart et al. 1993). Consequently, T cells become massively superinfected with FeLV-T, which may explain the immunosuppressive effects of this virus (Donahue et al. 1991; Reinhart et al. 1993). Furthermore, FeLV-T is not interfered with by FeLV subgroup A, B, or C viruses, which has led to the proposal that FeLV-T may use a unique receptor (Kristal et al. 1993; Moser et al. 1998; Reinhart et al. 1993). However, an effort to clone an FeLV-T receptor yielded only an FeLV-B-related SU glycoprotein fragment termed FELIX (Anderson et al. 2000) that binds to Pit1 and facilitates FeLV-T infection by a *trans*-complementation mechanism that is discussed below (see Sect. 8.3).

5
Threshold Effects of Receptor Concentrations on γ-Retroviral Infections

The γ-retrovirus receptors were all cloned based on transfection or transduction of receptor-encoding nucleic acid sequences from susceptible species into cells that are resistant to the corresponding viruses. An expectation of this strategy is that the resistant cells used for the cloning must lack functional receptors for the virus. Although this has generally been true, several important and informative exceptions have been reported. One exception concerns the resistance of CHO cells to amphotropic MuLVs (A-MuLV), which was initially interpreted to suggest that the CHO Pit2 protein was inactive in mediating infection by this virus (Chaudry et al. 1999; Miller and Miller 1992; Wilson et al. 1994). In contrast, E36 cells, which also were derived from a Chinese hamster, are susceptible to A-MuLVs. Furthermore, the E36 Pit 2 protein differs from that of CHO cells and was found to confer susceptibility to A-MuLVs when it was expressed in CHO cells (Wilson et al. 1994). Subsequently, it was unexpectedly found that the CHO Pit 2 protein is also an active receptor for A-MuLVs when its cDNA is transfected into CHO cells (Tailor et al. 2000a). Another example occurs with FeLV-C, which naturally infects human cells but not NIH/3T3 or *Mus dunni* mouse fibroblasts (Tailor et al. 1999c, 2000a). Indeed, human FLVCR1 was cloned on the basis of its ability to confer susceptibility of NIH/3T3 cells to FeLV-C (Tailor et al. 2000a). Consequently, it was surprising to find that the FLVCR1 ortholog cloned from *Mus dunni* fibroblasts also efficiently facilitated FeLV-C infections when it was overexpressed in *Mus dunni* fibroblasts (Tailor et al. 2000a). These and an additional example (Chung et al. 1999) strongly suggest that potentially active receptors may completely fail to mediate γ-retrovirus infections when they are expressed at low subthreshold levels and that they can mediate infections efficiently when they are overexpressed in the same cells from which they were originally derived.

Two general models have been invoked to explain such threshold requirements of receptor concentrations for infections. According to one model, there may be interfering retroviral-related SU glycoproteins or other receptor-masking substances that are endogenously expressed in the cells that are resistant to infection. Such interfering substances would block infections if they were present in excess of the receptor, but the receptor would become active if it was expressed in excess of the mask (Tailor et al. 2000a). Consistent with this idea, inhibitory substances have been identified in conditioned media from some cell cultures (Miller and Miller 1992, 1993). Furthermore, endogenously inherited Env glycoproteins are often synthesized in small amounts and they can interfere with infections of some γ-retroviruses (Bassin et al. 1982; Ikeda and Sugimura 1989; Kozak 1985; Lyu and Kozak 1996; Lyu et al. 1999; Ruscetti et al. 1981, 1985).

According to a second model, a receptor may be inherently weak in its ability to associate with a virus, so that it would mediate infection efficiently only when it is expressed at high concentrations. Furthermore, if infection requires a complex containing multiple receptors, as is believed to be the case for several enveloped viruses (Battini eta l. 1995; Blumenthal et al. 1996; Damico and Bates 2000; Danieli et al. 1996; Ellens et al. 1990; Kuhlmann et al. 2000; Salaün et al. 2002), a plot of virus titer versus receptor concentration would have a sigmoidal or stepwise shape, with negligible infectivity at low receptor concentrations and efficient infectivity above the transitional concentration (Damico and Bates 2000; Kuhmann et al. 2000; Platt et al. 2001). Precedent for this model is provided by studies of HIV-1 (Kuhmann et al. 2000; Platt et al. 2001). For example, the G163R substitution in human CCR5 causes a large reduction in its affinity for HIV-1 (Kuhmann et al. 2000; Siciliano et al. 1999). This mutant coreceptor is therefore inactive at low concentrations, but it is almost as active as wild-type CCR5 at high concentrations (Kuhmann et al. 2000). Furthermore, the G163R substitution is not anomalous because it naturally occurs in African green monkey CCR5 and it does not interfere with chemokine signaling or with infections by the simian immunodeficiency viruses that are endemic in those monkeys (Siciliano et al. 1999). Mathematical analyses of these sigmoidal shaped curves support the conclusion that a minimal complex of four to six CCR5s is necessary for HIV-1 infections (Kuhmann et al. 2000; Platt et al. 2001). Other studies also suggested that multiple Env glycoproteins function cooperatively in retroviral infections (Bachrach et al. 2000; Rein et al. 1998; Salzwedel and Berger 2000; Zhao et al. 1997).

6
Receptor Transport Activities Are Not Required for γ-Retrovirus Infections

Despite the fact that γ-retrovirus infections often inhibit superinfection efficiencies by 3–4 orders of magnitude, cell surface receptor concentrations usually appear to be downmodulated only partially (by ~60%–90%) (Wang et al. 1992). This downmodulation is partly caused by association of newly synthesized receptors and Env glycoproteins in the rough endoplasmic reticulum, which blocks their processing to cell surfaces, and partly by enhancement of receptor endocytosis (Heard and Danos 1991; Jobbagy et al. 2000; Kim and Cunningham 1993). In addition, production and shedding of SU glycoproteins by the infected cells causes saturation of the residual cell surface receptors and this evidently contributes to the interference. Because this saturation does not completely block transport activity of the receptor, residual transport occurs, and it is likely that this ameliorates pathogenic effects and enhances survival and replication of the infected cells. Thus it appears that a limitation in loss of the normal transport function of the receptor has probably been advantageous for γ-retrovirus replication. However, there are alternative compensatory mechanisms to protect infected cells from loss of the transporter/receptor. For example, downmodulation of Pit1 transport activity causes upregulation of Pit2 expression and vice versa (Chien et al. 1997; Kavanaugh et al. 1994a). Similarly, in other cases there are redundant mechanisms for transport of key solutes. It should be noted in this context that ASCT1 and ASCT2 transport an overlapping but nonidentical set of neutral amino acids, with the major difference being the exclusive transport of glutamine by ASCT2 (Kekuda et al. 1996, 1997). Thus downmodulation of ASCT2 cannot be fully compensated by upregulation of ASCT1.

Several studies have suggested that γ-retroviral receptor function does not require transporter activity. In the case of mouse CAT1, mutation of a conserved glutamic acid at position 107 in a hydrophobic transmembrane region to an aspartic acid (i.e., E107D) completely eliminated transport activity without significantly inhibiting infections by E-MuLVs (Wang et al. 1994). In the case of human Pit2, recent mutagenesis studies demonstrated the same conclusion (Bottger and Pedersen 2002). Moreover, we recently found that the ASCT2 protein consists of multiple isoforms that have diverse truncations at their amino-terminal ends (Tailor et al. 2001). The ASCT2 isoforms are translationally initiated by a leaky scanning process (Kozak 1999) at a series of CUG and GUG codons that occur in optimal Kozak consensus sequence contexts and that are situated downstream of the normal AUG initiation codon that occurs in a suboptimal and inefficient sequence context. Thus leaky scanning results in the synthesis of multiple ASCT2 isoforms that have substantial truncations at their amino termini. Interestingly, truncated human ASCT2 isoforms lacking at least 23 amino acids from their amino termini were active both in transport and in retroviral reception, whereas an isoform with a 79-amino acid truncation that eliminated the first TM sequence was active in viral reception but not in amino acid transport (Tailor et al. 2001).

A related question concerns the effects of SU glycoprotein binding on the transporter functions of the receptor. This has been most extensively studied in the case of E-MuLV interactions with the mouse facilitative transporter of cationic amino acids (mCAT1) (Wang et al. 1992). Extracellular addition of a saturating concentration of the SU glycoprotein gp70 derived from the Friend strain of E-MuLV had no effect on K_m values but caused a substantial (~25%) inhibition in the V_{max} for mCAT1-mediated uptake of Arg without any effect on mCAT-1 mediated Arg export from the cells. As expected, the gp70 did not bind to control nonrodent cells (mink CCL64 cells) and it had no effect on Arg uptake or export from cells that lacked mCAT1. A four-state alternating gate model for Arg transport by mCAT1 that can explain these results is diagrammed in Fig. 2A. The basic concept is that extracellular Arg binds to mCAT1 (A-B transition) to induce a conformational change (B-C transition) that enables release of Arg into the cytosol (C-D transition) and that the empty transporter then undergoes an additional conformational change (D-A transition) that restores mCAT1 to its original state A. Net import of Arg requires clockwise cycling between these states, whereas efflux of Arg requires counterclockwise cycling. In either cycling direction, the rate-limiting step for almost all transporters is the conformational reorientation of the empty transporter (i.e., A←→D transition), whereas the solute binding and release steps occur at least 100 times more rapidly. Strong evidence supporting this idea in the case of CAT1 derives from the occurrence of *trans*-stimulation (Christensen 1989; White 1985; White et al. 1982). Specifically, the presence of extracellular unlabeled Arg greatly stimulates CAT1-mediated efflux of intracellular l-[^{3}H]Arg, implying that the reversible exchanger partial cycle (D←→C←→B←→A) is much faster than the full efflux cycle that includes the A→D conformational change. Similarly, influx of l-[^{3}H]Arg into cells is greatly *trans*-stimulated by preloading of the cells with unlabeled Arg (Christensen 1989; White 1985; White et al. 1982), implying that the D→A conformational change is rate-limiting for the full import cycle. Because E-MuLV gp70 slows net uptake of Arg but has no affect on K_m, it was inferred from transition-state rate theory (Tinoco et al. 1978) that its binding onto mCAT1 stabilizes structure D more than it stabilizes the D←→A transition state. Conversely, because gp70 had no effect on Arg export, it was inferred that its binding equally stabilizes structure A and the A←→D transition state. Thus, as diagrammed in Fig. 2B, gp70 binding increases the energy barrier for the D→A conformational change but has no effect on the energy barrier for the A→D conformational change. The basic conclusion of this study was that E-MuLV gp70 binds more strongly to the mCAT1 conformations that have the Arg binding site exposed to the cytosol than to the A-D transition

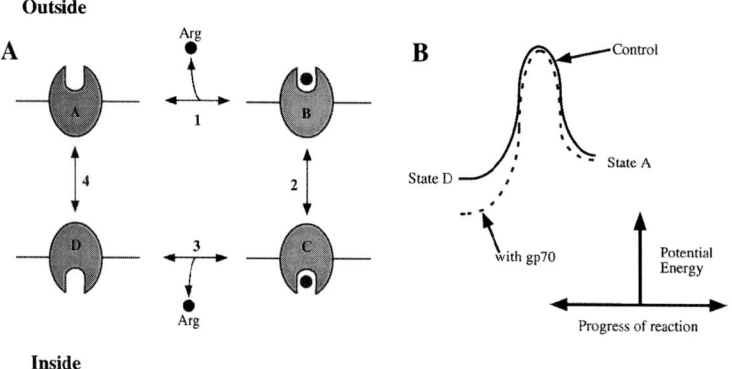

Fig. 2A, B Four-state model of the arginine transporter function of CAT-1 and interpretation of the gp70 inhibitory effects. **A** The four-state model is shown. In the import cycle (*clockwise*), state A binds extracellular Arg to form the Arg-B complex. The transporter then changes conformation to form Arg-C from which the amino acid can dissociate into the cytoplasm to form the empty D state. The final step in the import cycle occurs by conformational change of D to regenerate A. The Arg export cycle operates in the *counterclockwise* direction. Substantial evidence (Christensen 1989; White 1985) suggests that the D to A transition is the rate-limiting step of the amino acid import cycle and that the opposite A to D transition rate-limits the export cycle. This evidence derives in part from the existence of *trans*-stimulation. **B** Effects of gp70 binding are interpreted in terms of the energetics of the D to A transition, because these are believed to be the rate-limiting steps of the import and export cycles. The basic interpretation is that gp70 binding to CAT-1 stabilizes state D and has relatively little effect on state A or on the A-D transition state. In the *curve*, the *ordinate scale* represents the potential energy, and the *abscissa* represents the progress of the reaction. Because by transition state theory the rate of any reaction is proportional to the probability of reaching the transition state and because this probability is related by the Boltzmann distribution to the energy required (Tinoco et al. 1978), this model predicts that gp70 would inhibit the Arg import cycle (i.e., D to A transition) but have no effect on the Arg export cycle (i.e., limited by the A to D transition) (see also Wang et al. 1991). These results suggest that gp70 binds with higher affinity to the mCAT1 conformations that have the amino acid binding site exposed to the cytosol and with lower affinity to the conformations that allow Arg binding from the extracellular medium

state or to the mCAT1 conformations that have the Arg binding site accessible to the extracellular medium. Importantly, this apparent difference in gp70 affinities for the distinct mCAT1 conformations is clearly insufficient to freeze the transporter so that it cannot transport essential amino acids. Conversely, the changes in the free energy of gp70 binding that accompany the transport cycle are also clearly insufficient to induce release of the bound gp70. These results suggest that the interaction of gp70 with mCAT1 is dynamic and that it perturbs but does not block the amino acid transport cycle.

7
Host Range Control of γ-Retrovirus Entry into Cells

7.1
Previous Hypotheses and Recent Alternative Interpretations

The sections below review evidence concerning the interactions of γ-retroviruses with their cell surface receptors and the coevolutionary changes in the viral SU glycoproteins and receptors that have influenced viral host ranges. Although this evidence previously seemed fragmentary and confusing, we believe that recent investigations have substantially clarified this subject. In this section we describe our overall perspective concerning these issues.

We believe that host range control of γ-retrovirus infections can best be understood from a coevolutionary perspective. Clearly, it is disadvantageous for a species to harbor a horizontally transmitted and/or endogenously inherited infectious retrovirus. Indeed, it is well known that host proteins necessary for infections of parasites, bacteria, and viruses or for immunity become highly polymorphic at functionally important sites (Hill 1998; Murphy 1993; Penn et al. 2002). Accordingly, the critical sites in cell surface receptors for viruses have become highly polymorphic, with high ratios of nonsynonymous to synonymous nucleotide substitutions suggestive of strong selection for changes in the amino acid sequence and with extensive and variable glycosylation in these regions (Feigelstock et al. 1998; Hill 1998). An example occurs in the CCR5 sequences of African green monkeys, which are believed to have been chronically infected at high frequencies ($\sim$60% of adults) with immunodeficiency viruses (SIVagm) since ancient times before dispersal of these monkeys throughout Africa (Kuhlmann et al. 2001). Similarly, viruses also often become polymorphic because of the selection of mutants able to overcome these host barriers (Taplitz and Coffin 1997; Wilson et al. 2000). An example of such γ-retrovirus diversity occurs in the xenotropic-polytropic family of MuLVs. The X-receptors of mice are highly polymorphic, with many European mice being resistant to X-MuLVs but susceptible to P-MuLVs and with most wild mice being susceptible to both X-MuLVs and P-MuLVs or sometimes resistant to both (Kozak 1983; Kozak and O'Neill 1987; Lyu and Kozak 1996; Lyu et al. 1999; Marin et al. 1999). Presumably, the diversity of these viruses has coevolved to contend with this host diversity.

The receptors that have been successfully exploited by γ-retroviruses and the characteristics of the viral-receptor interactions appear to reflect this coevolutionary "arms race." From the perspective of the virus, survival seems to have depended on several factors. First, it has been advantageous for the virus to make functionally redundant interactions with several sites in the receptor, so that single-receptor mutations cannot generally cause host escape (Platt et al. 2001). As a consequence, in comparisons of receptor orthologs from susceptible and resistant species, it has usually been found that multiple-amino acid substitutions are required to inactivate the susceptible ortholog, whereas single changes at different positions often suffice to convert the resistant ortholog into a functional receptor (Dreyer et al. 2000; Eiden et al. 1993, 1994, 1996; Lundorf et al. 1998, 1999; Marin et al. 1999, 2000). Presumably for the same reason, it has been useful for the viruses to recognize two closely related receptors such as Pit1 and Pit2, ASCT1 and ASCT2, or PHuR-A1 and PHuR-A2 (see Fig. 1A) in a redundant or partially redundant manner. In this circumstance, mutations in a single receptor confer only a small survival advantage to the host and this reduces penetrance of the mutation into the species and provides a better opportunity for compensatory viral adaptations. Finally, it appears to have been advantageous for the viruses to interact with sites in the receptors that are important for the protein's normal function, presumably because these sites are relatively conserved and their mutation would cause a substantial loss of fitness to the host species. As a result, we believe that it has been difficult for the hosts to mutate the primary viral attachment site(s) in the receptors. Consequently, we believe that the resistance mutations in the receptors have largely been restricted to the nearby regions that control viral access to the primary viral attachment sites. Thus we hypothesize that these hypervariable sites in the receptors are negative control regions rather than primary viral interaction sites. These negative control regions often contain bulky residues, including sites for N-linked glycosylation, that may interfere with viral access to the receptors (Chabot et al. 2000; Eiden et al. 1994; Lavillette et al. 2002a; Marin et al. 2000; Wentworth and Holmes 2001). A model for the γ-retroviral receptors is shown in Fig. 3, with a conserved viral attachment site within a hypervariable negative-control access channel that may be heavily glycosylated. We emphasize that this basic model does not require that the viral attachment site be situated within a channel, because the negative control region could presumably function by other mechanisms.

It is helpful to compare this model with assumptions that have previously dominated this field. Specifically, the most common strategy for analyzing host range control of γ-retroviral receptors has been to compare the sequences of receptor orthologs from a susceptible and a resistant species and to then generate chimeras and/or substitution mutations between these orthologs to identify the active site(s) necessary for infection. Moreover, it has generally been assumed that the sequence differences between the orthologous proteins occur at the active sites for virus attachment. On the contrary, we are proposing that the divergent areas are generally negative control sequences that occur adjacent to the primary virus interaction site(s). According to our interpretation, the primary attachment sites are generally conserved in the receptor orthologs from susceptible and resistant species and they would therefore have been overlooked in the previous investigations. Consistent with our model, the hypervariable sequences in the receptor orthologs uniformly occur adjacent to sequences that are very highly conserved. Furthermore, the degree of diversity within the hypervariable sequences is often so great that common features cannot be discerned in these regions of receptors from distinct susceptible species.

The common occurrence of variably situated N-linked oligosaccharides within the hypervariable sequences of γ-retrovirus receptors from different species is also compatible with our interpretation that these are negative control regions rather than primary virus binding sites. Indeed, there is evidence in several cases that these N-linked oligosaccharides negatively influence viral receptor function (Chabot et al. 2000; Eiden et al. 1994; Kuhmann et al. 2001; Lavillette et al. 2002a; Marin et al. 2000; Wentworth and Holmes 2001). These N-linked oligosaccharides often inhibit but do not completely block receptor function, and in some cases full blockade requires cooperative inhibition by more than one N-linked oligosaccharide (Marin et al. 2000).

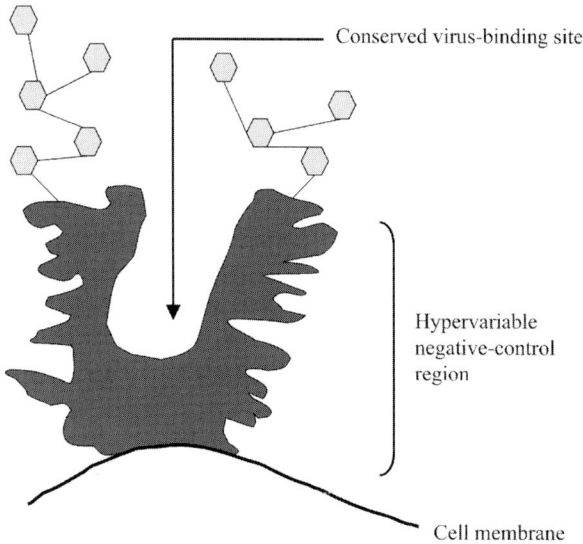

Fig. 3 A model of the γ-retroviral binding sites in the cell surface receptors. The model proposes that the viral binding site(s) occur in conserved sequences that are surrounded by hypervariable negative control regions that inhibit access of virus to the receptor. These negative control regions often contain N-linked oligosaccharides, which are depicted in *open stick* forms

7.2
Mouse CAT1, the Receptor for Ecotropic MuLVs

The mouse receptor for E-MuLVs was the first retroviral receptor that was molecularly cloned in a seminal investigation by Albritton and Cunningham (Albritton et al. 1989). It was later shown to be a broadly expressed transporter for the cationic amino acids Lys, Arg, and ornithine (Kim et al. 1991; Wang et al. 1991) that closely corresponds to the y^+ transport system previously characterized by extensive physiological studies (Christensen 1989; White 1985; White et al. 1982). These correspondent features include its Na^+ independence, amino acid specificity, *trans*-stimulation properties (see Sect. 6), and surprising ability to transport homoserine only in the presence of Na^+ (Christensen 1989; Wang et al. 1991; White 1985; White et al. 1982). This latter feature suggests that a Na^+-homoserine complex can mimic a cationic amino acid in the CAT1 active site. CAT1 is a glycoprotein that has both amino and carboxyl termini in the cytosol and is believed to contain 12 or 14 TM sequences and 6–7 extracellular (ECL) loops (Albritton et al. 1989, 1993; Kavanaugh et al. 1994b). CAT1 may have evolved by duplication of a smaller half-protein (Kavanaugh et al. 1994b).

After the molecular cloning and functional identification of mouse CAT1, other CAT family members were identified. These include CAT2α (in lymphocytes) and CAT2β (in liver), which are identical except for a divergent region of 43 amino acids that is encoded by alternatively spliced exons (Closs et al. 1993a–c; Kavanaugh et al. 1994c). Consistent with the fact that liver lacks a high-affinity uptake system for Arg, these CAT2 isoforms differ greatly in their K_m values for Arg, with CAT2α having a K_m of 38 μM and CAT2β having a K_m of 2.7 mM (Closs et al. 1993a,b; Kavanaugh et al. 1994c). Because liver contains urea cycle enzymes for conversion of Arg to urea, its lack of a high-affinity uptake system prevents Arg depletion from blood and preserves its supply to other tissues. Neither mouse CAT2 isoform is active as a receptor for E-MuLVs, but mouse CAT1/CAT2 chimeras are active receptors if they contain mouse CAT1 ECL3 (Closs et al. 1993b; Kavanaugh et al. 1994c). Conversely, in these same chimeras, the K_m for Arg is determined exclusively by the alternatively spliced exon of the CAT2 mRNAs (Closs et al. 1993b; Kavanaugh et al. 1994c). Furthermore, an additional transporter termed CAT3 has been identified (Hosokawa et al. 1997; Ito and Groudine 1997). Although CAT3 is normally synthesized exclusively in the brain, CAT1 knockout mice appear to express CAT3 in other tissues (Nicholson et al. 1998). Mouse CAT3 has been reported to have weak activity as a receptor for E-MuLVs (Masuda et al. 1999).

Consistent with the fact that E-MuLVs can only infect mice and rats, it is not surprising that human CAT1, which is 87% identical to mCAT1, is inactive as a viral receptor when it is expressed in naturally resistant cells. This enabled two groups to construct human-mouse CAT1 chimeras and to establish that the ECL3 region of mCAT1 is necessary for E-MuLV infections (Albritton et al. 1993; Yoshimoto et al. 1993). Consistent with the hypothesis that it is a battlefield in host-virus coevolution, the ECL3 sequences of CAT1 proteins are hypervariable in comparison to other regions; they contain proven sites for N-linked glycosylation (Albritton et al. 1993; Kim and Cunningham 1993; Yoshimoto et al. 1993); and they contain portions with a relatively high ratio of nonsynonymous to synonymous nucleotide sequence changes, implying that they have been under strong negative selection pressure in rodents. Fig-

```
              210  214       222 223      229   235 237   242
               |   |          |   |        |     |   |     |
    mCAT1    VKGSIKNWQLTEK---N̊FS---CNNN̊DTNVKYG-EGGFMP
    MDTF     ....V........---...---........G......
    CHO-K1   ...........EDFL.R.SPL.G.......H.-......
    BHK 21   ...........EDFL.SPSAPLG..........-......
    Rat      .....E......----.K.SPL.G..........-......
    Mink     ...........EDFQ.T.SHR.LS...KQGTLGA.....
    Human    ....V.......EDFG.T.GPL.L....KEGKPGV.....
```

Fig. 4 Comparison of hypervariable ECL3 sequences of the mouse CAT1 receptor with corresponding orthologous sequences of other species. The region shown has a major effect on binding and infectivity of ecotropic host-range MuLVs. Sites for N-linked glycosylation are shown with *asterisks*. Consistent with Fig. 3, the variable sequences are surrounded by highly conserved regions

ure 4 compares the ECL3 sequences of CAT1 proteins from NIH Swiss mice with the corresponding sequences of Asian wild mice (*Mus dunni*), Chinese (CHO) and Syrian (BHK-21) hamsters, rats, mink, and humans, with the underlined regions denoting the Asn-X-Ser/Thr consensus sites for N-linked glycosylation. The hypervariable sequences are bordered on both sides by highly conserved ECL3 sequences that are presumably important for normal transporter function.

Although previous comparative studies of mCAT1 with the CAT1 orthologs shown in Fig. 4 were interpreted based on the assumption that the functionally important sequence differences occur at sites for direct binding of E-MuLVs, we believe that the evidence is more consistent with the model described above in Sect. 7.1 and in Fig. 3, which proposes that the divergent sequences are principally negative control regions that restrict viral access to relatively conserved viral attachment site(s). For example, initial comparisons of mCAT1 with human CAT1 by chimera constructions and site-directed mutagenesis implied that the YGE sequence (positions 235–237) in mCAT1 might be most important. Thus substitution of YGE for PGV in the human sequence resulted in a partially active receptor when it was expressed at high levels in the cells (Albritton et al. 1993; Yoshimoto et al. 1993). However, in the same studies the mCAT1 residues N232, V233, and E237 and the deletion shown in that region also made important contributions compared with the human counterpart sequences (Yoshimoto et al. 1993). Although the *Mus dunni* CAT1 protein has two differences in this ECL3 region (I214V and G inserted within YGE to make a YGGE), it is an excellent receptor for the Rauscher strain of E-MuLV but is inactive as a receptor for Moloney E-MuLV (Eiden et al. 1993). Reversal of the change at position 214 converted the *Mus dunni* CAT1 into an active receptor for Moloney MuLV (Eiden et al. 1993). Subsequently, the same group found that treatment of *Mus dunni* fibroblasts with tunicamycin, an inhibitor of N-linked glycosylation, also made the cells susceptible to Moloney MuLV and that elimination of the N-linked oligosaccharide at the NDT site by mutagenesis had the same effect (Eiden et al. 1994). Thus *Mus dunni* CAT1 can be converted into an active receptor for Moloney MuLV either by reversing the I214V substitution or by eliminating the distal N-linked oligosaccharide at position 229. The results further suggest that the N-linked oligosaccharide at position 229 is inhibitory for viral reception but its influence depends on the remainder of the ECL3 sequence and on the particular virus strain that is analyzed. Although CHO-K1 and BHK-21 hamster cells are resistant to E-MuLVs, they become highly susceptible when treated with tunicamycin (Masuda et al. 1996; Miller and Miller 1992; Wilson and Eiden 1991), strongly suggesting that N-linked glycosylation at position 229 also inhibits receptor function of these hamster CAT1 proteins. Moreover the CHO-K1 CAT1 contains HGE rather than YGE, suggesting that Y235 is not essential for E-MuLV infections. Interestingly, when the Friend strain of E-MuLV replicates in rats, neurotropic variants form that can bind more strongly to rat CAT1 than to mouse CAT1 (Masuda et al. 1996a,b; Park et al. 1994). Studies of the adapted neurotropic virus PVC-211 also showed that it efficiently infects CHO-K1 and BHK-21 cells in the absence of tunicamycin (Masuda et al. 1996b). Thus the inhibitory effect of glycosylation at position 229 in the CHO-K1 and BHK-21 receptors can also be overcome by viral mutations in SU (Masuda et al. 1996b). Other interesting neurotropic variants of E-MuLVs have been identified and analyzed in other laboratories (see, e.g., Chung et al. 1999; Lynch et al. 1994; Park et al. 1994; Saha and Wong 1992; Shikova et al. 1993; Takase-Yoden and Watanabe 1999). Considered together, these results suggest that sequence differences throughout ECL3 (at least between the positions numbered 214–237 in Fig. 4) influence viral receptor function. It is very difficult to ascertain from current data whether any mCAT1 amino acids in divergent regions of ECL3 play a direct role in viral binding or whether they are merely less inhibitory than alternative sequences in CAT1 orthologs from resistant species. However, it is clear that some sequences in this region (e.g., the sites of glycosylation) have negative modulatory effects on infectivity. Moreover, it seems very likely that the divergent sequences have been selected during evolution of mice and other species for their inhibitory effects on viral replication and pathogenesis.

Infectivities of E-MuLVs can also be restricted by endogenously inherited Env glycoproteins. For example, the Fv-4 resistance allele of mice encodes a secreted E-MuLV-related SU glycoprotein that binds to mCAT1 and interferes with viruses that use that receptor (Gardner et al. 1986; Ikeda and Sugimura 1989; Taylor et al. 2001).

7.3
Pit 1 and Pit 2 Receptors

Pit1 and Pit2 are closely related (~60% identity) type III Na^+-dependent phosphate transporters that are widely expressed in somatic cells (Johann et al. 1993; Kavanaugh et al. 1994a; Miller et al. 1994; Miller and Miller 1994; Overbaugh et al. 2001; Werner et al. 1998). They differ almost completely in sequence from type I and II Na^+-phosphate symporters that function in the apical membranes of epithelial cells to control phosphate reuptake from bile, urine, and intestines (Werner et al. 1998). Indeed, Pit1 and Pit2 are the major transporters that mediate phosphate flux between blood and tissues. A notable exception is erythrocytes that transport phosphate via the Cl^-/HCO_3^- exchanger (Wehrle and Pedersen 1989; Werner et al. 1998). This exception may be important because retrovirus entry into enucleated erythrocytes would be wasteful. Depletion of extracellular phosphate causes enhanced expression of Pit1 and Pit2, and inhibition of either transporter also causes upregulation of the other (Chien et al. 1997; Kavanaugh et al. 1994a). The Pit proteins may have originated by duplication of a smaller half-protein progenitor (Salaun et al. 2001).

Initially, human Pit1 was cloned as the receptor for the GALV group of γ-retroviruses, which includes woolly monkey viruses (O'Hara et al. 1990), and it was later also identified as the receptor for the B-subgroup of feline leukemia viruses (Takeuchi et al. 1992) and for the 10A1 MuLV (Miller and Miller 1994; Wilson et al. 1994). On the basis of chimera and mutagenesis comparisons of human Pit1 with Pit1 orthologs from *Neurospora crassa* and European mice, which cannot function as receptors for GALV, it was inferred that an important region for GALV interaction with human Pit1 occurs in a hydrophilic sequence of nine amino acids at positions 550–558 called region A that is hypervariable in different species (see Fig. 5). An extended region A of 13 amino acids between positions 546 and 558 was later found to be critical for infections by FeLV-B (see Fig. 5) (Dreyer et al. 2000). In addition, other regions of the human Pit1 receptor have also been shown to be very important for both GALV and FeLV-B, although relative contributions of these different regions can depend on the virus isolate and on the overall receptor chimera that is analyzed (Chaudry and Eiden 1997; Leverett et al. 1998; Lundorf et al. 1999; Tailor and Kabat 1997; Tailor et al. 2000b). Subsequently, human Pit2 was identified as a receptor for A-MuLVs and it was also found that the 10A1 recombinant isolate of MuLV can utilize both human Pit1 and Pit2 (Miller and Miller 1994; Wilson et al. 1994, 1995). Chimera and mutagenesis studies also indicated that the regions of human Pit2 that contribute to A-MuLV infections generally correspond to the sites in Pit1 that are used by FeLV-B, including the extended region A (Dreyer et al. 2000; Lundorf et al. 1999; Pedersen et al. 1995; Tailor and Kabat 1997).

One approach that has been used to address the above issues was based on the observation that chimeric FeLV-B/A-MuLV Env glycoproteins that were spliced between the VRA-VRB variable loops of SU (these loops contribute to receptor recognition properties of γ-retroviruses; Battini et al. 1992, 1995)) were unable to use either human Pit1 or Pit2 but were able to efficiently use certain Pit1/Pit2 chimeras (Tailor and Kabat 1997, 2000b). By analyzing various combinations of Env chimeras and site-directed mutants for abilities to use distinct Pit1/Pit2 chimeric receptors, evidence was obtained concerning the regions in the Env glycoproteins that functionally interact with specific sites of human Pit1 and Pit2. Interestingly, these results suggested that FeLV-B and A-MuLV SU glycoproteins interact with their receptors at precisely correspondent contact sites in the same overall orientations (Tailor and Kabat 1997, 2000b). However, differences between viral strains can affect the absolute and relative energetic contributions of specific contact sites. We believe that, considered together, the evidence in this field supports the conclusion that the viruses that use Pit1 and Pit2 interact with them in the same orientation at a correspondent contact surface, consistent with the idea that these viruses formed by divergent evolution from a common origin.

In accordance with this idea and with the model described in Fig. 3, recent evidence strongly suggests that the viruses originally identified as being specific for Pit1 or Pit2 actually are generally rather promiscuous

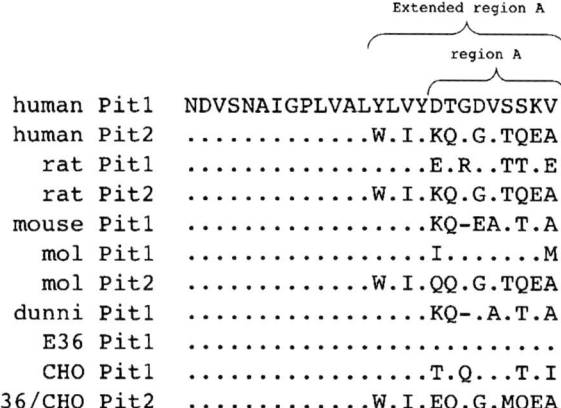

Fig. 5 Comparison of an important hypervariable region in the Pit1 and Pit2 proteins of different mammalian species. The sequences indicated as *region A* and *extended region A* have been shown to have a major influence on ability of the corresponding proteins to function as γ-retroviral receptors. It is generally believed that Pit1 and Pit2 have identical topologies, consistent with their common function as highly homologous Na^+-phosphate symporters, and that the sequences indicated comprise an extracellular loop (ECL4) that interacts with the viruses. However, this hypothesis has not been proven unambiguously. Moreover, other regions (e.g., ECL2) of the Pit proteins also contribute to the interactions with viruses. The variable sequences occur amid highly conserved regions

in their abilities to use both receptors. Thus, for example, FeLV-B uses both Pit1 and Pit2 in domestic cats, with distinct FeLV-B isolates differing somewhat in their abilities to use feline Pit2 (Boomer et al. 1997; Sugai et al. 2001). Furthermore, the abilities of FeLV-B viruses to use feline Pit2 seem to be acquired by selection during their replication in vivo (Anderson et al. 2001). In addition, some FeLV-B isolates can even use hamster Pit2 (Boomer et al. 1997). Similarly, GALV can use hamster Pit1 and Pit2 (Wilson et al. 1994) and Japanese feral mouse Pit1 and Pit2 (Schneiderman et al. 1996; Wilson et al. 1994). A single amino acid change in human Pit2 enables it to function as a receptor for GALV (Eiden et al. 1996), and a single amino acid insertion in region A of murine Pit1 makes it a functional receptor for A-MuLVs (Lundorf et al. 1998). Interestingly, a Pit ortholog in the fungus *Neurospora crassa* was recently shown to function as a receptor for the 10A1 MuLV (L. Pedersen, personal communication). This evidence strongly supports the hypothesis (see Sect. 7.1 and Fig. 3) that the viruses that use Pit1 and/or

Pit2 recognize common features in these proteins but inhibitory sequence changes during evolution have partially or fully restricted infections by particular viruses. This interpretation is also supported by evidence that the divergent extended A regions of Pit1 and Pit2 are bordered by highly conserved areas (see Fig. 5) and by mutagenesis studies that imply that individual amino acids in the divergent region are unnecessary for infections (Chaudry and Eiden 1997).

7.4
Xenotropic and Polytropic MuLVs

The interactions of these closely related viruses with X-receptors of mice provides an excellent illustration of host-virus coevolution and of host range control. As mentioned above, X-MuLVs were initially termed xenotropic because they cannot infect inbred strains of mice derived from European origins (Levy 1978). However, X-MuLVs are frequently endogenously inherited in these inbred mice and they are sometimes expressed during their lifetimes (Kozak and O'Neill 1987; Levy 1978). In addition, X-MuLVs can infect many wild strains of mice such as *Mus spretus* and *Mus dunni* (Kozak 1985). In contrast, polytropic MuLVs (MCFs) efficiently infect almost all mice and they are often highly pathogenic (Cloyd et al. 1980; Hartley et al. 1977; Kabat 1989; Kozak 1985; Rosenberg and Jolicoeur 1997; Ruscetti et al. 1981; Stoye et al. 1991). Certain mice are, nevertheless, resistant to MCFs and/or to X-MuLVs because of endogenous interfering Env glycoproteins (Bassin et al. 1982; Jung et al. 2002; Kozak 1985; Lyu and Kozak 1996; Lyu et al. 1999; Ruscetti et al. 1981, 1985), transcriptional repression (Aaronson and Stephenson 1973; Levy 1978), and/or production of a serum lipoprotein factor that specifically inactivates these viruses (Levy 1978; Wu et al. 2002). Although it is unknown how this lipoprotein factor specifically inactivates X-MuLVs and P-MuLVs, it is interesting that a lipoprotein can also inactivate hepatitis C virus (Enjoji et al. 2000). In addition, *Mus castaneus* mice are completely resistant to X-MuLVs and P-MuLVs primarily because of a small deletion mutation in their X-receptor gene (Marin et al. 1999). However, *Mus castaneus* mice also inherit an X-MuLV-related Env glycoprotein (Lyu and Kozak 1996; Lyu et al. 1999). As determined by genetic crosses, this Env glycoprotein interferes with infections mediated by X-receptors from wild mice that interact with the X-MuLV Env but not with infections mediated by X-receptors from European mice that cannot interact with X-MuLVs. Thus this Env glycoprotein blocks MCF and X-MuLV infections in *Mus castaneus* x *Mus spretus* F1 hybrids, but does not block MCF infections of *Mus castaneus* x *Mus musculus* F1 hybrids (Lyu and Kozak 1996; Lyu et al. 1999). This supports the idea that interference requires strong binding of an interfering Env glycoprotein to the receptor that occurs in the specific animal. Furthermore, hamster cells are resistant to infections by both X-MuLVs and MCFs (Marin et al. 1999; Miller and Miller 1992).

Interestingly, when expressed in CHO cells the X-receptors from these European and Asian strains of mice and from hamster, mink, and humans conferred viral susceptibilities that were identical to the susceptibilities of the cells used for the X-receptor cDNA isolations (Marin et al. 1999). Thus xenotropism in this system is caused by inherent properties of the X-receptor orthologs. Figure 6 compares the sequences of these X-receptors in their critical presumptive ECL3 and ECL4 regions. These regions of the X-receptors contain consensus sites for N-linked glycosylation and are much more polymorphic than other regions of the proteins (see Marin et al. 1999).

X-receptors were recently cloned independently by three groups (Battini et al. 1999; Tailor et al. 1999a; Yang et al. 1999). Subsequently, a mutagenesis study was done to identify sequences responsible for the ability of X-MuLVs to use the *Mus dunni* X-receptor but not the NIH Swiss mouse ortholog (Marin et al. 1999). Interestingly, it was found that the NIH Swiss X-receptor contains two key differences (identified in Fig. 6 as K500E in ECL3 and T582Δ in ECL4) that are both necessary to prevent its utilization by X-MuLVs. Thus reversal of either of these mutations is sufficient to enable use of the NIH Swiss X-receptor by X-MuLVs. Conversely, both K500E and T582Δ must be substituted into the *Mus dunni* protein to prevent its use by X-MuLVs. These results suggest that X-MuLVs interact with different sites in the X-receptor, so that elimination of both sites in the *Mus dunni* protein is needed for resistance to infection. Furthermore, neither the K500E nor the T582Δ mutation had any effect on MCF infections, implying that MCFs rely on sites in the X-receptors that are unimportant for X-MuLVs and vice versa. It is noteworthy, however, that residues corresponding K500 and T582 both occur in the hamster X-receptor and that K500 occurs in the *Mus castaneus* X-receptor, despite the fact that they cannot mediate X-MuLV infections. Consequently, the latter X-receptors must contain other in-

```
                                                                    ECL 3
Human X-MLV   LKWDESKGLLPNSEESGICHKYTYGVRAIVQCIPAWLRFIQCCLRRYRDTKRAFPHLVNAGKYSTFFM
                                       *
NIH Swiss     ..........................DPQ.PEF....S.........................N.R......T
M. dunni      ..........................DPQ.PEF....S................................T
SC-1          ..........................DPQ.PEF....S..........................R.....T
M.spretus     ..........................DPQ.PEF....S..........................R.....T
M.castanteus  ..........................DPQ.PEF....S..........................R.....T
Hamster       ........*.................DPQ.PEF..R.S..........................R.....T
              ....N.S...................DLQ.PEF..R.............................R.....T
Mink          ......G...................PE..........S..............V.................T

              VTFAALYSTHKERGHSDTMVFFYLWIVFYIISSCYTLIWDLKMDWGLFDKNAGENTFLREEIVYPQKAYY
                          ◆ 500
                           *
Human X-MLV   ......E.QN............V.......VF.C...................................
NIH Swiss     ........QN............V.......VF.C...................................
M. dunni      ......................V.......VF.C...................................
SC-1          ........QN............V.......VF.C...................................
M.spretus     ........QN............V.......VF.C...................................
M.castanteus  ........Q.............V..L....V..CA..................................
Hamster       ..............................C................................P..R..
Mink

                                           ECL 4
                                            ◆ 582
Human X-MLV   YCAIIEDVILRFAWTIQISITSTTLLPHSGDIIATVFAPLEVFRRFVWNFF
NIH Swiss     ..............................A-.FK..V.N..........
M. dunni      ..............................A..FK..V............
SC-1          ..............................A..FK..V...........L
M.spretus     ..............................A..FK..V............
M.castanteus  ........................I.....A----.V.............
Hamster       ..............................A.AFQ..V............
Mink          ..T...................V........M..................
```

hibitory mutation(s) that override the permissive effects of K500 and/or T582.

A striking aspect of this system is that MCFs cause only weak interference to superinfections, whereas X-MuLVs cause strong interference that seems to depend on the presence of K500 and to a lesser extent on T582 (Marin et al. 1999). Accordingly, MCFs, which seem to ignore K500 and T582, have only weak interference and massively superinfect cells in culture and in vivo, which likely contributes to their pathogenic effects (Chesebro and Wehrly 1985; Herr and Gilbert 1984; Kozak 1985; Marin et al. 1999; Temin 1988; Yoshimura et al. 2001). An hypothesis that could explain these results is that mutations in the X-receptors of European mice corresponding to K500E and T582Δ (perhaps in cooperation with other changes) enabled the mice to escape from X-MuLVs and that P-MuLVs then evolved to overcome these host barriers by changing their *env* genes. However, because the K500E and T582Δ receptor mutations are probably inhibitory barriers that reduce accessibility of the viruses, the MCFs bind weakly and cause negligible interference. These data appear to support a ratchet model of coevolution in which polymorphisms in receptors lead to compensatory adaptations in the viruses in an endless progression that results in increasing diversity of the host receptors and of the viruses.

7.5
The RD114 Superfamily of Retroviruses

The RD114 superfamily, which generally use human ASCT2 as a common receptor (Blond et al. 2000; Lavillette et al. 2002a; Marin et al. 2000; Rasko et al. 1999; Tailor et al. 1999b), is the most widely dispersed interference group of retroviruses. This group includes not only the RD114 feline endogenous virus but also BaEV, HERV-W, type D primate retro-

---

Fig. 6 Comparison of an important region in the X-receptors that mediates infections by X-MuLVs and P-MuLVs (*MCFs*). Hypervariable regions identified as *ECL3* and *ECL4* are believed to control infections by these viruses, with the sequences indicated by *diamonds* (identified at positions 500 and 582) being especially important. Identical residues are indicated by *dots* and deletions by *dashes*. The TM regions in the human sequence are *underlined*. Sites for N-linked glycosylation are indicated with *asterisks*

viruses, and avian REVs and SNVs (Gautier et al. 2000; Kewalramani et al. 1992; Koo et al. 1991, 1992; Lavillette et al. 2002a; Marin et al. 2000; Sommerfelt and Weiss 1990). Strong evidence suggests that the *env* genes of these viruses evolved by divergent evolution from a common origin (Benit et al. 2001; Boeke and Stoye 1997). In particular, it is believed that the avian group formed by a rare zoonosis from a primate progenitor into a bird (Barbacid et al. 1979; Kewalramani et al. 1992; Koo et al. 1991, 1992) and that RD114 may also have arisen by infection of a cat by a primate γ-retrovirus related to BaEV (Barbacid et al. 1979; van der Kuyl et al. 1999). Consistent with the hypothesis that they had a common origin, these viruses all contain an immunosuppressive domain in TM (Benit et al. 2001; van der Kuyl et al. 1997); they all lack the PHQ motif for transactivation that occurs near the amino terminus of SU in other γ-retroviruses; and they all interact with the same region of the receptors (see below). This viral superfamily probably also includes many additional members that have not yet been analyzed for their receptor usages, including, for example, the HERV-F family that is very similar to HERV-W (Benit et al. 2001). This system has provided particularly strong evidence that the viruses have evolved to recognize conserved amino acids in the receptor that are difficult for the host to mutate without loss of fitness, and that the host response has been to drastically alter nearby regions that can interfere with access of virus to the recognition site, as proposed in Fig. 3. These host changes include insertions and deletions and additions of bulky N-linked oligosaccharides. Because the viruses recognize highly conserved sequences, they are generally capable of using both ASCT2 and the related transporter ASCT1 (Lavillette et al. 2002a; Marin et al. 2000). The ASCT transporters are members of the glutamate transporter superfamily, which have been extensively investigated for their topology and structure (Brocke et al. 2002; Kanai 1997; Seal et al. 2000; Slotboom et al. 1999; Utsunomiya-Tate et al. 1996; Zerangue and Kavanaugh 1996). These transporters all contain an associated Cl^- anion channel that is gated open in the presence of a transported amino acid. However, the Cl^- flux is uncoupled from the amino acid flux (Broer et al. 2000; Slotboom et al. 1999; Zerangue and Kavanaugh 1996).

The human ASCT2 receptor was originally cloned from cDNA libraries based on the natural resistance of NIH Swiss mouse fibroblasts to RD114 (Rasko et al. 1999; Tailor et al. 1999b). Consistent with this strategy, the mouse ASCT2 ortholog was found to be inactive as a receptor for RD114 (Marin et al. 2000, 2003). By using human/mouse ASCT2 chimeras it was then found that the critical sequence difference occurred in ECL2, which is shown in Fig. 7. Specifically, it was found that region C in the carboxyl-terminal portion of ECL2 in human ASCT2 was necessary for infections by RD114, BaEV, and type D primate retroviruses and that substitution of this region into mouse ASCT2 generated an active receptor for all of these viruses (Marin et al. 2003). Interestingly, this ECL2 region is hypervariable compared with other regions of the human and mouse ASCT2 proteins (see Fig. 7).

Despite the general use of human ASCT2 as a common receptor, the viruses of this interference group have distinct host ranges. For example, BaEV and HERV-W efficiently infect mouse cells. Furthermore, RD114 and type D primate retroviruses can also infect mouse cells that have been pretreated with tunicamycin to eliminate N-linked oligosaccharides (Marin et al. 2000). Interestingly, hamster cells are resistant to all viruses of this superfamily including BaEV and HERV-W, but the hamster cells also become susceptible after treatment with tunicamycin (Marin et al. 2003). Further studies showed that mouse ASCT2 is not a receptor for BaEV and that N-deglycosylated mutants of mouse ASCT2 also are nonfunctional as receptors for BaEV, RD114, or type D primate retroviruses. These viral host range properties were explained by the finding that human and mouse ASCT1, which are approximately 58% identical to human ASCT2, are strong receptors for BaEV and HERV-W but not for RD114 or type D viruses. Furthermore, N-deglycosylation of the mouse ASCT1 C-region by mutagenesis converted it into a strong receptor for all of the viruses including RD114 and type D primate viruses (Lavillette et al. 2002a; Marin et al. 2000, 2003).

Figure 7 compares the ECL2 sequences of human and mouse ASCT2 and ASCT1 and of the hamster ASCT1 protein. Significantly, the only two N-linked glycosylation sites in mouse and human ASCT1 occur within ECL2 region C, and elimination of either of these sites by mutagenesis is sufficient to activate mouse ASCT1 as a receptor for RD114 and the type D viruses (Marin et al. 2000). Thus the two N-linked oligosaccharides in mouse ASCT1 collaborate to block interaction with RD114 and type D viruses, and neither one alone is sufficient. However, these two oligosaccharides are unable to block interactions with BaEV and HERV-W. Interestingly, hamster ASCT1 contains a third N-linked oligosaccharide in ECL2 region C (see Fig. 7) and this oligosaccharide by itself is sufficient to prevent infection of all the viruses in this super-

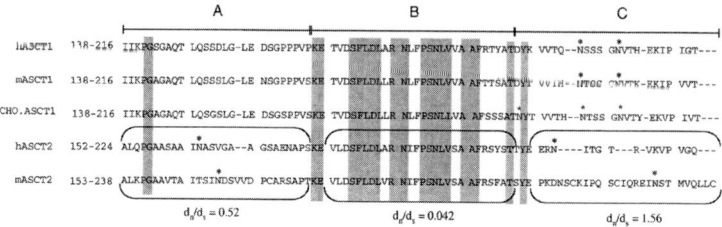

Fig. 7 Comparison of the critical ECL3 regions of ASCT1 and ASCT2 proteins from different species. Chimera and site-directed mutagenesis studies indicated that region C within ECL3 is critical for control of the viral receptor functions of these proteins. Amino acids that are identical in all of the proteins are shown by *shading*. Sites for N-linked glycosylation have been proven to occur and are indicated by *asterisks*. The ratios of nonsynonymous to synonymous nucleotide sequence substitutions in the cDNAs (i.e., the dn/ds ratios) of the human and mouse ASCT2 sequences are indicated below the protein sequences. These ratios confirm that region C has been under strong evolutionary pressure to diverge and that the adjacent region B has been under strong positive selection pressure to be retained. This supports other evidence that region C has been a battlefield in host-virus coevolution and that the N-linked glycosylations in this region negatively influence viral utilization. Despite the enormous diversity in region C of these ASCT1 and ASCT2 proteins, many γ-retroviruses efficiently and promiscuously use them as receptors (see text). These results strongly support the model in Fig. 3, implying that the viruses recognize conserved sequences that are situated amid hypervariable negative control regions

family (Marin et al. 2003). This additional N-linked oligosaccharide occurs in CHO ASCT1 between two highly conserved amino acids that are not only common to ASCT1 and ASCT2 proteins of both humans and mice but are also conserved in all other members of the glutamate transporter superfamily. Thus the hypervariable region C occurs adjacent to a highly conserved region that is likely to be important for normal transporter function. Although all of the viruses in this interference group have a substantial ability to use both ASCT2 and ASCT1 when the latter is N-deglycosylated, the HERV-W Env is especially promiscuous because it alone can also use N-deglycosylated mouse ASCT2 as a receptor (Lavillette et al. 2002a). Such broad abilities of viruses to use ASCT1 and ASCT2 proteins as receptors is surprising, particularly because common features cannot be discerned within the critical control region C (see Fig. 7). The only reasonable interpretation in our opinion is that the viruses recognize invariant features in ECL2 that are highly conserved and that the variable region C is a negative control area that modulates viral reception by steric hindrance and other inhibitory mechanisms, as proposed by the model in Fig. 3.

A corollary of this interpretation is that it has been advantageous for mammals to change region C of ECL2 and to conserve the adjacent region B. In agreement with this hypothesis, the ratios of nonsynonymous to synonymous nucleotide substitutions determined by a comparison of the human and mouse ASCT2 cDNAs is 0.125 for the complete coding sequences and 0.52, 0.042, and 1.56 for the A, B, and C regions of ECL2, respectively, as shown in Fig. 7. This analysis supports the conclusions that ASCT2 is an important protein that has been conserved throughout evolution, that region B in ECL2 has been under especially strong selection pressure to remain conserved, and, conversely, that region C has been under extremely strong pressure to diverge in its amino acid sequence, presumably because of viral attack. These results strongly support the general interpretations outlined above in Sect. 7.1 and in Fig. 3.

7.6
The FeLV-C Receptor

The receptor for FeLV-C, FLVCR1, was recently cloned from human and domestic cat cDNA libraries (Quigley et al. 2000; Tailor et al. 1999c). It is a member of the major facilitator superfamily (MFS) of transporters that contains 12 TM domains and is weakly homologous to MFS transporters for small organic anions such as glycerol-3-phosphate and glucarate. MFS transporters contain common features including 12–14 TM domains, a large hydrophilic loop between TM6 and TM7, and a conserved sequence between TM2 and TM3 (Pao et al. 1998). FLVCR1 has been classified as MFS subfamily member 28 of unknown function. Other MFS subfamilies include the widely studied 12-TM glucose transporters.

Because the SU envelopes of FeLV-C evolve in vivo from FeLV-A by accumulation of a few mutations in one disulfide-bonded loop that has been implicated in receptor interactions (Brojatsch et al. 1992; Rigby et al. 1992), it was proposed that the receptor for FeLV-A might be an MFS transporter that is closely related to FLVCR1 (Tailor et al. 1999c). Consistent with this hypothesis, a 70-kDa protein of unknown function has been implicated as a FeLV-A receptor (Ghosh et al. 1992). Similarly, small adaptive changes in disulfide-bonded loop regions of SU cause slight shifts of coreceptor specificities of HIV-1 (Chabot and Broder 2000; Connor et al. 1997; Glushakova et al. 1998; Littman 1998; Platt et al. 2001) and of other retroviruses (Masuka et al. 1996a,b; Taplitz and Coffin 1997). On the basis of these considerations, a human protein termed FLVCR2 that is closely related to FLVCR1 (52% amino acid identity) was recently cloned (C. Tailor, manuscript in preparation). Human FLVCR2 is a weak receptor for FeLV-C but does not mediate infections by FeLV-A, which was expected because human cells are resistant to FeLV-A. Because FeLV-A is principally infectious for feline cells, it will be important to clone the feline ortholog of FLVCR2 to determine whether it is a receptor for FeLV-A. Based on their similarities, chimeras of the human FLVCR1 and FLVCR2 proteins were generated. Their analysis identified ECL6 of FLVCR1 as a critical region for FeLV-C receptor function (C. Tailor, manuscript in preparation). This region is highly diverse compared with other regions of FLVCR1 and FLVCR2 and differs at 7 of 10 amino acids.

7.7
A Pair of PERV-A Receptors

Recently, Ericsson et al. (C. Patience, personal communication) molecularly cloned two closely related human proteins, PHuR-A1 and PHuR-A2, that function as receptors for PERV-A and are widely expressed in human tissues, consistent with previous viral susceptibility studies (Takeuchi et al. 1998; Wilson et al. 2000). These novel receptors have unknown functions and have hydrophobicity profiles suggesting that they contain 10–11 TM domains, consistent with the other receptors for γ-retroviruses, which also contain multiple TM sequences. The widespread expression of these receptors in human tissues is of special concern because of the use of pig organs for xenotransplantation. The use by PERV-A of the closely related receptor pairs PHuR-A1 and PHuR-A2 is intriguing in view of the other examples of receptor pairs (e.g., Pit1 and Pit2, ASCT1 and ASCT2, FLVCR1 and FLVCR2) discussed above.

8
The Role(s) of Receptors in γ-Retrovirus Infections

8.1
General Issues

As discussed in the sections below, the interactions of retroviruses with cell surfaces involve multiple steps, including adsorption from the extracellular medium, binding of Env glycoproteins to receptors, cooperative interactions between Env glycoproteins within the trimeric SU-TM complexes and between trimers (i.e., cross-talk), and irreversible conformational changes of the Env glycoproteins that lead to the formation of a membrane fusion pore. Although receptors appear to be essential for the overall process, they seem to be expendable for many of the individual steps. For example, in some situations γ-retroviruses can infect cells that lack the cognate receptor (Barnett and Cunningham 2001; Barnett et al. 2001; Innes et al. 1990; Lavillette et al. 2002b; Sharma et al. 1997, 2000). Furthermore, the viral adsorption process seems to occur independently of the receptors (Andreadis et al. 2000; Pizzato et al. 1999, 2001; Sharma et al. 2000), and it is also unclear whether the receptors perform a hit-and-run function or whether they participate in the final membrane fusion steps. Because these issues are critical for understanding the roles of receptors, we will discuss them briefly.

8.2
Adsorption onto Cell Surfaces

Adsorption of viruses onto cultured cells from the medium is usually a very slow and inefficient process, principally because of the slow rates of their diffusion into contact with the cell surfaces (Allison and Valentine 1960; Andreadis et al. 2000; Valentine and Allison 1959). In general, the rate of contact cannot be significantly enhanced by mixing or stirring because the boundary layer of relatively stationary fluid that surrounds walls or other large objects (e.g., cells) in flowing liquids is substantial compared with the rate of virus diffusion, so that the stirring does not increase the concentration of virus that surrounds this boundary zone (Allison and Valentine 1960; Palsson and Andreadis 1997; Valentine and Allison 1959).

In the case of retroviruses, it has become especially clear that adsorption is a severely limiting step in infection of cultured cells. In classic studies in which virus samples were incubated with cells for several hours before washing with fresh medium and subsequently detecting the foci of infection, it was estimated that only 1/1,000 or fewer of the virions in the medium were infectious. In contrast to previous interpretations, recent studies suggested that this low infectivity-to-virion ratio is principally caused by the inefficiency of adsorption (Andreadis et al. 2000). Accordingly, serial incubation of a virus-containing medium for 2-h periods with sequential cell cultures results in the same titers in each of the cultures after correction for spontaneous viral decay (Kabat et al. 1994). Furthermore, centrifuging the virus down onto the cultured cells (i.e., spinoculation) often increases retroviral titers by 1–2 orders of magnitude (Bahnson et al. 1995; Damico and Bates 2000; Forestell et al. 1996; O'Doherty et al. 2000).

Recently, it has become possible to count retrovirions adsorbed onto cell surfaces by confocal immunofluoresence microscopy or by quantitative PCR methods (Marechal et al. 2001; O'Doherty et al. 2000; Pizzato et al. 1999). Such studies have demonstrated that receptors for viral entry are irrelevant for initial adsorption of retrovirions onto surfaces of most cells (Pizzato et al. 1999, 2001). On the contrary, the initial steps of virus attachment seem to more critically depend on accessory cellular binding substances such as heparan sulfates, integrins, or lectins including DC-SIGN (Bounou et al. 2002; Guibinga et al. 2002; Jinno-Oue et al. 2001; Lee et al. 2001; Mondor et al. 1998; Saphire et al. 2001; Zhang et al. 2002). By forming multivalent weak reversible bonds with such abundant cell surface components, a virus would become efficiently bound in a manner that would allow it to graze until it makes appropriate contact with a true receptor (Haywood 1994; Park et al. 2000). A similar grazing or rolling process occurs when lymphocyte selectins contact their carbohydrate ligands in the capillary endothelium (Li et al. 1996a,b; McEver et al. 1995). In essence, the accessory binding factors would be expected to more efficiently attach the virus onto the cell surface in a manner that allows it to move, thus enabling it to make improved and repetitive contacts with a small number of receptors. Formation of such "capture complexes" (Park et al. 2000), may be especially important for viruses such as FeLV-T, MCFs, SNVs, and primary patient isolates of HIV-1 that bind to their receptors with very low affinities. By a similar mechanism, heparan sulfates enhance chemokine and growth factor signaling processes

(Aviezer et al. 1994; Bounou et al. 2002; Jinno-Oue et al. 2001; Lee et al. 2001; Park et al. 2000; Schlessinger et al. 1995). Binding of the PVC-211 neurotropic variant of Friend E-MuLV onto heparan sulfates is also believed to increase its infection of brain capillary endothelial cells (Jinno-Oue et al. 2001). In this context it should be recognized that a small number of cell surface receptors (e.g., 10^3 per cell) is theoretically capable of efficiently capturing any tight-binding ligand that diffuses onto the cell surface, so that accessory binding substances would not necessarily enhance attachment of a high-affinity virus or hormonal ligand to its receptor (Berg and Purcell 1977). Bacteriophage lambda is an example of a virus that binds efficiently onto its receptor even when the receptor concentration is low (Schwartz 1975, 1976). However, such accessory associations can be critically important for viruses or other ligands that bind only weakly and reversibly onto their receptors. Such ligands would be more likely to dissociate from the cells if they were not anchored to the binding substances.

8.3
Binding to Receptors Initiates a Pathway of Cooperative Interactions Between Env Glycoproteins

Recent evidence has suggested that assembly of a complex containing several receptors may be a prerequisite for the membrane fusion step of retrovirus infections and that multiple Env molecules cooperatively participate in this process. For example, several Env glycoprotein trimers appear to be necessary for retroviral infectivity (Bachrach et al. 2000; Frey et al. 1995; Layne et al. 1990). In the case of HIV-1, the presence of more than one CD4 in contact with the virus enhances the infectivity dramatically and reduces the concentration of coreceptor needed for infection (Platt et al. 1998). Further investigation of this system has implied that a critical complex containing approximately four to six coreceptors is a requirement for infection, although it is not known whether this complex performs a transient role and then disperses or is maintained throughout the membrane fusion process (Kuhmann et al. 2000; Platt et al. 2001). Despite some uncertainties, several lines of evidence have suggested that three to six hemagglutin trimers may cooperatively participate in the influenza A virus-mediated membrane fusion reaction (Blumenthal et al. 1996; Boulay et al. 1988; Danieli et al. 1996; Ellens et al. 1990; Gunther-Ausborn et al. 2000) and that multiple envelope glycoprotein trimers are required for rabies virus-mediated membrane fusion (Roche and Gaudin 2002). Receptor clusters also appear to enhance infectivities of MuLVs (Battini et al. 1995; Davey et al. 1999; Salaün et al. 2002; Valsesia-Wittmann et al. 1997). In the case of ALV-A, titration studies by Damico and Bates also strongly support the idea that a multivalent Env-receptor complex is essential for infection (Damico and Bates 2000).

Cooperative interactions have also been reported between the monomeric units of the SU-TM trimeric complexes. Infectious γ-retrovirions can be produced by cells that coexpress two mutant Env glycoproteins that are individually incapable of forming infectious virus pseudotypes (Zhao et al. 1997). For example, a MuLV mutant with a defect in SU that prevents receptor attachment was complemented by a fusion-defective TM mutant (Rein et al. 1998; Zhao et al. 1997). Similar studies with HIV-1 implied that binding to CD4 and to coreceptors can involve different monomers within the Env trimeric complexes (Salzwedel and Berger 2000). However, the latter investigation was based on syncytia assays and was done with cells that expressed very high concentrations of the Env glycoproteins. The basic conclusion of these investigations was that two Env monomers that are defective at different stages of the fusion pathway can form heterotrimers that work in concert to mediate fusion. In agreement with these ideas, Env glycoprotein trimers function as concerted units in inserting the amino termini of their TM subunits into target cell membranes (Carr et al. 1997; Carr and Kim 1993; Chan et al. 1997; Li et al. 1996; Salzwedel and Berger 2000; Wahlberg et al. 1992; Zhao et al. 1997, 1998). This conformational change initially produces a trimeric coil that undergoes a further conformational change to form a six-stranded coiled coil (Carr and Kim 1993; Chan et al. 1997).

Recent investigations have also strongly suggested that intertrimer cooperative interactions may also be prerequisite for membrane fusion mediated by γ-retroviruses (Barnett and Cunningham 2001; Barnett et al. 2001, 2002; Lavillette et al. 2000, 2001, 2002b). This line of inquiry was initiated by studies of Bae et al. (1997) of a conserved PHQ motif that occurs near the amino-terminal ends of SU glycoproteins in all γ-retroviruses with the exception of those that use ASCT1 or ASCT2 as receptors. In addition, the motif is modified in the PERV viruses, being SHK and PHR for PERV-A and PERV-B, respectively (Patience et al. 2001; Takeuchi et al. 1998). Mutation of this PHQ motif blocked membrane fusion but had no effect on receptor attachment (Bae et al. 1997;

Lavillette et al. 2002b; Zavorotinskaya and Albritton 1999). Subsequently, Lavillette and coworkers (2000) discovered that noninfectious γ-retrovirions lacking this histidine could be transactivated by addition to the cultured cells of a soluble SU or of an amino-terminal fragment of SU called the receptor-binding domain (RBD) (Battini et al. 1992, 1995, 1998). Initially, it was found that transactivation requires the use of cells that contain receptors for both the ΔHis virus and for the RBD but that the receptor specificity of the RBD need not match that of the ΔHis virus (Barnett and Cunningham 2001; Barnett et al. 2001, 2002; Lavillette et al. 2000, 2001). Thus, for example, a Friend E-MuLV RBD can trans-complement ΔHis viruses derived from A-MuLV, MCF, X-MuLV, FeLV-B, or FeLV-T (Barnett and Cunningham 2001; Barnett et al. 2001, 2002; Lavillette et al. 2000). Similarly, an A-MuLV RBD can at least weakly transactivate ΔHis E-MuLV (Lavillette et al. 2000, 2001) and ΔHis FeLV-B (D. Lavillette, unpublished observation). FeLV-T can be transactivated by FELIX, FeLV-B, or MuLV-E (Anderson et al. 2000; Barnett et al. 2002; Lauring et al. 2001, 2002). Despite such examples of cross-reactivity, transcomplementation reactions are often nonreciprocal or even specific (Barnett and Cunningham 2001; Farrell et al. 2002). For example, complementation of fusion-defective PHQ motif mutants of GALV requires a GALV RBD (Farrell et al. 2002). Further investigations of transcomplementation have suggested the hypothesis that receptor engagement of a retroviral SU glycoprotein may induce exposure of the amino terminal PHQ motif (or a site that is controlled by this motif) and a region termed C2 in the carboxyl-terminal portion of the SU and that these exposed sites in nearby trimers may then associate in a manner that is essential for the membrane fusion reaction (Barnett and Cunningham 2001; Barnett et al. 2002; Lavillette et al. 2001, 2002b). Because transcomplementation can be achieved by a soluble RBD, it is clear that the activation can occur from outside of the virus-associated ΔHis Env trimer. This implies that the natural process of γ-retroviral infection may involve corresponding intertrimer interactions on the viral surface.

Although initial studies indicated that transcomplementation required association of both the RBD and the ΔHis virus with their cognate receptors, as mentioned above, recent investigations demonstrated that several γ-retroviruses with mutant or recombinant Env glycoproteins can be transactivated in the absence of their receptors, as long as the receptor for the RBD is present (Barnett and Cunningham 2001; Barnett et al. 2001, 2002; Lavillette et al. 2002b). For example, Cunningham and coworkers reported that γ-retroviruses with a deletion of sequences needed for receptor binding can be transactivated by RBDs bound to their cognate receptor (Barnett and Cunningham 2001; Barnett et al. 2001, 2002). A likely interpretation is that the C2 Env regions in those mutant and recombinant viruses may be exposed in the absence of a receptor. In this circumstance, binding of an RBD to its receptor can enable it to transactivate a virus that is not attached to a receptor.

Recent studies by Overbaugh and coworkers have demonstrated that similar transactivation processes can occur in natural infections by γ-retroviruses. Specifically, they found that infections by the immunosuppressive FeLV-T virus, which has a Pro in place of His in its PHQ motif (Donahue et al. 1991; Overbaugh et al. 1988), require transactivation either by a soluble FeLV-B-related SU glycoprotein termed FELIX that is endogenously expressed in cat T cells or by an FeLV-B SU glycoprotein (Anderson et al. 2000; Lauring et al. 2001, 2002). These transactivations require the natural FeLV-B receptor Pit1 (Anderson et al. 2000; Lauring et al. 2001). The FeLV-T SU glycoprotein binds with negligible affinity to susceptible cells (Donahue et al. 1991; Kristal et al. 1993; Lauring et al. 2001; Moser et al. 1998; Reinhard et al. 1993; Rohn et al. 1998), and it is consequently unclear whether FeLV-T can be transactivated in the absence of a primary receptor or might also interact with Pit1. The former possibility is supported by recent evidence that FeLV-T can be transactivated by a MuLV-E RBD in cells that contain mouse CAT1 but lack functional Pit1 receptors (Barnett et al. 2002). Similarly, it was recently found that MCFs can infect cells that lack functional X-receptors if they are transactivated by the Friend E-MuLV RBD (J. Cunningham, personal communication). As described above in Sect. 4.2, MCFs naturally occur only in mice that also contain replicating E-MuLVs (Fischinger et al. 1978; Kabat 1989; Rosenberg and Jolicoeur 1997; Stoye et al. 1991). Presumably, MCFs may have the C2 region of their SU glycoproteins in an exposed conformation in the absence of X-receptors. Interestingly, both FeLV-T and MCFs are examples of γ-retroviruses that emerge late in natural infections initiated by other viruses (FeLV-A and E-MuLV, respectively), that bind to receptors weakly or negligibly, and that cause massive superinfections with cytopathic consequences (Donahue et al. 1991; Hartley et al. 1977; Herr and Gilbert 1984; Marin et al. 1999; Moser et al. 1998; Rohn et al. 1998; Yoshimura et al. 2001). Transactivation is clearly a powerful means for such retroviruses to overcome interference barriers in chronically infected animals.

Although it seems likely that such a fundamental mechanism of viral activation by receptors must have been highly selected during evolution, we emphasize that transcomplementation has not yet been reported for other genera of retroviruses or even for all γ-retroviruses. For example, the PHQ motif is absent in the RD-114 and BaEV family of γ-retroviruses that use ASCT1 and ASCT2 as their receptors and it is substantially altered in the PERV viruses.

The evidence reviewed in this section provides very strong support for the hypothesis that attachment of γ-retroviruses to their receptors initiates a pathway that obligatorily contains intermediate steps. These intermediate steps very likely include viral association with multiple receptors, cooperative conformational changes within Env glycoprotein trimers, and cross-talk between Env trimers on the viral surfaces. A hallmark of an obligatory pathway is that blockage of intermediate steps causes a failure in the process. The transcomplementation evidence supports this idea because it suggests that a failure in Env-Env cross-talk prevents membrane fusion. Indeed, this evidence suggests that virus binding to receptors does not directly induce irreversible structural changes in SU-TM complexes as was previously believed. Rather, it implies that the binding to receptors induces SU-SU interactions that are prerequisites for later steps in a highly coordinated membrane fusion pathway. We anticipate that similar intermediate steps are likely to be involved in infections by other groups of retroviruses and perhaps in infections by other membrane-enveloped viruses.

9
Summary

Evidence obtained during the last few years has greatly extended our understanding of the cell surface receptors that mediate infections of retroviruses and has provided many surprising insights. In contrast to other cell surface components such as lectins or proteoglycans that influence infections indirectly by enhancing virus adsorption onto specific cells, the true receptors induce conformational changes in the viral envelope glycoproteins that are essential for infection. One surprise is that all of the cell surface receptors for γ-retroviruses are proteins that have multiple TM sequences, compatible with their identification in known instances as transporters of important solutes. In striking contrast, almost all other animal viruses use receptors that exclusively have single TM sequences, with the sole proven exception we know of being the coreceptors used by lentiviruses. This dichotomy strongly suggests that virus genera have been prevented because of their previous evolutionary adaptations from switching their specificities between single-TM and multi-TM receptors. This evidence also implies that γ-retroviruses formed by divergent evolution from a common origin millions of years ago and that individual viruses have occasionally jumped between species (zoonoses) while retaining their commitment to use the orthologous receptor of the new host. Another surprise is that many γ-retroviruses use not just one receptor but pairs of closely related receptors as alternatives. This appears to have enhanced viral survival by severely limiting the likelihood of host escape mutations. All of the receptors used by γ-retroviruses contain hypervariable regions that are often heavily glycosylated and that control the viral host range properties, consistent with the idea that these sequences are battlegrounds of viral host coevolution. However, in contrast to previous assumptions, we propose that γ-retroviruses have become adapted to recognize conserved sites that are important for the receptor's natural function and that the hypervariable sequences have been elaborated by the hosts as defense bulwarks that surround the conserved viral attachment sites. Previously, it was believed that binding to receptors directly triggers a series of conformational changes in the viral envelope glycoproteins that culminate in fusion of the viral and cellular membranes. However, new evidence suggests that γ-retroviral association with receptors triggers an obligatory interaction or cross-talk between envelope glycoproteins on the viral surface. If this intermediate step is prevented, infection fails. Conversely, in several circumstances this cross-talk can be induced in the absence of a cell surface receptor for the virus, in which case infection can proceed efficiently. This new evidence strongly implies that the role of cell surface receptors in infections of γ-retroviruses (and perhaps of other enveloped viruses) is more complex and interesting than was previously imagined.

Recently, another gammaretroviral receptor with multiple transmembrane sequences was cloned. See Prassolov, Y., Zhang, D., Ivanov, D., Lohler, J., Ross, S.R., and Stocking, C. Sodium-dependent myo-inositol transporter 1 is a receptor for Mus cervicolor M813 murine leukemia virus.

Acknowledgements. Our work in this field and in preparation of this manuscript has been supported by NIH Grants CA-25810 and CA-67358. The first three authors contributed equally to this review. These contributions included helping to identify key issues, reviewing drafts, and assisting with figures and references. We thank Eric Barklis for reviewing an early draft and Gloria Ellis for excellent assistance in preparing the manuscript and in organizing the reference files. We apologize to the many authors of important original contributions that were not directly cited. In addition, we thank James Cunningham, Lene Pederson, and Clive Patience for allowing us to mention their important results.

References

Aaronson SA, and Stephenson JR (1973) Independent segregation of loci for activation of biologically distinguishable RNA C-type viruses in mouse cells. Proc Natl Acad Sci USA 70:2055–2058

Abkowitz JL, Holly RD, and Adamson JW (1987) Retrovirus-induced feline pure red cell aplasia: the kinetics of erythroid marrow failure. J Cell Physiol 132:571–577

Abkowitz JL, Holly RD, and Grant CK (1987) Retrovirus-induced feline pure red cell aplasia. Hematopoietic progenitors are infected with feline leukemia virus and erythroid burst-forming cells are uniquely sensitive to heterologous complement. J Clin Invest 80:1056–1063

Adkins HB, Blacklow SC, and Young JA (2001) Two functionally distinct forms of a retroviral receptor explain the nonreciprocal receptor interference among subgroups B, D, and E avian leukosis viruses. J Virol 75:3520–3526

Adkins HB, Brojatsch J, Naughton J, Rolls MM, Pesola JM, and Young JA (1997) Identification of a cellular receptor for subgroup E avian leukosis virus. Proc Natl Acad Sci USA 94:11617–11622

Agnello V, Abel G, Elfahal M, Knight GB, and Zhang QX (1999) Hepatitis C virus and other flaviviridae viruses enter cells via low density lipoprotein receptor. Proc Natl Acad Sci USA 96:12766–12771

Albritton LM, Kim JW, Tseng L, and Cunningham JM (1993) Envelope-binding domain in the cationic amino acid transporter determines the host range of ecotropic murine retroviruses. J Virol 67:2091–2096

Albritton LM, Tseng L, Scadden D, and Cunningham JM (1989) A putative murine ecotropic retrovirus receptor gene encodes a multiple membrane-spanning protein and confers susceptibility to virus infection. Cell 57:659–666

Allison AC, and Valentine RC (1960) Virus particle adsorption. II. Adsorption of vaccinia and fowl plague viruses to cells in suspension. Biochim Biophys Acta 40:393–399

Alvarez CP, Lasala F, Carrillo J, Muniz O, Corbi AL, and Delgado R (2002) C-type lectins DC-SIGN and L-SIGN mediate cellular entry by Ebola virus in cis and in trans. J Virol 76:6841–6844

Anderson MM, Lauring AS, Burns CC, and Overbaugh J (2000) Identification of a cellular cofactor required for infection by feline leukemia virus. Science 287:1828–1830

Anderson MM, Lauring AS, Robertson S, Dirks C, and Overbaugh J (2001) Feline pit2 functions as a receptor for subgroup b feline leukemia viruses. J Virol 75:10563–10572

Andreadis S, Lavery T, Davis HE, Le Doux JM, Yarmush ML, and Morgan JR (2000) Toward a more accurate quantitation of the activity of recombinant retroviruses: alternatives to titer and multiplicity of infection [corrected and republished article originally printed in J Virol 2000 Feb;74(3):1258-66]. J Virol 74:3431–3439

Aviezer D, Hecht D, Safran M, Eisinger M, David G, and Yayon A (1994) Perlecan, basal lamina proteoglycan, promotes basic fibroblast growth factor-receptor binding, mitogenesis, and angiogenesis. Cell 79:1005–1013

Bachrach E, Marin M, Pelegrin M, Karavanas G, and Piechaczyk M (2000) Efficient cell infection by Moloney murine leukemia virus-derived particles requires minimal amounts of envelope glycoprotein. J Virol 74:8480–8486

Bae Y, Kingsman SM, and Kingsman AJ (1997) Functional dissection of the Moloney murine leukemia virus envelope protein gp70. J Virol 71:2092–2099

Bahnson AB, Dunigan JT, Baysal BE, Mohney T, Atchison RW, Nimgaonkar MT, Ball ED, and Barranger JA (1995) Centrifugal enhancement of retroviral mediated gene transfer. J Virol Methods 54:131–143

Ban J, Portetelle D, Altaner C, Horion B, Milan D, Krchnak V, Burny A, and Kettmann R (1993) Isolation and characterization of a 2.3-kilobase-pair cDNA fragment encoding the binding domain of the bovine leukemia virus cell receptor. J Virol 67:1050–1057

Baranowski E, Ruiz-Jarabo CM, and Domingo E (2001) Evolution of cell recognition by viruses. Science 292:1102–1105

Barbacid M, Hunter E, and Aaronson SA (1979) Avian reticuloendotheliosis viruses: evolutionary linkage with mammalian type C retroviruses. J Virol 30:508–514

Barnett AL, and Cunningham JM (2001) Receptor binding transforms the surface subunit of the mammalian C-type retrovirus envelope protein from an inhibitor to an activator of fusion. J Virol 75:9096–9105

Barnett AL, Davey RA, and Cunningham JM (2001) Modular organization of the Friend murine leukemia virus envelope protein underlies the mechanism of infection. Proc Natl Acad Sci USA 98:4113–4118

Barnett AL, Wensel WL, Fass D, and Cunningham JM (2002) Structure and mechanism of a "co-receptor" for infection by a pathogenic feline retrovirus. J Virol. In press

Bassin RH, Ruscetti S, Ali I, Haapala DK, and Rein A (1982) Normal DBA/2 mouse cells synthesize a glycoprotein which interferes with MCF virus infection. Virology 123:139–151

Bates P, Young JA, and Varmus HE (1993) A receptor for subgroup A Rous sarcoma virus is related to the low density lipoprotein receptor. Cell 74:1043–1051

Battini JL, Danos O, and Heard JM (1998) Definition of a 14-amino-acid peptide essential for the interaction between the murine leukemia virus amphotropic envelope glycoprotein and its receptor. J Virol 72:428–435

Battini JL, Danos O, and Heard JM (1995) Receptor-binding domain of murine leukemia virus envelope glycoproteins. J Virol 69:713–719

Battini JL, Heard JM, and Danos O (1992) Receptor choice determinants in the envelope glycoproteins of amphotropic, xenotropic, and polytropic murine leukemia viruses. J Virol 66:1468–1475

Battini JL, Rasko JE, and Miller AD (1999) A human cell-surface receptor for xenotropic and polytropic murine leukemia viruses: possible role in G protein-coupled signal transduction. Proc Natl Acad Sci USA 96:1385–1390

Beaumont T, van Nuenen A, Broersen S, Blattner WA, Lukashov VV, and Schuitemaker H (2001) Reversal of human immunodeficiency virus type 1 IIIB to a neutralization-resistant phenotype in an accidentally infected laboratory worker with a progressive clinical course. J Virol 75:2246–2252

Bechtel MK, Hayes KA, Mathes LE, Pandey R, Stromberg PC, and Roy-Burman P (1999) Recombinant feline leukemia virus (FeLV) variants establish a limited infection with altered cell tropism in specific-pathogen-free cats in the absence of FeLV subgroup A helper virus. Vet Pathol 36:91–99

Benit L, Dessen P, and Heidmann T (2001) Identification, phylogeny, and evolution of retroviral elements based on their envelope genes. J Virol 75:11709–11719

Berg HC, and Purcell EM (1977) Physics of chemoreception. Biophys J 20:193–219

Blaak H, van't Wout AB, Brouwer M, Hooibrink B, Hovenkamp E, and Schuitemaker H (2000) In vivo HIV-1 infection of $CD45RA^+CD4^+$ T cells is established primarily by syncytium-inducing variants and correlates with the rate of $CD4^+$ T cell decline. Proc Natl Acad Sci USA 97:1269–1274

Bleul CC, Wu L, Hoxie JA, Springer TA, and Mackay CR (1997) The HIV coreceptors CXCR4 and CCR5 are differentially expressed and regulated on human T lymphocytes. Proc Natl Acad Sci USA 94:1925–1930

Blond JL, Lavillette D, Cheynet V, Bouton O, Oriol G, Chapel-Fernandes S, Mandrand B, Mallet F, and Cosset FL (2000) An envelope glycoprotein of the human endogenous retrovirus HERV-W is expressed in the human placenta and fuses cells expressing the type D mammalian retrovirus receptor. J Virol 74:3321–3329

Blumenthal R, Sarkar DP, Durell S, Howard DE, and Morris SJ (1996) Dilation of the influenza hemagglutinin fusion pore revealed by the kinetics of individual cell-cell fusion events. J Cell Biol 135:63–71

Boeke JD, and Stoye JP 1997. Retrotransposons, endogenous retroviruses, and the evolution of retroelements, p. 343–435. *In* JM Coffin, Hughes SH, and Varmus HE (eds), Retroviruses. Cold Spring Harbor Laboratory Press, Plainview, New York

Bonham L, Wolgamot G, and Miller AD (1997) Molecular cloning of *Mus dunni* endogenous virus: an unusual retrovirus in a new murine viral interference group with a wide host range. J Virol 71:4663–4670

Boomer S, Eiden M, Burns CC, and Overbaugh J (1997) Three distinct envelope domains, variably present in subgroup B feline leukemia virus recombinants, mediate Pit1 and Pit2 receptor recognition. J Virol 71:8116–8123

Boomer S, Gasper P, Whalen LR, and Overbaugh J (1994) Isolation of a novel subgroup B feline leukemia virus from a cat infected with FeLV-A. Virology 204:805–810

Borza CM, and Hutt-Fletcher LM (2002) Alternate replication in B cells and epithelial cells switches tropism of Epstein Barr virus. Nat Med 8:594–599

Bottger P, and Pedersen L (2002) Two highly conserved glutamate residues critical for type III sodium-dependent phosphate transport revealed by uncoupling transport function from retroviral receptor function. J Biol Chem. In press

Boulay F, Doms RW, Webster RG, and Helenius A (1988) Posttranslational oligomerization and cooperative acid activation of mixed influenza hemagglutinin trimers. J Cell Biol 106:629–639

Bounou S, Leclerc JE, and Tremblay MJ (2002) Presence of host ICAM-1 in laboratory and clinical strains of human immunodeficiency virus type 1 increases virus infectivity and CD4(+)-T- cell depletion in human lymphoid tissue, a major site of replication in vivo. J Virol 76:1004–1014

Bour S, Perrin C, and Strebel K (1999) Cell surface CD4 inhibits HIV-1 particle release by interfering with Vpu activity. J Biol Chem 274:33800–33806

Brelot A, Heveker N, Pleskoff O, Sol N, and Alizon M (1997) Role of the first and third extracellular domains of CXCR-4 in human immunodeficiency virus coreceptor activity. J Virol 71:4744–4751

Brocke L, Bendahan A, Grunewald M, and Kanner BI (2002) Proximity of two oppositely oriented reentrant loops in the glutamate transporter GLT-1 identified by paired cysteine mutagenesis. J Biol Chem 277:3985–3992

Broer A, Wagner C, Lang F, and Broer S (2000) Neutral amino acid transporter ASCT2 displays substrate-induced Na^+ exchange and a substrate-gated anion conductance. Biochem J 346:705–710

Brojatsch J, Kristal BS, Viglianti GA, Khiroya R, Hoover EA, and Mullins JI (1992) Feline leukemia virus subgroup C phenotype evolves through distinct alterations near the N terminus of the envelope surface glycoprotein. Proc Natl Acad Sci USA 89:8457–8461

Brojatsch J, Naughton J, Rolls MM, Zingler K, and Young JA (1996) CAR1, a TNFR-related protein, is a cellular receptor for cytopathic avian leukosis-sarcoma viruses and mediates apoptosis. Cell 87:845–855

Burrage TG, Tignor GH, and Smith AL (1985) Rabies virus binding at neuromuscular junctions. Virus Res 2:273–289

Camerini D, Su HP, Gamez-Torre G, Johnson ML, Zack JA, and Chen IS (2000) Human immunodeficiency virus type 1 pathogenesis in SCID-hu mice correlates with syncytium-inducing phenotype and viral replication. J Virol 74:3196–3204

Cantin R, Fortin JF, Lamontagne G, and Tremblay M (1997) The presence of host-derived HLA-DR1 on human immunodeficiency virus type 1 increases viral infectivity. J Virol 71:1922–1930

Carr CM, Chaudhry C, and Kim PS (1997) Influenza hemagglutinin is spring-loaded by a metastable native conformation. Proc Natl Acad Sci USA 94:14306–14313

Carr CM, and Kim PS (1993) A spring-loaded mechanism for the conformational change of influenza hemagglutinin. Cell 73:823–832

Chabot DJ, and Broder CC (2000) Substitutions in a homologous region of extracellular loop 2 of CXCR4 and CCR5 alter coreceptor activities for HIV-1 membrane fusion and virus entry. J Biol Chem 275:23774–23782

Chabot DJ, Chen H, Dimitrov DS, and Broder CC (2000) N-linked glycosylation of CXCR4 masks coreceptor function for CCR5-dependent human immunodeficiency virus type 1 isolates. J Virol 74:4404–4413

Chan DC, Fass D, Berger JM, and Kim PS (1997) Core structure of gp41 from the HIV envelope glycoprotein. Cell 89:263–273

Chaudry GJ, and Eiden MV (1997) Mutational analysis of the proposed gibbon ape leukemia virus binding site in Pit1 suggests that other regions are important for infection. J Virol 71:8078–8081

Chaudry GJ, Farrell KB, Ting YT, Schmitz C, Lie SY, Petropoulos CJ, and Eiden MV (1999) Gibbon ape leukemia virus receptor functions of type III phosphate transporters from CHOK1 cells are disrupted by two distinct mechanisms. J Virol 73:2916–2920

Chen BK, Gandhi RT, and Baltimore D (1996) CD4 down-modulation during infection of human T cells with human immunodeficiency virus type 1 involves independent activities of *vpu*, *env*, and *nef*. J Virol 70:6044–6053

Chen WY, and Townes TM (2000) Molecular mechanism for silencing virally transduced genes involves histone deacetylation and chromatin condensation. Proc Natl Acad Sci USA 97:377–382

Chesebro B, and Wehrly K (1985) Different murine cell lines manifest unique patterns of interference to superinfection by murine leukemia viruses. Virology 141:119–129

Chesebro B, Wehrly K, Nishio J, and Evans L (1984) Leukemia induction by a new strain of Friend mink cell focus-inducing virus: synergistic effect of Friend ecotropic murine leukemia virus. J Virol 51:63–70

Chien ML, Foster JL, Douglas JL, and Garcia JV (1997) The amphotropic murine leukemia virus receptor gene encodes a 71-kilodalton protein that is induced by phosphate depletion. J Virol 71:4564–4570

Choe H, Farzan M, Sun Y, Sullivan N, Rollins B, Ponath PD, Wu L, Mackay CR, LaRosa G, Newman W, Gerard N, Gerard C, and Sodroski J (1996) The beta-chemokine receptors CCR3 and CCR5 facilitate infection by primary HIV-1 isolates. Cell 85:1135–1148

Christensen HN (1989) Distinguishing amino acid transport systems of a given cell or tissue. Methods Enzymol 173:576–616

Chung M, Kizhatil K, Albritton LM, and Gaulton GN (1999) Induction of syncytia by neuropathogenic murine leukemia viruses depends on receptor density, host cell determinants, and the intrinsic fusion potential of envelope protein. J Virol 73:9377–9385

Closs EI, Albritton LM, Kim JW, and Cunningham JM (1993a) Identification of a low affinity, high capacity transporter of cationic amino acids in mouse liver. J Biol Chem 268:7538–7544

Closs EI, Lyons CR, Kelly C, and Cunningham JM (1993b) Characterization of the third member of the MCAT family of cationic amino acid transporters. Identification of a domain that determines the transport properties of the MCAT proteins. J Biol Chem 268:20796–20800

Closs EI, Rinkes IH, Bader A, Yarmush ML, and Cunningham JM (1993c) Retroviral infection and expression of cationic amino acid transporters in rodent hepatocytes. J Virol 67:2097–2102

Cloyd MW, Hartley JW, and Rowe WP (1980) Lymphomagenicity of recombinant mink cell focus-inducing murine leukemia viruses. J Exp Med 151:542–552

Coffin JM 1992. Structure and classification of retroviruses, p. 19–50. *In* JA Levy (ed.), The Retroviridae, vol. 1. Penum Press, New York

Connor RI, Sheridan KE, Ceradini D, Choe S, and Landau NR (1997) Change in coreceptor use correlates with disease progression in HIV-1-infected individuals. J Exp Med 185:621–628

Corbin A, Richardson J, Denesvre C, Pozo F, Ellerbrok H, and Sitbon M (1994) The envelopes of two ecotropic murine leukemia viruses display distinct efficiencies in retroviral vaccination by interference. Virology 202:70–75

Cornelissen M, Mulder-Kampinga G, Veenstra J, Zorgdrager F, Kuiken C, Hartman S, Dekker J, van der Hoek L, Sol C, Coutinho R, and et al. (1995) Syncytium-inducing (SI) phenotype suppression at seroconversion after intramuscular inoculation of a non-syncytium-inducing/SI phenotypically mixed human immunodeficiency virus population. J Virol 69:1810–1818

Cortes MJ, Wong-Staal F, and Lama J (2002) Cell surface CD4 interferes with the infectivity of HIV-1 particles released from T cells. J Biol Chem 277:1770–1779

Damico R, and Bates P (2000) Soluble receptor-induced retroviral infection of receptor-deficient cells. J Virol 74:6469–6475

Damico RL, Crane J, and Bates P (1998) Receptor-triggered membrane association of a model retroviral glycoprotein. Proc Natl Acad Sci USA 95:2580–2585

Danieli T, Pelletier SL, Henis YI, and White JM (1996) Membrane fusion mediated by the influenza virus hemagglutinin requires the concerted action of at least three hemagglutinin trimers. J Cell Biol 133:559–569

Davey RA, Zuo Y, and Cunningham JM (1999) Identification of a receptor-binding pocket on the envelope protein of friend murine leukemia virus. J Virol 73:3758–3763

Dean GA, Groshek PM, Mullins JI, and Hoover EA (1992) Hematopoietic target cells of anemogenic subgroup C versus nonanemogenic subgroup A feline leukemia virus. J Virol 66:5561–5568

Delassus S, Sonigo P, and Wain-Hobson S (1989) Genetic organization of gibbon ape leukemia virus. Virology 173:205–213

Delwart EL, and Panganiban AT (1989) Role of reticuloendotheliosis virus envelope glycoprotein in superinfection interference. J Virol 63:273–280

Deng H, Liu R, Ellmeier W, Choe S, Unutmaz D, Burkhart M, Di Marzio P, Marmon S, Sutton RE, Hill CM, Davis CB, Peiper SC, Schall TJ, Littman DR, and Landau NR (1996) Identification of a major co-receptor for primary isolates of HIV-1. Nature 381:661–666

Domingo E, Webster RG, and Holland JJ (eds.) 1999 Origin and Evolution of Viruses. Academic Press, San Diego, California

Donahue PR, Quackenbush SL, Gallo MV, deNoronha CM, Overbaugh J, Hoover EA, and Mullins JI (1991) Viral genetic determinants of T-cell killing and immunodeficiency disease induction by the feline leukemia virus FeLV-FAIDS. J Virol 65:4461–4469

Doranz BJ, Baik SS, and Doms RW (1999) Use of a gp120 binding assay to dissect the requirements and kinetics of human immunodeficiency virus fusion events. J Virol 73:10346–10358

Doranz BJ, Rucker J, Yi Y, Smyth RJ, Samson M, Peiper SC, Parmentier M, Collman RG, and Doms RW (1996) A dual-tropic primary HIV-1 isolate that uses fusin and the beta-chemokine receptors CKR-5, CKR-3, and CKR-2b as fusion cofactors. Cell 85:1149-1158

Dragic T, Litwin V, Allaway GP, Martin SR, Huang Y, Nagashima KA, Cayanan C, Maddon PJ, Koup RA, Moore JP, and Paxton WA (1996) HIV-1 entry into CD4+ cells is mediated by the chemokine receptor CC- CKR-5. Nature 381:667-673

Dreyer K, Pedersen FS, and Pedersen L (2000) A 13-amino-acid Pit1-specific loop 4 sequence confers feline leukemia virus subgroup B receptor function upon Pit2. J Virol 74:2926-2929

Edinger AL, Amedee A, Miller K, Doranz BJ, Endres M, Sharron M, Samson M, Lu ZH, Clements JE, Murphey-Corb M, Peiper SC, Parmentier M, Broder CC, and Doms RW (1997) Differential utilization of CCR5 by macrophage and T cell tropic simian immunodeficiency virus strains. Proc Natl Acad Sci USA 94:4005-4010

Eiden MV, Farrell K, Warsowe J, Mahan LC, and Wilson CA (1993) Characterization of a naturally occurring ecotropic receptor that does not facilitate entry of all ecotropic murine retroviruses. J Virol 67:4056-4061

Eiden MV, Farrell K, and Wilson CA (1994) Glycosylation-dependent inactivation of the ecotropic murine leukemia virus receptor. J Virol 68:626-631

Eiden MV, Farrell KB, and Wilson CA (1996) Substitution of a single amino acid residue is sufficient to allow the human amphotropic murine leukemia virus receptor to also function as a gibbon ape leukemia virus receptor. J Virol 70:1080-1085

Ellens H, Bentz J, Mason D, Zhang F, and White JM (1990) Fusion of influenza hemagglutinin-expressing fibroblasts with glycophorin-bearing liposomes: role of hemagglutinin surface density. Biochemistry 29:9697-9707

Enjoji M, Nakamuta M, Kinukawa N, Sugimoto R, Noguchi K, Tsuruta S, Iwao M, Kotoh K, Iwamoto H, and Nawata H (2000) Beta-lipoproteins influence the serum level of hepatitis C virus. Med Sci Monit 6:841-844

Farrell KB, Ting YT, and Eiden MV (2002) Fusion-defective gibbon ape leukemia virus vectors can be rescued by homologous but not heterologous soluble envelope proteins. J Virol 76:4267-4274

Fass D, Davey RA, Hamson CA, Kim PS, Cunningham JM, and Berger JM (1997) Structure of a murine leukemia virus receptor-binding glycoprotein at 2.0 angstrom resolution. Science 277:1662-1666

Feigelstock D, Thompson P, Mattoo P, and Kaplan GG (1998) Polymorphisms of the hepatitis A virus cellular receptor 1 in African green monkey kidney cells result in antigenic variants that do not react with protective monoclonal antibody 190/4. J Virol 72:6218-6222

Feng Y, Broder CC, Kennedy PE, and Berger EA (1996) HIV-1 entry cofactor: functional cDNA cloning of a seven-transmembrane, G protein-coupled receptor. Science 272:872-877

Fischinger PJ, Blevins CS, and Dunlop NM (1978) Genomic masking of nondefective recombinant murine leukemia virus in Moloney virus stocks. Science 201:457-459

Fischinger PJ, Nomura S, and Bolognesi DP (1975) A novel murine oncornavirus with dual eco- and xenotropic properties. Proc Natl Acad Sci USA 72:5150-5155

Flint SJ, Enquist LW, Krug RM, Racaniello VR, and Skalka AM 2000a. Virus attachment to host cells, p. 101-131, Principles of virology: molecular biology, pathogensis and control. ASM Press, Washington D.C

Flint SJ, Enquist LW, Krug RM, Racaniello VR, and Skalka AM 2000b. Virus entry into cells, p. 133-161, Principles of virology: molecular biology, pathogensis and control. ASM Press, Washington D.C

Forestell SP, Dando JS, Bohnlein E, and Rigg RJ (1996) Improved detection of replication-competent retrovirus. J Virol Methods 60:171-178

Fortin JF, Cantin R, Lamontagne G, and Tremblay M (1997) Host-derived ICAM-1 glycoproteins incorporated on human immunodeficiency virus type 1 are biologically active and enhance viral infectivity. J Virol 71:3588-3596

Frey S, Marsh M, Gunther S, Pelchen-Matthews A, Stephens P, Ortlepp S, and Stegmann T (1995) Temperature dependence of cell-cell fusion induced by the envelope glycoprotein of human immunodeficiency virus type I. J Virol 69:1462-1472

Gardner M, Dandekar S, and Cardiff R (1986) Molecular mechanism of an ecotropic MuLV restriction gene Akvr-1/FV-4 in California wild mice. Curr Top Microbiol Immunol 127:338-345

Gautier R, Jiang A, Rousseau V, Dornburg R, and Jaffredo T (2000) Avian reticuloendotheliosis virus strain A and spleen necrosis virus do not infect human cells. J Virol 74:518-522

Geijtenbeek TB, Kwon DS, Torensma R, van Vliet SJ, van Duijnhoven GC, Middel J, Cornelissen IL, Nottet HS, KewalRamani VN, Littman DR, Figdor CG, and van Kooyk Y (2000) DC-SIGN, a dendritic cell-specific HIV-1-binding protein that enhances trans-infection of T cells. Cell 100:587-597

Ghosh AK, Bachmann MH, Hoover EA, and Mullins JI (1992) Identification of a putative receptor for subgroup A feline leukemia virus on feline T cells. J Virol 66:3707-3714

Gilbert JM, Hernandez LD, Balliet JW, Bates P, and White JM (1995) Receptor-induced conformational changes in the subgroup A avian leukosis and sarcoma virus envelope glycoprotein. J Virol 69:7410-7415

Gilbert JM, Mason D, and White JM (1990) Fusion of Rous sarcoma virus with host cells does not require exposure to low pH. J Virol 64:5106-5113

Glushakova S, Grivel JC, Fitzgerald W, Sylwester A, Zimmerberg J, and Margolis LB (1998) Evidence for the HIV-1 phenotype switch as a causal factor in acquired immunodeficiency. Nat Med 4:346-349

Golovkina TV, Dzuris J, van den Hoogen B, Jaffe AB, Wright PC, Cofer SM, and Ross SR (1998) A novel membrane protein is a mouse mammary tumor virus receptor. J Virol 72:3066-3071

Guibinga GH, Miyanohara A, Esko JD, and Friedmann T (2002) Cell surface heparan sulfate is a receptor for attachment of envelope protein-free retrovirus-like particles and VSV-G pseudotyped MLV-derived retrovirus vectors to target cells. Mol Ther 5:538-546

Gunther-Ausborn S, Schoen P, Bartoldus I, Wilschut J, and Stegmann T (2000) Role of hemagglutinin surface density in the initial stages of influenza virus fusion: lack of evidence for cooperativity. J Virol 74:2714-2720

Hartley JW, Wolford NK, Old LJ, and Rowe WP (1977) A new class of murine leukemia virus associated with development of spontaneous lymphomas. Proc Natl Acad Sci USA 74:789-792

Haywood AM (1994) Virus receptors: binding, adhesion strengthening, and changes in viral structure. J Virol 68:1-5

Heard JM, and Danos O (1991) An amino-terminal fragment of the Friend murine leukemia virus envelope glycoprotein binds the ecotropic receptor. J Virol 65:4026–4032

Hernandez LD, Hoffman LR, Wolfsberg TG, and White JM (1996) Virus-cell and cell-cell fusion. Annu Rev Cell Dev Biol 12:627–661

Herr W, and Gilbert W (1984) Free and integrated recombinant murine leukemia virus DNAs appear in preleukemic thymuses of AKR/J mice. J Virol 50:155–162

Higginbottom A, Quinn ER, Kuo CC, Flint M, Wilson LH, Bianchi E, Nicosia A, Monk PN, McKeating JA, and Levy S (2000) Identification of amino acid residues in CD81 critical for interaction with hepatitis C virus envelope glycoprotein E2. J Virol 74:3642–3649

Hill AV (1998) The immunogenetics of human infectious diseases. Annu Rev Immunol 16:593–617

Hoffman TL, Canziani G, Jia L, Rucker J, and Doms RW (2000) A biosensor assay for studying ligand-membrane receptor interactions: binding of antibodies and HIV-1 Env to chemokine receptors. Proc Natl Acad Sci USA 97:11215–11220

Holmen SL, Melder DC, and Federspiel MJ (2001) Identification of key residues in subgroup A avian leukosis virus envelope determining receptor binding affinity and infectivity of cells expressing chicken or quail Tva receptor. J Virol 75:726–737

Hosokawa H, Sawamura T, Kobayashi S, Ninomiya H, Miwa S, and Masaki T (1997) Cloning and characterization of a brain-specific cationic amino acid transporter. J Biol Chem 272:8717–8722

Hunter E 1997. Viral entry and receptors, p. 71–120. *In* JM Coffin, Hughes SH, and Varmus HE (eds), Retroviruses. Cold Spring Harbor Laboratory Press, Plainview, New York

Hunter E, Casey J, Hahn B, Hayami M, Korber B, Kurth R, Neil JC, Rethwilm A, Sonigo P, and Stoye JP 2000. Retroviridae, p. 369–387. *In* MHV van Regenmortel, Fauquet CM, Bishop DHL, Carstens EB, Estes MK, Lemon SM, Maniloff J, Mayo MA, McGeoch DJ, Pringle CR, and Wickner RB (eds), Virus Taxonomy Seventh Report of the International Committee on Taxonomy of Viruses. Academic Press, London

Hunter E, and Swanstrom R (1990) Retrovirus envelope glycoproteins. Curr Top Microbiol Immunol 157:187–253

Ikeda H, and Sugimura H (1989) *Fv-4* resistance gene: a truncated endogenous murine leukemia virus with ecotropic interference properties. J Virol 63:5405–5412

Innes CL, Smith PB, Langenbach R, Tindall KR, and Boone LR (1990) Cationic liposomes (Lipofectin) mediate retroviral infection in the absence of specific receptors. J Virol 64:957–961

Ito K, and Groudine M (1997) A new member of the cationic amino acid transporter family is preferentially expressed in adult mouse brain. J Biol Chem 272:26780–26786

Jin MJ, Hui H, Robertson DL, Muller MC, Barre-Sinoussi F, Hirsch VM, Allan JS, Shaw GM, Sharp PM, and Hahn BH (1994) Mosaic genome structure of simian immunodeficiency virus from west African green monkeys. EMBO J 13:2935–2947

Jinno-Oue A, Oue M, and Ruscetti SK (2001) A unique heparin-binding domain in the envelope protein of the neuropathogenic PVC-211 murine leukemia virus may contribute to its brain capillary endothelial cell tropism. J Virol 75:12439–12445

Jobbagy Z, Garfield S, Baptiste L, Eiden MV, and Anderson WB (2000) Subcellular redistribution of Pit-2 P_i transporter/amphotropic leukemia virus (A-MuLV) receptor in A-MuLV-infected NIH 3T3 fibroblasts: involvement in superinfection interference. J Virol 74:2847–2854

Johann SV, van Zeijl M, Cekleniak J, and O'Hara B (1993) Definition of a domain of GLVR1 which is necessary for infection by gibbon ape leukemia virus and which is highly polymorphic between species. J Virol 67:6733–6736

Jung A, Maier R, Vartanian JP, Bocharov G, Jung V, Fischer U, Meese E, Wain-Hobson S, and Meyerhans A (2002) Recombination: Multiply infected spleen cells in HIV patients. Nature 418:144

Jung YT, Lyu MS, Buckler-White A, and Kozak CA (2002) Characterization of a polytropic murine leukemia virus proviral sequence associated with the virus resistance gene Rmcf of DBA/2 mice. J Virol 76:8218–8224

Kabat D (1989) Molecular biology of Friend viral erythroleukemia. Curr Top Microbiol Immunol 148:1–42

Kabat D, Kozak SL, Wehrly K, and Chesebro B (1994) Differences in CD4 dependence for infectivity of laboratory-adapted and primary patient isolates of human immunodeficiency virus type 1. J Virol 68:2570–2577

Kanai Y (1997) Family of neutral and acidic amino acid transporters: molecular biology, physiology and medical implications. Curr Opin Cell Biol 9:565–572

Katen LJ, Januszeski MM, Anderson WF, Hasenkrug KJ, and Evans LH (2001) Infectious entry by amphotropic as well as ecotropic murine leukemia viruses occurs through an endocytic pathway. J Virol 75:5018–5026

Kavanaugh MP, Miller DG, Zhang W, Law W, Kozak SL, Kabat D, and Miller AD (1994a) Cell-surface receptors for gibbon ape leukemia virus and amphotropic murine retrovirus are inducible sodium-dependent phosphate symporters. Proc Natl Acad Sci USA 91:7071–7075

Kavanaugh MP, Wang H, Boyd CAR, North RA, and Kabat D (1994b) Cell surface receptor for ecotropic host-range mouse retroviruses: A cationic amino acid transporter. Arch Virol 9:485–494

Kavanaugh MP, Wang H, Zhang Z, Zhang W, Wu YN, Dechant E, North RA, and Kabat D (1994c) Control of cationic amino acid transport and retroviral receptor functions in a membrane protein family. J Biol Chem 269:15445–15450

Kekuda R, Prasad PD, Fei YJ, Torres-Zamorano V, Sinha S, Yang-Feng TL, Leibach FH, and Ganapathy V (1996) Cloning of the sodium-dependent, broad-scope, neutral amino acid transporter Bo from a human placental choriocarcinoma cell line. J Biol Chem 271:18657–18661

Kekuda R, Torres-Zamorano V, Fei YJ, Prasad PD, Li HW, Mader LD, Leibach FH, and Ganapathy V (1997) Molecular and functional characterization of intestinal Na^+-dependent neutral amino acid transporter B0. Am J Physiol 272:G1463–G1472

Keshet E, and Temin HM (1979) Cell killing by spleen necrosis virus is correlated with a transient accumulation of spleen necrosis virus DNA. J Virol 31:376–388

Kewalramani VN, Panganiban AT, and Emerman M (1992) Spleen necrosis virus, an avian immunosuppressive retrovirus, shares a receptor with the type D simian retroviruses. J Virol 66:3026-3031

Khan AS (1984) Nucleotide sequence analysis establishes the role of endogenous murine leukemia virus DNA segments in formation of recombinant mink cell focus- forming murine leukemia viruses. J Virol 50:864-871

Kielian M, and Helenius A 1986. Entry of alphaviruses. In S Schlesinger, and Schlesinger MJ (eds), The Togaviridae and Flaviviridae. Plenum

Kim JW, Closs EI, Albritton LM, and Cunningham JM (1991) Transport of cationic amino acids by the mouse ecotropic retrovirus receptor. Nature 352:725-728

Kim JW, and Cunningham JM (1993) N-linked glycosylation of the receptor for murine ecotropic retroviruses is altered in virus-infected cells. J Biol Chem 268:16316-16320

Kizhatil K, and Albritton LM (1997) Requirements for different components of the host cell cytoskeleton distinguish ecotropic murine leukemia virus entry via endocytosis from entry via surface fusion. J Virol 71:7145-7156

Koo HM, Brown AM, Ron Y, and Dougherty JP (1991) Spleen necrosis virus, an avian retrovirus, can infect primate cells. J Virol 65:4769-4776

Koo HM, Gu J, Varela-Echavarria A, Ron Y, and Dougherty JP (1992) Reticuloendotheliosis type C and primate type D oncoretroviruses are members of the same receptor interference group. J Virol, 66:3448-3454

Kozak CA (1983) Genetic mapping of a mouse chromosomal locus required for mink cell focus-forming virus replication. J Virol 48:300-303

Kozak CA (1985) Susceptibility of wild mouse cells to exogenous infection with xenotropic leukemia viruses: control by a single dominant locus on chromosome 1. J Virol 55:690-695

Kozak CA, and O'Neill RR (1987) Diverse wild mouse origins of xenotropic, mink cell focus-forming, and two types of ecotropic proviral genes. J Virol 61:3082-3088

Kozak M (1999) Initiation of translation in prokaryotes and eukaryotes. Gene 234:187-208

Kreisberg JF, Kwa D, Schramm B, Trautner V, Connor R, Schuitemaker H, Mullins JI, van't Wout AB, and Goldsmith MA (2001) Cytopathicity of human immunodeficiency virus type 1 primary isolates depends on coreceptor usage and not patient disease status. J Virol 75:8842-8847

Kristal BS, Reinhart TA, Hoover EA, and Mullins JI (1993) Interference with superinfection and with cell killing and determination of host range and growth kinetics mediated by feline leukemia virus surface glycoproteins. J Virol 67:4142-4153

Kuhmann SE, Madani N, Diop OM, Platt EJ, Morvan J, Muller-Trutwin MC, Barre-Sinoussi F, and Kabat D (2001) Frequent substitution polymorphisms in African green monkey CCR5 cluster at critical sites for infections by simian immunodeficiency virus SIVagm, implying ancient virus-host coevolution. J Virol 75:8449-8460

Kuhmann SE, Platt EJ, Kozak SL, and Kabat D (2000) Cooperation of multiple CCR5 coreceptors is required for infections by human immunodeficiency virus type 1. J Virol 74:7005-7015

Kwa D, Vingerhoed J, Boeser-Nunnink B, Broersen S, and Schuitemaker H (2001) Cytopathic effects of non-syncytium-inducing and syncytium-inducing human immunodeficiency virus type 1 variants on different CD4(+)-T-cell subsets are determined only by coreceptor expression. J Virol 75:10455–10459

Lama J, Mangasarian A, and Trono D (1999) Cell-surface expression of CD4 reduces HIV-1 infectivity by blocking Env incorporation in a Nef- and Vpu-inhibitable manner. Curr Biol 9:622–631

Lauring AS, Anderson MM, and Overbaugh J (2001) Specificity in receptor usage by T-cell-tropic feline leukemia viruses: implications for the in vivo tropism of immunodeficiency-inducing variants. J Virol 75:8888–8898

Lauring AS, Cheng HH, Eiden MV, and Overbaugh J (2002) Genetic and biochemical analyses of receptor and cofactor determinants for T-cell-tropic feline leukemia virus infection. J Virol 76:8069–8078

Lavillette D, Boson B, Russell SJ, and Cosset FL (2001) Activation of membrane fusion by murine leukemia viruses is controlled in cis or in trans by interactions between the receptor-binding domain and a conserved disulfide loop of the carboxy terminus of the surface glycoprotein. J Virol 75:3685–3695

Lavillette D, Marin M, Ruggieri A, Mallet F, Cosset FL, and Kabat D (2002a) The envelope glycoprotein of human endogenous retrovirus type W uses a divergent family of amino acid transporters/cell surface receptors. J Virol 76:6442–6452

Lavillette D, Ruggieri A, Boson B, Maurice M, and Cosset FL (2002b) Relationship between SU subdomains that regulate the receptor-mediated transition from the native (fusion-Inhibited) to the fusion-active conformation of the murine leukemia virus glycoprotein. J Virol 76:9673–9685

Lavillette D, Ruggieri A, Russell SJ, and Cosset FL (2000) Activation of a cell entry pathway common to type C mammalian retroviruses by soluble envelope fragments. J Virol 74:295–304

Layne SP, Merges MJ, Dembo M, Spouge JL, and Nara PL (1990) HIV requires multiple gp120 molecules for CD4-mediated infection. Nature 346:277–279

Lee B, Leslie G, Soilleux E, O'Doherty U, Baik S, Levroney E, Flummerfelt K, Swiggard W, Coleman N, Malim M, and Doms RW (2001) cis Expression of DC-SIGN allows for more efficient entry of human and simian immunodeficiency viruses via CD4 and a coreceptor. J Virol 75:12028–12038

Lee B, Sharron M, Montaner LJ, Weissman D, and Doms RW (1999) Quantification of CD4, CCR5, and CXCR4 levels on lymphocyte subsets, dendritic cells, and differentially conditioned monocyte-derived macrophages. Proc Natl Acad Sci USA 96:5215–5220

Lee EJ, Kaminchik J, and Hankins WD (1984) Expression of xenotropic-like env RNA sequences in normal DBA/2 and NZB mouse tissues. J Virol 51:247–250

Leverett BD, Farrell KB, Eiden MV, and Wilson CA (1998) Entry of amphotropic murine leukemia virus is influenced by residues in the putative second extracellular domain of its receptor, Pit2. J Virol 72:4956–4961

Levy JA (1978) Xenotropic type C viruses. Curr Top Microbiol Immunol 79:111–213

Levy JA (1973) Xenotropic viruses: murine leukemia viruses associated with NIH swiss, NZB, and other mouse strains. Science 182:1151–1153

Li F, Erickson HP, James JA, Moore KL, Cummings RD, and McEver RP (1996a) Visualization of P-selectin glycoprotein ligand-1 as a highly extended molecule and mapping of protein epitopes for monoclonal antibodies. J Biol Chem 271:6342–6348

Li F, Wilkins PP, Crawley S, Weinstein J, Cummings RD, and McEver RP (1996b) Post-translational modifications of recombinant P-selectin glycoprotein ligand-1 required for binding to P- and E-selectin. J Biol Chem 271:3255–3264

Li YY, O'Donnell MA, and Perez LG (1996c) Coexpression of a nonsyncytium inducer HIV-1 glycoprotein inhibits syncytium formation by another HIV-1 Env protein. Virology 215:197–202

Lin CL, Sewell AK, Gao GF, Whelan KT, Phillips RE, and Austyn JM (2000) Macrophage-tropic HIV induces and exploits dendritic cell chemotaxis. J Exp Med 192:587–594

Linenberger ML, and Abkowitz JL (1995) Haematological disorders associated with feline retrovirus infections. Baillieres Clin Haematol 8:73–112

Linenberger ML, and Abkowitz JL (1992) In vivo infection of marrow stromal fibroblasts by feline leukemia virus. Exp Hematol 20:1022–1027

Linenberger ML, and Abkowitz JL (1992) Studies in feline long-term marrow culture: hematopoiesis on normal and feline leukemia virus infected stromal cells. Blood 80:651–662

Littman DR (1998) Chemokine receptors: keys to AIDS pathogenesis? Cell 93:677–680

Liu R, Paxton WA, Choe S, Ceradini D, Martin SR, Horuk R, MacDonald ME, Stuhlmann H, Koup RA, and Landau NR (1996) Homozygous defect in HIV-1 coreceptor accounts for resistance of some multiply-exposed individuals to HIV-1 infection. Cell 86:367–377

Lu Z, Berson JF, Chen Y, Turner JD, Zhang T, Sharron M, Jenks MH, Wang Z, Kim J, Rucker J, Hoxie JA, Peiper SC, and Doms RW (1997) Evolution of HIV-1 coreceptor usage through interactions with distinct CCR5 and CXCR4 domains. Proc Natl Acad Sci USA 94:6426–6431

Lundorf MD, Pedersen FS, O'Hara B, and Pedersen L (1999) Amphotropic murine leukemia virus entry is determined by specific combinations of residues from receptor loops 2 and 4. J Virol 73:3169–3175

Lundorf MD, Pedersen FS, O'Hara B, and Pedersen L (1998) Single amino acid insertion in loop 4 confers amphotropic murine leukemia virus receptor function upon murine Pit1. J Virol 72:4524–4527

Lynch WP, Brown WJ, Spangrude GJ, and Portis JL (1994) Microglial infection by a neurovirulent murine retrovirus results in defective processing of envelope protein and intracellular budding of virus particles. J Virol 68:3401–3409

Lyu MS, and Kozak CA (1996) Genetic basis for resistance to polytropic murine leukemia viruses in the wild mouse species *Mus castaneus*. J Virol 70:830–833

Lyu MS, Nihrane A, and Kozak CA (1999) Receptor-mediated interference mechanism responsible for resistance to polytropic leukemia viruses in *Mus castaneus*. J Virol 73:3733–3736

Mang R, Goudsmit J, and van der Kuyl AC (1999) Novel endogenous type C retrovirus in baboons: complete sequence, providing evidence for baboon endogenous virus gag-pol ancestry. J Virol 73:7021–7026

Marechal V, Prevost MC, Petit C, Perret E, Heard JM, and Schwartz O (2001) Human immunodeficiency virus type 1 entry into macrophages mediated by macropinocytosis. J Virol 75:11166–11177

Marin M, Lavillette D, Kelly SM, and Kabat D (2003) N-linked glycosylation and sequence changes in a critical negative control region of the ASCT1 and ASCT2 neutral amino acid transporters determines their retroviral receptor functions. J Virol. In press

Marin M, Tailor CS, Nouri A, and Kabat D (2000) Sodium-dependent neutral amino acid transporter type 1 is an auxiliary receptor for baboon endogenous retrovirus. J Virol 74:8085–8093

Marin M, Tailor CS, Nouri A, Kozak SL, and Kabat D (1999) Polymorphisms of the cell surface receptor control mouse susceptibilities to xenotropic and polytropic leukemia viruses. J Virol 73:9362–9368

Martin J, Herniou E, Cook J, O'Neill RW, and Tristem M (1999) Interclass transmission and phyletic host tracking in murine leukemia virus-related retroviruses. J Virol 73:2442–2449

Mason PW, Rieder E, and Baxt B (1994) RGD sequence of foot-and-mouth disease virus is essential for infecting cells via the natural receptor but can be bypassed by an antibody-dependent enhancement pathway. Proc Natl Acad Sci USA 91:1932–1936

Masuda M, Hanson CA, Alvord WG, Hoffman PM, and Ruscetti SK (1996a) Effects of subtle changes in the SU protein of ecotropic murine leukemia virus on its brain capillary endothelial cell tropism and interference properties. Virology 215:142–151

Masuda M, Hanson CA, Hoffman PM, and Ruscetti SK (1996b) Analysis of the unique hamster cell tropism of ecotropic murine leukemia virus PVC-211. J Virol 70:8534–8539

Masuda M, Kakushima N, Wilt SG, Ruscetti SK, Hoffman PM, and Iwamoto A (1999) Analysis of receptor usage by ecotropic murine retroviruses, using green fluorescent protein-tagged cationic amino acid transporters. J Virol 73:8623–8629

Masuda M, Remington MP, Hoffman PM, and Ruscetti SK (1992) Molecular characterization of a neuropathogenic and nonerythroleukemogenic variant of Friend murine leukemia virus PVC-211. J Virol 66:2798–2806

McClure MO, Sommerfelt MA, Marsh M, and Weiss RA (1990) The pH independence of mammalian retrovirus infection. J Gen Virol 71:767–773

McEver RP, Moore KL, and Cummings RD (1995) Leukocyte trafficking mediated by selectin-carbohydrate interactions. J Biol Chem 270:11025–11028

Meola A, Sbardellati A, Bruni Ercole B, Cerretani M, Pezzanera M, Ceccacci A, Vitelli A, Levy S, Nicosia A, Traboni C, McKeating J, and Scarselli E (2000) Binding of hepatitis C virus E2 glycoprotein to CD81 does not correlate with species permissiveness to infection. J Virol 74:5933–5938

Miller AD, Bonham L, Alfano J, Kiem HP, Reynolds T, and Wolgamot G (1996) A novel murine retrovirus identified during testing for helper virus in human gene transfer trials. J Virol 70:1804–1809

Miller DA, and Wolgamot G (1997) Murine retroviruses use at least six different receptors for entry in *Mus dunni* cells. J Virol 71:4531–4535

Miller DG, Edwards RH, and Miller AD (1994) Cloning of the cellular receptor for amphotropic murine retroviruses reveals homology to that for gibbon ape leukemia virus. Proc Natl Acad Sci USA 91:78–82

Miller DG, and Miller AD (1994) A family of retroviruses that utilize related phosphate transporters for cell entry. J Virol 68:8270–8276

Miller DG, and Miller AD (1993) Inhibitors of retrovirus infection are secreted by several hamster cell lines and are also present in hamster sera. J Virol 67:5346–5352

Miller DG, and Miller AD (1992) Tunicamycin treatment of CHO cells abrogates multiple blocks to retrovirus infection, one of which is due to a secreted inhibitor. J Virol 66:78–84

Mondor I, Moulard M, Ugolini S, Klasse PJ, Hoxie J, Amara A, Delaunay T, Wyatt R, Sodroski J, and Sattentau QJ (1998) Interactions among HIV gp120, CD4, and CXCR4: dependence on CD4 expression level, gp120 viral origin, conservation of the gp120 COOH- and NH_2-termini and V1/V2 and V3 loops, and sensitivity to neutralizing antibodies. Virology 248:394–405

Mondor I, Ugolini S, and Sattentau QJ (1998) Human immunodeficiency virus type 1 attachment to HeLa CD4 cells is CD4 independent and gp120 dependent and requires cell surface heparans. J Virol 72:3623–3634

Moore JP, Trkola A, and Dragic T (1997) Co-receptors for HIV-1 entry. Curr Opin Immunol 9:551–562

Moser M, Burns CC, Boomer S, and Overbaugh J (1998) The host range and interference properties of two closely related feline leukemia variants suggest that they use distinct receptors. Virology 242:366–377

Mothes W, Boerger AL, Narayan S, Cunningham JM, and Young JA (2000) Retroviral entry mediated by receptor priming and low pH triggering of an envelope glycoprotein. Cell 103:679–689

Murakami T, and Freed EO (2000) The long cytoplasmic tail of gp41 is required in a cell type-dependent manner for HIV-1 envelope glycoprotein incorporation into virions. Proc Natl Acad Sci USA 97:343–348

Murphy PM (1993) Molecular mimicry and the generation of host defense protein diversity. Cell 72:823–826

Neil JC, Fulton R, Rigby M, and Stewart M (1991) Feline leukaemia virus: generation of pathogenic and oncogenic variants. Curr Top Microbiol Immunol 171:67–93

Nicholson B, Sawamura T, Masaki T, and MacLeod CL (1998) Increased Cat3-mediated cationic amino acid transport functionally compensates in Cat1 knockout cell lines. J Biol Chem 273:14663–14666

O'Doherty U, Swiggard WJ, and Malim MH (2000) Human immunodeficiency virus type 1 spinoculation enhances infection through virus binding. J Virol 74:10074–10080

O'Hara B, Johann SV, Klinger HP, Blair DG, Rubinson H, Dunn KJ, Sass P, Vitek SM, and Robins T (1990) Characterization of a human gene conferring sensitivity to infection by gibbon ape leukemia virus. Cell Growth Differ 1:119–127

O'Neill RR, Khan AS, Hoggan MD, Hartley JW, Martin MA, and Repaske R (1986) Specific hybridization probes demonstrate fewer xenotropic than mink cell focus-forming murine leukemia virus env-related sequences in DNAs from inbred laboratory mice. J Virol 58:359–366

Olah Z, Lehel C, Anderson WB, Eiden MV, and Wilson CA (1994) The cellular receptor for gibbon ape leukemia virus is a novel high affinity sodium-dependent phosphate transporter. J Biol Chem 269:25426–25431

Oldstone MB, Lewicki H, Thomas D, Tishon A, Dales S, Patterson J, Manchester M, Homann D, Naniche D, and Holz A (1999) Measles virus infection in a transgenic model: virus-induced immunosuppression and central nervous system disease. Cell 98:629–640

Onions D, Jarrett O, Testa N, Frassoni F, and Toth S (1982) Selective effect of feline leukaemia virus on early erythroid precursors. Nature 296:156–158

Ott D, Friedrich R, and Rein A (1990) Sequence analysis of amphotropic and 10A1 murine leukemia viruses: close relationship to mink cell focus-inducing viruses. J Virol 64:757–766

Overbaugh J, Donahue PR, Quackenbush SL, Hoover EA, and Mullins JI (1988) Molecular cloning of a feline leukemia virus that induces fatal immunodeficiency disease in cats. Science 239:906–910

Overbaugh J, Miller AD, and Eiden MV (2001) Receptors and entry cofactors for retroviruses include single and multiple transmembrane-spanning proteins as well as newly described glycophosphatidylinositol-anchored and secreted proteins. Microbiol Mol Biol Rev 65:371–389

Overbaugh J, Riedel N, Hoover EA, and Mullins JI (1988) Transduction of endogenous envelope genes by feline leukaemia virus in vitro. Nature 332:731–734

Palsson B, and Andreadis S (1997) The physico-chemical factors that govern retrovirus-mediated gene transfer. Exp Hematol 25:94–102

Pao SS, Paulsen IT, and Saier MH, Jr. (1998) Major facilitator superfamily. Microbiol Mol Biol Rev 62:1–34

Park BH, Matuschke B, Lavi E, and Gaulton GN (1994) A point mutation in the env gene of a murine leukemia virus induces syncytium formation and neurologic disease. J Virol 68:7516–7524

Park PW, Reizes O, and Bernfield M (2000) Cell surface heparan sulfate proteoglycans: selective regulators of ligand-receptor encounters. J Biol Chem 275:29923–29926

Parker JS, Murphy WJ, Wang D, O'Brien SJ, and Parrish CR (2001) Canine and feline parvoviruses can use human or feline transferrin receptors to bind, enter, and infect cells. J Virol 75:3896–3902

Patience C, Switzer WM, Takeuchi Y, Griffiths DJ, Goward ME, Heneine W, Stoye JP, and Weiss RA (2001) Multiple groups of novel retroviral genomes in pigs and related species. J Virol 75:2771–2775

Pavlicek A, Paces J, Elleder D, and Hejnar J (2002) Processed pseudogenes of human endogenous retroviruses generated by LINEs: their integration, stability, and distribution. Genome Res 12:391–399. 2002

Pedersen L, Johann SV, van Zeijl M, Pedersen FS, and O'Hara B (1995) Chimeras of receptors for gibbon ape leukemia virus/feline leukemia virus B and amphotropic murine leukemia virus reveal different modes of receptor recognition by retrovirus. J Virol 69:2401–2405

Penn DJ, Damjanovich K, and Potts WK (2002) MHC heterozygosity confers a selective advantage against multiple-strain infections. Proc Natl Acad Sci USA 99: 11260–11264

Petracca R, Falugi F, Galli G, Norais N, Rosa D, Campagnoli S, Burgio V, Di Stasio E, Giardina B, Houghton M, Abrignani S, and Grandi G (2000) Structure-function analysis of hepatitis C virus envelope-CD81 binding. J Virol 74:4824–4830

Picard L, Simmons G, Power CA, Meyer A, Weiss RA, and Clapham PR (1997) Multiple extracellular domains of CCR-5 contribute to human immunodeficiency virus type 1 entry and fusion. J Virol 71:5003–5011

Piguet V, Chen YL, Mangasarian A, Foti M, Carpentier JL, and Trono D (1998) Mechanism of Nef-induced CD4 endocytosis: Nef connects CD4 with the mu chain of adaptor complexes. EMBO J 17:2472–2481

Piguet V, Schwartz O, Le Gall S, and Trono D (1999) The downregulation of CD4 and MHC-I by primate lentiviruses: a paradigm for the modulation of cell surface receptors. Immunol Rev 168:51–63

Pileri P, Uematsu Y, Campagnoli S, Galli G, Falugi F, Petracca R, Weiner AJ, Houghton M, Rosa D, Grandi G, and Abrignani S (1998) Binding of hepatitis C virus to CD81. Science 282:938–941

Pizzato M, Blair ED, Fling M, Kopf J, Tomassetti A, Weiss RA, and Takeuchi Y (2001) Evidence for nonspecific adsorption of targeted retrovirus vector particles to cells. Gene Ther 8:1088–1096

Pizzato M, Marlow SA, Blair ED, and Takeuchi Y (1999) Initial binding of murine leukemia virus particles to cells does not require specific Env-receptor interaction. J Virol 73:8599–8611

Platt EJ, Kuhmann SE, Rose PP, and Kabat D (2001) Adaptive mutations in the V3 loop of gp120 enhance fusogenicity of human immunodeficiency virus type 1 and enable use of a CCR5 coreceptor that lacks the amino-terminal sulfated region. J Virol 75:12266–12278

Platt EJ, Wehrly K, Kuhmann SE, Chesebro B, and Kabat D (1998) Effects of CCR5 and CD4 cell surface concentrations on infections by macrophagetropic isolates of human immunodeficiency virus type 1. J Virol 72:2855–2864

Pöhlmann S, Baribaud F, Lee B, Leslie GJ, Sanchez MD, Hiebenthal-Millow K, Munch J, Kirchhoff F, and Doms RW (2001a) DC-sign interactions with human immunodeficiency virus type 1 and 2 and simian immunodeficiency virus. J Virol 75:4664–4672

Pöhlmann S, Soilleux EJ, Baribaud F, Leslie GJ, Morris LS, Trowsdale J, Lee B, Coleman N, and Doms RW (2001b) DC-SIGNR, a DC-SIGN homologue expressed in endothelial cells, binds to human and simian immunodeficiency viruses and activates infection in trans. Proc Natl Acad Sci USA 98:2670–2675

Pollakis G, Kang S, Kliphuis A, Chalaby MI, Goudsmit J, and Paxton WA (2001) N-linked glycosylation of the HIV-1 gp120 envelope glycoprotein as a major determinant of CCR5 and CXCR4 Co-receptor utilization. J Biol Chem 16:16

Polzer S, Dittmar MT, Schmitz H, Meyer B, Muller H, Krausslich HG, and Schreiber M (2001) Loss of N-linked glycans in the V3-loop region of gp120 is correlated to an enhanced infectivity of HIV-1. Glycobiology 11:11–19

Pontow S, and Ratner L (2001) Evidence for common structural determinants of human Immunodeficiency virus type 1 coreceptor activity provided through functional analysis of CCR5/CXCR4 chimeric coreceptors. J Virol 75:11503–11514

Portis JL, McAtee FJ, and Evans LH (1985) Infectious entry of murine retroviruses into mouse cells: evidence of a postadsorption step inhibited by acidic pH. J Virol 55:806–812

Prassolov V, Hein S, Ziegler M, Ivanov D, Munk C, Lohler J, and Stocking C (2001) *Mus cervicolor* murine leukemia virus isolate M813 belongs to a unique receptor interference group. J Virol 75:4490–4498

Quigley JG, Burns CC, Anderson MM, Lynch ED, Sabo KM, Overbaugh J, and Abkowitz JL (2000) Cloning of the cellular receptor for feline leukemia virus subgroup C (FeLV-C), a retrovirus that induces red cell aplasia [published erratum appears in Blood 2000 Jul 1;96(1):8]. Blood 95:1093–1099

Ragheb JA, and Anderson WF (1994) pH-independent murine leukemia virus ecotropic envelope-mediated cell fusion: implications for the role of the R peptide and p12E TM in viral entry. J Virol 68:3220–3231

Rai SK, Duh FM, Vigdorovich V, Danilkovitch-Miagkova A, Lerman MI, and Miller AD (2001) Candidate tumor suppressor HYAL2 is a glycosylphosphatidylinositol (GPI)-anchored cell-surface receptor for jaagsiekte sheep retrovirus, the envelope protein of which mediates oncogenic transformation. Proc Natl Acad Sci USA 98:4443–4448

Rasko JE, Battini JL, Gottschalk RJ, Mazo I, and Miller AD (1999) The RD114/simian type D retrovirus receptor is a neutral amino acid transporter. Proc Natl Acad Sci USA 96:2129–2134

Redmond S, Peters G, and Dickson C (1984) Mouse mammary tumor virus can mediate cell fusion at reduced pH. Virology 133:393–402

Rein A, and Schultz A (1984) Different recombinant murine leukemia viruses use different cell surface receptors. Virology 136:144–152

Rein A, Yang C, Haynes JA, Mirro J, and Compans RW (1998) Evidence for cooperation between murine leukemia virus Env molecules in mixed oligomers. J Virol 72:3432–3435

Reinhart TA, Ghosh AK, Hoover EA, and Mullins JI (1993) Distinct superinfection interference properties yet similar receptor utilization by cytopathic and noncytopathic feline leukemia viruses. J Virol 67:5153–5162

Rigby MA, Rojko JL, Stewart MA, Kociba GJ, Cheney CM, Rezanka LJ, Mathes LE, Hartke JR, Jarrett O, and Neil JC (1992) Partial dissociation of subgroup C phenotype and in vivo behaviour in feline leukaemia viruses with chimeric envelope genes. J Gen Virol 73:2839–2847

Robertson DL, Sharp PM, McCutchan FE, and Hahn BH (1995) Recombination in HIV-1. Nature 374:124–126

Roche S, and Gaudin Y (2002) Characterization of the equilibrium between the native and fusion-inactive conformation of rabies virus glycoprotein indicates that the fusion complex is made of several trimers. Virology 297:128–135

Rogers GN, Daniels RS, Skehel JJ, Wiley DC, Wang XF, Higa HH, and Paulson JC (1985) Host-mediated selection of influenza virus receptor variants. Sialic acid-alpha 2,6Gal-specific clones of A/duck/Ukraine/1/63 revert to sialic acid-alpha 2,3Gal-specific wild type in ovo. J Biol Chem 260:7362–7367

Rohn JL, Moser MS, Gwynn SR, Baldwin DN, and Overbaugh J (1998) In vivo evolution of a novel, syncytium-inducing and cytopathic feline leukemia virus variant. J Virol 72:2686–2696

Rojko JL, Cheney CM, Gasper PW, Hamilton KL, Hoover EA, Mathes LE, and Kociba GJ (1986) Infectious feline leukaemia virus is erythrosuppressive in vitro. Leuk Res 10:1193–1199

Rojko JL, Hartke JR, Cheney CM, Phipps AJ, and Neil JC (1996) Cytopathic feline leukemia viruses cause apoptosis in hemolymphatic cells. Prog Mol Subcell Biol 16:13–43

Rosenberg N, and Jolicoeur P 1997. Retroviral pathogenesis, p. 71–120. In JM Coffin, Hughes SH, and Varmus HE (eds), Retroviruses. Cold Spring Harbor Laboratory Press, Plainview, New York

Ross SR, Schofield JJ, Farr CJ, and Bucan M (2002) Mouse transferrin receptor 1 is the cell entry receptor for mouse mammary tumor virus. Proc Natl Acad Sci USA 99:12386–12390

Ross TM, Oran AE, and Cullen BR (1999) Inhibition of HIV-1 progeny virion release by cell-surface CD4 is relieved by expression of the viral Nef protein. Curr Biol 9:613–621

Roy-Burman P (1995) Endogenous env elements: partners in generation of pathogenic feline leukemia viruses. Virus Genes 11:147–161

Ruscetti S, Davis L, Fcild J, and Oliff A (1981) Friend murine leukemia virus-induced leukemia is associated with the formation of mink cell focus-inducing viruses and is blocked in mice expressing endogenous mink cell focus-inducing xenotropic viral envelope genes. J Exp Med 154:907–920

Ruscetti S, Matthai R, and Potter M (1985) Susceptibility of BALB/c mice carrying various DBA/2 genes to development of Friend murine leukemia virus-induced erythroleukemia. J Exp Med 162:1579–1587

Saha K, and Wong PK (1992) ts1, a temperature-sensitive mutant of Moloney murine leukemia virus TB, can infect both CD4+ and CD8+ T cells but requires CD4+ T cells in order to cause paralysis and immunodeficiency. J Virol 66:2639–2646

Salaün C, Gyan E, Rodrigues P, and Heard JM (2002) Pit2 assemblies at the cell surface are modulated by extracellular inorganic phosphate concentration. J Virol 76:4304–4311

Salaun C, Rodrigues P, and Heard JM (2001) Transmembrane topology of pit-2, a phosphate transporter-retrovirus receptor. J Virol 75:5584–5592

Salzwedel K, and Berger EA (2000) Cooperative subunit interactions within the oligomeric envelope glycoprotein of HIV-1: functional complementation of specific defects in gp120 and gp41. Proc Natl Acad Sci USA 97:12794–12799

Saphire AC, Bobardt MD, and Gallay PA (1999) Host cyclophilin A mediates HIV-1 attachment to target cells via heparans. EMBO J 18:6771–6785

Saphire AC, Bobardt MD, Zhang Z, David G, and Gallay PA (2001) Syndecans serve as attachment receptors for human immunodeficiency virus type 1 on macrophages. J Virol 75:9187–9200

Scarlatti G, Tresoldi E, Bjorndal A, Fredriksson R, Colognesi C, Deng HK, Malnati MS, Plebani A, Siccardi AG, Littman DR, Fenyo EM, and Lusso P (1997) In vivo evolution of HIV-1 co-receptor usage and sensitivity to chemokine-mediated suppression. Nat Med 3:1259–1265

Schlessinger J, Lax I, and Lemmon M (1995) Regulation of growth factor activation by proteoglycans: what is the role of the low affinity receptors? Cell 83:357–360

Schneiderman RD, Farrell KB, Wilson CA, and Eiden MV (1996) The Japanese feral mouse Pit1 and Pit2 homologs lack an acidic residue at position 550 but still function as gibbon ape leukemia virus receptors: implications for virus binding motif. J Virol 70:6982–6986

Schramm B, Penn ML, Speck RF, Chan SY, De Clercq E, Schols D, Connor RI, and Goldsmith MA (2000) Viral entry through CXCR4 is a pathogenic factor and therapeutic target in human immunodeficiency virus type 1 disease. J Virol 74:184–192

Schubert U, Anton LC, Bacik I, Cox JH, Bour S, Bennink JR, Orlowski M, Strebel K, and Yewdell JW (1998) CD4 glycoprotein degradation induced by human immunodeficiency virus type 1 Vpu protein requires the function of proteasomes and the ubiquitin-conjugating pathway. J Virol 72:2280–2288

Schwartz M (1976) The adsorption of coliphage lambda to its host: effect of variations in the surface density of receptor and in phage-receptor affinity. J Mol Biol 103:521–536

Schwartz M (1975) Reversible interaction between coliphage lambda and its receptor protein. J Mol Biol 99:185–201

Seal RP, Leighton BH, and Amara SG (2000) A model for the topology of excitatory amino acid transporters determined by the extracellular accessibility of substituted cysteines. Neuron 25:695–706

Sharma S, Miyanohara A, and Friedmann T (2000) Separable mechanisms of attachment and cell uptake during retrovirus infection. J Virol 74:10790–10795

Sharma S, Murai F, Miyanohara A, and Friedmann T (1997) Noninfectious virus-like particles produced by Moloney murine leukemia virus-based retrovirus packaging cells deficient in viral envelope become infectious in the presence of lipofection reagents. Proc Natl Acad Sci USA 94:10803–10808

Sheets RL, Pandey R, Jen WC, and Roy-Burman P (1993) Recombinant feline leukemia virus genes detected in naturally occurring feline lymphosarcomas. J Virol 67:3118–3125

Sheets RL, Pandey R, Klement V, Grant CK, and Roy-Burman P (1992) Biologically selected recombinants between feline leukemia virus (FeLV) subgroup A and an endogenous FeLV element. Virology 190:849–855

Shikova E, Lin YC, Saha K, Brooks BR, and Wong PK (1993) Correlation of specific virus-astrocyte interactions and cytopathic effects induced by ts1, a neurovirulent mutant of Moloney murine leukemia virus. J Virol 67:1137–1147

Siciliano SJ, Kuhmann SE, Weng Y, Madani N, Springer MS, Lineberger JE, Danzeisen R, Miller MD, Kavanaugh MP, DeMartino JA, and Kabat D (1999) A critical site in the core of the CCR5 chemokine receptor required for binding and infectivity of human immunodeficiency virus type 1. J Biol Chem 274:1905–1913

Siess DC, Kozak SL, and Kabat D (1996) Exceptional fusogenicity of Chinese hamster ovary cells with murine retroviruses suggests roles for cellular factor(s) and receptor clusters in the membrane fusion process. J Virol 70:3432–3439

Skehel JJ, Bizebard T, Bullough PA, Hughson FM, Knossow M, Steinhauer DA, Wharton SA, and Wiley DC 1995. Membrane fusion by influenza hemagglutinin, p. 573–580, Cold Spring Harbor Symposia on Quantitative Biology, vol. 55. Cold Spring Harbor Laboratory Press

Skehel JJ, and Wiley DC (2000) Receptor binding and membrane fusion in virus entry: the influenza hemagglutinin. Annu Rev Biochem 69:531-569

Slotboom DJ, Konings WN, and Lolkema JS (1999) Structural features of the glutamate transporter family. Microbiol Mol Biol Rev 63:293-307

Sommerfelt MA (1999) Retrovirus receptors. J Gen Virol 80:3049-3064

Sommerfelt MA, and Weiss RA (1990) Receptor interference groups of 20 retroviruses plating on human cells. Virology 176:58-69

Speck RF, Wehrly K, Platt EJ, Atchison RE, Charo IF, Kabat D, Chesebro B, and Goldsmith MA (1997) Selective employment of chemokine receptors as human immunodeficiency virus type 1 coreceptors determined by individual amino acids within the envelope V3 loop. J Virol 71:7136-7139

Stewart MA, Warnock M, Wheeler A, Wilkie N, Mullins JI, Onions DE, and Neil JC (1986) Nucleotide sequences of a feline leukemia virus subgroup A envelope gene and long terminal repeat and evidence for the recombinational origin of subgroup B viruses. J Virol 58:825-834

Stoye JP, Moroni C, and Coffin JM (1991) Virological events leading to spontaneous AKR thymomas. J Virol 65:1273-1285

Sugai J, Eiden M, Anderson MM, Van Hoeven N, Meiering CD, and Overbaugh J (2001) Identification of envelope determinants of feline leukemia virus subgroup B that permit infection and gene transfer to cells expressing human Pit1 or Pit2. J Virol 75:6841-6849

Suzuki Y, Ito T, Suzuki T, Holland RE, Jr., Chambers TM, Kiso M, Ishida H, and Kawaoka Y (2000) Sialic acid species as a determinant of the host range of influenza A viruses [In Process Citation]. J Virol 74:11825-11831

Suzuki Y, Kato H, Naeve CW, and Webster RG (1989) Single-amino-acid substitution in an antigenic site of influenza virus hemagglutinin can alter the specificity of binding to cell membrane-associated gangliosides. J Virol 63:4298-4302

Tailor CS, and Kabat D (1997) Variable regions A and B in the envelope glycoproteins of feline leukemia virus subgroup B and amphotropic murine leukemia virus interact with discrete receptor domains. J Virol 71:9383-9391

Tailor CS, Marin M, Nouri A, Kavanaugh MP, and Kabat D (2001) Truncated forms of the dual function human ASCT2 neutral amino acid transporter/retroviral receptor are translationally initiated at multiple alternative CUG and GUG codons. J Biol Chem 276:27221-27230

Tailor CS, Nouri A, and Kabat D (2000a) Cellular and species resistances to murine amphotropic, Gibbon ape, and feline subgroup C leukemia viruses are strongly influenced by receptor expression levels and by receptor masking mechanisms. J Virol 74:9797-9801

Tailor CS, Nouri A, and Kabat D (2000b) A comprehensive approach to mapping the interacting surfaces of murine amphotropic and feline subgroup B leukemia viruses with their cell surface receptors. J Virol 74:237-244

Tailor CS, Nouri A, Lee CG, Kozak C, and Kabat D (1999a) Cloning and characterization of a cell surface receptor for xenotropic and polytropic murine leukemia viruses. Proc Natl Acad Sci USA 96:927-932

Tailor CS, Nouri A, Zhao Y, Takeuchi Y, and Kabat D (1999b) A sodium-dependent neutral-amino-acid transporter mediates infections of feline and baboon endogenous retroviruses and simian type D retroviruses. J Virol 73:4470-4474

Tailor CS, Takeuchi Y, O'Hara B, Johann SV, Weiss RA, and Collins MK (1993) Mutation of amino acids within the gibbon ape leukemia virus (GALV) receptor differentially affects feline leukemia virus subgroup B, simian sarcoma-associated virus, and GALV infections. J Virol 67:6737–6741

Tailor CS, Willett BJ, and Kabat D (1999c) A putative cell surface receptor for anemia-inducing feline leukemia virus subgroup C is a member of a transporter superfamily. J Virol 73:6500–6505

Takase-Yoden S, and Watanabe R (1999) Contribution of virus-receptor interaction to distinct viral proliferation of neuropathogenic and nonneuropathogenic murine leukemia viruses in rat glial cells. J Virol 73:4461–4464

Takeuchi Y, Patience C, Magre S, Weiss RA, Banerjee PT, Le Tissier P, and Stoye JP (1998) Host range and interference studies of three classes of pig endogenous retrovirus. J Virol 72:9986–9991

Takeuchi Y, Vile RG, Simpson G, O'Hara B, Collins MK, and Weiss RA (1992) Feline leukemia virus subgroup B uses the same cell surface receptor as gibbon ape leukemia virus. J Virol 66:1219–1222

Taplitz RA, and Coffin JM (1997) Selection of an avian retrovirus mutant with extended receptor usage. J Virol 71:7814–7819

Tatsuo H, Ono N, Tanaka K, and Yanagi Y (2000) SLAM (CDw150) is a cellular receptor for measles virus. Nature 406:893–897

Taylor GM, Gao Y, and Sanders DA (2001) Fv-4: identification of the defect in env and the mechanism of resistance to ecotropic murine leukemia virus. J Virol 75:11244–11248

Temin HM (1988) Mechanisms of cell killing/cytopathic effects by nonhuman retroviruses. Rev Infect Dis 10:399–405

Testa NG, Onions D, Jarrett O, Frassoni F, and Eliason JF (1983) Haemopoietic colony formation (BFU-E, GM-CFC) during the development of pure red cell hypoplasia induced in the cat by feline leukaemia virus. Leuk Res 7:103–116

Thoulouze MI, Lafage M, Schachner M, Hartmann U, Cremer H, and Lafon M (1998) The neural cell adhesion molecule is a receptor for rabies virus. J Virol 72:7181–7190

Tinoco I, Sauer K, and Wang JC 1978. Transition-state theory, p. 294–298, Physical chemistry: Principles and applications in biological sciences. Prentice-Hall, Inc., Englewood Cliffs

Tomonaga K, and Coffin JM (1998) Structure and distribution of endogenous nonecotropic murine leukemia viruses in wild mice. J Virol 72:8289–8300

Torres-Zamorano V, Leibach FH, and Ganapathy V (1998) Sodium-dependent homo- and hetero-exchange of neutral amino acids mediated by the amino acid transporter ATB degree. Biochem Biophys Res Commun 245:824–829

Ugolini S, Mondor I, and Sattentau QJ (1999) HIV-1 attachment: another look. Trends Microbiol 7:144–149

Unutmaz D, and Littman DR (1997) Expression pattern of HIV-1 coreceptors on T cells: implications for viral transmission and lymphocyte homing. Proc Natl Acad Sci USA 94:1615–1618

Utsunomiya-Tate N, Endou H, and Kanai Y (1996) Cloning and functional characterization of a system ASC-like Na^+-dependent neutral amino acid transporter. J Biol Chem 271:14883–14890

Valentine RC, and Allison AC (1959) Virus particle adsorption. I. Theory of adsorption and experiments on attachment of particles to non-biological surfaces. Biochim Biophys Acta 34:10–23

Valsesia-Wittmann S, Morling FJ, Hatziioannou T, Russell SJ, and Cosset FL (1997) Receptor co-operation in retrovirus entry: recruitment of an auxiliary entry mechanism after retargeted binding. EMBO J 16:1214–1223

Van der Kuyl AC, Dekker JT, and Goudsmit J (1999) Discovery of a new endogenous type C retrovirus (FcEV) in cats: evidence for RD-114 being an FcEV(Gag-Pol)/baboon endogenous virus BaEV(Env) recombinant. J Virol 73:7994–8002

Van der Kuyl AC, Mang R, Dekker JT, and Goudsmit J (1997) Complete nucleotide sequence of simian endogenous type D retrovirus with intact genome organization: evidence for ancestry to simian retrovirus and baboon endogenous virus. J Virol 71:3666–3676

Vogt PK 1997. Historical introduction to the general properties of retroviruses, p. 1–26. In JM Coffin, Hughes SH, and Varmus HE (eds), Retroviruses. Cold Spring Harbor Laboratory Press, New York

Wahlberg JM, Bron R, Wilschut J, and Garoff H (1992) Membrane fusion of Semliki Forest virus involves homotrimers of the fusion protein. J Virol 66:7309–7318

Wang H, Dechant E, Kavanaugh M, North RA, and Kabat D (1992) Effects of ecotropic murine retroviruses on the dual-function cell surface receptor/basic amino acid transporter. J Biol Chem 267:23617–23624

Wang H, Kavanaugh MP, and Kabat D (1994) A critical site in the cell surface receptor for ecotropic murine retroviruses required for amino acid transport but not for viral reception. Virology 202:1058–1060

Wang H, Kavanaugh MP, North RA, and Kabat D (1991) Cell-surface receptor for ecotropic murine retroviruses is a basic amino-acid transporter. Nature 352:729–731

Wehrle JP, and Pedersen PL (1989) Phosphate transport processes in eukaryotic cells. J Membr Biol 111:199–213

Weiss RA 1992. Cellular receptors and viral glycoproteins involved in retrovirus entry, p. 3–90. In JA Levy (ed.), The Retroviruses, vol. 2. Plenum Press

Weller SK, Joy AE, and Temin HM (1980) Correlation between cell killing and massive second-round superinfection by members of some subgroups of avian leukosis virus. J Virol 33:494–506

Wentworth DE, and Holmes KV (2001) Molecular determinants of species specificity in the coronavirus receptor aminopeptidase N (CD13): influence of N-linked glycosylation. J Virol 75:9741–9752

Werner A, Dehmelt L, and Nalbant P (1998) Na^+-dependent phosphate cotransporters: the NaPi protein families. J Exp Biol 201:3135–3142

White J, Kartenbeck J, and Helenius A (1980) Fusion of Semliki forest virus with the plasma membrane can be induced by low pH. J Cell Biol 87:264–272

White JM 1995. Membrane fusion: The influenza paradigm, p. 581–588, Cold Spring Harbor Symposia on Quantitative Biology, vol. 60. Cold Spring Harbor Laboratory Press

White MF (1985) The transport of cationic amino acids across the plasma membrane of mammalian cells. Biochim Biophys Acta 822:355–374

White MF, Gazzola GC, and Christensen HN (1982) Cationic amino acid transport into cultured animal cells. I. Influx into cultured human fibroblasts. J Biol Chem 257:4443-4449

Wilk T, de Haas F, Wagner A, Rutten T, Fuller S, Flugel RM, and Lochelt M (2000) The intact retroviral Env glycoprotein of human foamy virus is a trimer. J Virol 74:2885-2887

Wilson CA, and Eiden MV (1991) Viral and cellular factors governing hamster cell infection by murine and gibbon ape leukemia viruses. J Virol 65:5975-5982

Wilson CA, Eiden MV, Anderson WB, Lehel C, and Olah Z (1995) The dual-function hamster receptor for amphotropic murine leukemia virus (MuLV), 10A1 MuLV, and gibbon ape leukemia virus is a phosphate symporter. J Virol 69:534-537

Wilson CA, Farrell KB, and Eiden MV (1994) Comparison of cDNAs encoding the gibbon ape leukaemia virus receptor from susceptible and non-susceptible murine cells. J Gen Virol 75:1901-1908

Wilson CA, Farrell KB, and Eiden MV (1994) Properties of a unique form of the murine amphotropic leukemia virus receptor expressed on hamster cells. J Virol 68:7697-7703

Wilson CA, Wong S, VanBrocklin M, and Federspiel MJ (2000) Extended analysis of the in vitro tropism of porcine endogenous retrovirus. J Virol 74:49-56

Wu T, Lee CG, Buckler-White A, and Kozak CA (2002) Genetic control of a mouse serum lipoprotein factor that inactivates murine leukemia viruses: evaluation of apolipoprotein f as a candidate. J Virol 76:2279-2286

Yang YL, Guo L, Xu S, Holland CA, Kitamura T, Hunter K, and Cunningham JM (1999) Receptors for polytropic and xenotropic mouse leukaemia viruses encoded by a single gene at Rmc1. Nat Genet 21:216-219

Yoshimoto T, Yoshimoto E, and Meruelo D (1993) Identification of amino acid residues critical for infection with ecotropic murine leukemia retrovirus. J Virol 67:1310-1314

Yoshimura FK, Wang T, and Nanua S (2001) Mink cell focus-forming murine leukemia virus killing of mink cells involves apoptosis and superinfection. J Virol 75:6007-6015

Young JA, Bates P, and Varmus HE (1993) Isolation of a chicken gene that confers susceptibility to infection by subgroup A avian leukosis and sarcoma viruses. J Virol 67:1811-1816

Zavorotinskaya T, and Albritton LM (1999) Suppression of a fusion defect by second site mutations in the ecotropic murine leukemia virus surface protein. J Virol 73:5034-5042

Zerangue N, and Kavanaugh MP (1996) ASCT-1 is a neutral amino acid exchanger with chloride channel activity. J Biol Chem 271:27991-27994

Zhang YJ, Hatziioannou T, Zang T, Braaten D, Luban J, Goff SP, and Bieniasz PD (2002) Envelope-dependent, cyclophilin-independent effects of glycosaminoglycans on human immunodeficiency virus type 1 attachment and infection. J Virol 76:6332-6343

Zhao Y, Lee S, and Anderson WF (1997) Functional interactions between monomers of the retroviral envelope protein complex. J Virol 71:6967-6972

Zhao Y, Zhu L, Benedict CA, Chen D, Anderson WF, and Cannon PM (1998) Functional domains in the retroviral transmembrane protein. J Virol 72:5392-5398

Alpharetrovirus Envelope–Receptor Interactions

R. J. O. Barnard · J. A. T. Young

McArdle Laboratories for Cancer Research, Department of Oncology,
University of Wisconsin Madison, 1400 University Ave, Madison, WI 53706, USA
E-mail: johnyoung@wisc.edu

1	Introduction	108
2	Viral Determinants of Host Range	109
2.1	The ASLV Envelope Glycoprotein	110
2.2	Host Range Determinants of ASLV Env.	111
3	Host Factors Influencing Infection: ASLV Receptors	113
3.1	ASLV Receptors	114
3.1.1	Subgroup A Viral Receptors: TVA800 and TVA950	114
3.1.2	ASLV-A Envelope–Receptor Interactions	116
3.1.3	Subgroup B, D and E Viral Receptors: TVB^{S1} and TVB^{S3}	119
3.1.4	ASLV-B Interaction with TVB^{S1}	120
3.1.5	Nonreciprocal Interference Pattern of TVB^{S1} with ASLV Subgroups B, D, and E	121
4	Viral Entry Mechanisms	122
4.1	ASLV-Receptor Interactions: Receptor Priming and Low-pH Activation	122
4.2	ASLV Env-Dependent Viral Fusion	124
5	GATE Proteins (General Adaptors for Targeted Virus Entry)	127
6	Conclusions	127
	References	129

Abstract Infection by all enveloped viruses occurs via the fusion of viral and cellular membranes and delivery of the viral nucleocapsid into the cell cytoplasm, after association of the virus with cognate receptors at the cell surface. This process is mediated by viral fusion proteins anchored in the viral envelope and can be defined based on the requirement for low pH to trigger membrane fusion. In viruses that utilize a pH-dependent entry mechanism, such as influenza virus, viral fusion is triggered by the acidic environment of intracellular organelles after uptake of the virus from the cell surface and trafficking to a low-pH compartment. In contrast, in viruses that utilize a pH-independent entry mechanism, such as most retroviruses, membrane fusion is triggered solely by the interaction of the envelope glycoprotein with cognate receptors, often at the cell surface. However, recent work has indicated that the alpharetrovirus, avian sarcoma and leukosis virus (ASLV), utilizes a novel entry mechanism that combines aspects of both pH-independent and pH-dependent entry. In ASLV infection, the interaction of the envelope glycoprotein (Env) with cognate receptors at the cell surface causes an initial conformational change that primes (activates) Env and renders it sensitive to subsequent low-pH triggering from an intracellular compartment. Thus unlike other pH-dependent viruses, ASLV Env is only sensitive to low-pH triggering following interaction with its cognate receptor. In this manuscript we review current research on ASLV Env–receptor interactions and focus on the specific molecular requirements of both the viral fusion protein and cognate receptors for ASLV entry. In addition, we review data pertaining to the novel two-step entry mechanism of ASLV entry and propose a model by which ASLV Env elicits membrane fusion.

1
Introduction

Attachment of viruses to the cell surface is the first stage in a sequence of events that lead to delivery of the viral core into the cell cytoplasm. In enveloped viruses, this process is initiated by interaction of viral membrane glycoproteins with specific cell surface receptors. Although adsorption of viruses to the surface of both susceptible and nonsusceptible cells can occur (Piranio 1967), viral penetration requires the expression of a cognate receptor on the target cell surface. Consequently, the choice of receptor and its abundance among species have a major influence in determining the host range of a virus. Furthermore, the tissue distribution of receptor-expressing cells within an organism can also influence viral pathogenesis (for a review, see Schneider-Schaulies 2000). After receptor binding, infection proceeds through a complex series of conformational changes in the envelope glycoprotein that ultimately lead to fusion of viral and cellular membranes and the introduction of the viral genome into the cell. For many viruses, such as Influenza A virus, the envelope glycoprotein is activated exclusively by the low-pH environment of an acidic organelle after uptake of the virus by receptor-mediated endocytosis. In contrast, the fusion proteins of pH-independent viruses, such as those of most retroviruses, are triggered solely by interaction with their cognate receptors, or in some cases also by coreceptors (for a review, see Eckert and Kim 2001). However, as discussed below, recent data obtained for the alpharetrovirus avian sarcoma and leukosis virus (ASLV) have revealed a third type of entry mechanism that utilizes aspects of both pH-dependent and pH-independent entry. Specifically, interaction with cell surface receptors primes the ASLV envelope glycoprotein (Env), rendering it sensitive to subsequent low-pH-dependent activation, presumably within an intracellular acidic compartment. This requirement for a prior receptor-priming step distinguishes ASLV Env from other pH-dependent viral fusion proteins that are activated by low pH alone (Mothes et al. 2000). At present, ASLV is the only virus known to use this novel two-step entry mechanism.

In this chapter, we review the current understanding of ASLV Env–receptor interactions and describe the specific domains within Env that determine the viral host range specificity. In addition, we discuss in detail the cellular molecular requirements for ASLV penetration, and data pertaining to the novel receptor-primed low-pH entry mechanism utilized by ASLV are reviewed. Furthermore, we discuss how an understanding of ASLV receptor–envelope interactions has led to novel strategies to redirect ASLV to utilize other cell surface molecules as receptors for infection.

2
Viral Determinants of Host Range

The avian retroviruses of the genus alpharetrovirus predominantly infect birds of the order Galliformes and are divided into ten subgroups (A–J) based on receptor specificity, sensitivity to neutralizing antibodies, and cross-interference of infection (Weiss 1993). Of these viruses, the Env-receptor interactions of ASLV subgroups A, B, D, and E (which infect animals of the *Gallus* species, predominantly the domestic chicken *Gallus gallus*) have been extensively studied and are the focus of this review. Two of these viral subgroups (B and D) cause cytopathic effects on infection of cultured avian cells, leading to the death of up to 40% of the cell population during the early (acute) phase of infection. In contrast, viruses of the other two subgroups (A and E) are noncytopathic and infection has no adverse effect on cell viability.

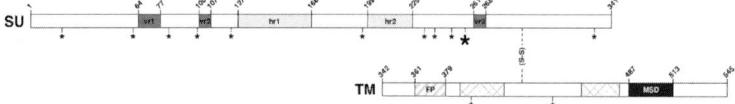

Fig. 1 Schematic of ASLV-A envelope glycoprotein. *vr*, variable region; *hr*, host range domain; *FP*, fusion peptide' *MSD*, membrane-spanning domain. The *hashed boxes* are heptad repeat domains. The *asterisks* indicate glycosylation sites. Glycosylation site 10, required for correct folding of the receptor binding domain (Delos et al. 2002), is represented by an *enlarged asterisk*. The *numbers* indicate amino acids in the processed protein. The signal peptide is not shown

2.1
The ASLV Envelope Glycoprotein

ASLV Env is translated from a spliced mRNA molecule that encodes a precursor polypeptide with the six N-terminal residues being derived from the *gag* gene (Schwarz et al. 1983). After removal of its 62-amino acid-long leader sequence, the envelope glycoprotein is synthesized as a precursor protein of 95 kDa (Pr95) that assembles as a homotrimer in the endoplasmic reticulum (ER) (Lee et al. 1979; Purchio et al. 1980; Hunter et al. 1983; Einfeld and Hunter 1988). Pr95 is proteolytically processed to form two subunits, gp85 (SU) and gp37 (TM), that remain linked by a disulfide bond (England et al. 1977; Moelling and Hayami 1977; Buchhagen and Hanafusa 1978; Klemenz and Digglemann 1978; Hunter et al. 1983; Perez and Hunter 1987; Einfeld and Hunter 1988; Dong et al. 1990). The SU subunit of ASLV Env contains between 10 and 14 consensus sites for N-linked glycosylation, depending on the viral subgroup. Of these sites, nine are absolutely conserved between subgroups A–E (Fig. 1). The trimer of heterodimers is then transported to the plasma membrane, where it is incorporated into budding virions (Einfeld and Hunter 1988).

The SU subunit contains the viral receptor-binding determinants. The TM subunit contains a C-terminal membrane-spanning domain that anchors Env to the viral membrane. In addition, this domain contains a conserved hydrophobic region located close to the N-terminus, which most likely constitutes a fusion peptide required for viral membrane fusion (Hernandez and White 1998; Balliet et al. 2000; Delos et al. 2000) and two heptad repeat domains. The N-terminal heptad repeat is juxtaposed to the putative fusion peptide, whereas the C-terminal heptad repeat lies close to the membrane-spanning domain (Fig. 1). It is thought that the association of these heptad repeat domains, to form a thermostable six-helix bundle (6HB), elicit fusion of the viral and cellular membranes (see Sect. 4.2 and Chambers et al. 1991; Skehel and Wiley 1998). Therefore, the overall organization of the ASLV envelope glycoprotein closely resembles that of other class I fusion proteins for example, influenza HA, HIV gp120/gp41, and Ebola virus GP1/GP2 (Chambers et al. 1991; Skehel and Wiley 1998; Weissenhorn et al. 1999). Interestingly, the ASLV TM subunit exhibits significant sequence and architectural homology to the Ebola virus GP2 (Volchkov et al. 1992; Gallaher 1996), suggesting that these viruses could utilize similar mechanisms of entry.

2.2
Host Range Determinants of ASLV Env

The receptor usage of the closely related ASLV family is determined solely by the viral envelope glycoprotein (Hanafusa 1965; Vogt 1965; Crittenden 1968; Joho et al. 1975; Coffin et al. 1978). The Env proteins of ASLV subgroups A–E contain five regions of variable amino acid sequence: three small variable regions (vr) termed vr1, vr2, and vr3 and two larger areas of sequence heterogeneity (host range or hr) termed hr1 and hr2 (Fig. 1) (Dorner et al. 1985; Bova et al. 1986, 1988). Furthermore, additional variability exists in the hr2 region among viruses of the same subgroup (Hara et al. 1996). The major determinants of host range specificity map to an area of the SU subunit that contains all five variable regions (Bova et al. 1988; Bova-Hill et al. 1991).

Several lines of evidence suggest that of these domains, hr1 and hr2 play the most important role in determining host range. First, substitution of the hr2 region of ASLV-B Env with the corresponding domain from ASLV-E resulted in a virus that could infect cells via both ASLV-B and ASLV-E receptors (Tsichlis and Coffin 1980; Tsichlis et al. 1980; Dorner et al. 1985, 1986). Second, alteration of specific residues in the hr1 region of ASLV-B with ASLV subgroup D-specific residues Asn-157, Pro-159, and Asp-160 also changed the host range of the virus (Bova-Hill et al. 1991). Third, ASLV virions selected to have an extended host range displayed modifications only to the hr1 and hr2 regions: ASLV-B virions grown alternately in permissive (ASLV-B receptor expressing) and then nonpermissive (ASLV-E receptor expressing) cells had specific alterations in the hr1 domain of Env (Leu-155 to Ser and Thr-156 to Ile) that allowed use of both ASLV-B and ASLV-E receptors (Taplitz and Coffin 1997); ASLV-A virions adapted to grow in the presence of a soluble form of the SU domain of ASLV-A Env exhibited a deletion of six amino acids in the hr1 region that resulted in an altered host range (Holmen and Federspiel 2000); ASLV-A variants selected to resist inhibition by a soluble form of the quail ASLV-A receptor had mutations of residues Tyr-142 and/or Glu-149 of the hr1 region of Env, resulting in virions with a decreased affinity for the quail, but not chicken, form of the subgroup A viral receptor (Holmen et al. 1999; Holmen et al. 2001).

Alteration of the vr1, vr2, and vr3 regions alone has no effect on viral host range (Dorner et al. 1985; Bova et al. 1986; Dorner and Coffin 1986; Bova et al. 1988; Bova-Hill et al. 1991). However, the vr3 domain has been found to influence receptor usage in the context of a chimeric ASLV-B/E Env protein, in which the hr2 from ASLV-E is combined with the vr1, vr2, and hr1 regions of ASLV-B. In this context, the vr3 region of ASLV-E narrowed the host range of the virus from that which utilizes ASLV-B or ASLV-E receptors to one that could infect cells only via ASLV-E receptors (Dorner and Coffin 1986). This data suggests that the vr3 domain plays an auxiliary role in determining host range. The reason for the sequence variability in the vr1 and vr2 regions of Env remains to be established. Although there is evidence these regions play a direct role in dictating receptor usage, it is possible that they could act to shield one or more conserved core structural elements of ASLV Env from neutralizing antibodies during persistent infection in vivo, in a manner similar to that proposed for some of the variable regions of HIV gp120 (Cao et al. 1997; Stamatotos and Cheng-Mayer 1998; Johnson and Desrosiers 2002). For example, these variable regions could act by restricting access of neutralizing antibodies raised against the conserved functional elements of ASLV Env that normally lie hidden in the native structure until activation of the envelope glycoprotein. On elucidation of the three-dimensional structure of the native form of ASLV Env, it would be interesting to see whether the vr1 and vr2 domains lie at the surface of Env, where they could potentially fulfill such a shielding role.

The fact that separate regions of Env (hr1, hr2, and possibly vr3) specify receptor usage indicates that these regions could come together to form a receptor-binding site. Consistent with this notion, residues of the hr1 and hr2 region of ASLV-B have been cross-linked to a 15-amino acid peptide that was previously shown to function as a minimal soluble viral receptor (see below) (T. Gibson and J.A.T Young, manuscript in preparation).

Interestingly, of the putative N-linked glycosylation sites in the SU subunit of Env, none is present in either of the receptor-binding regions (hr1 and hr2), suggesting that, as is the case for the interaction of HIV with its receptor during productive infection, oligosaccharides do not play a direct role in viral recognition of the cognate receptors (Kwong et al. 1998). Rigorous mutational analysis of the conserved consensus N-linked glycosylation sites in the SU subunit of ASLV-A revealed that glycosylation at either the second or sixth N-linked glycosylation position is required for the correct folding of Env (Delos et al. 2002). In addition, mutation of the tenth N-linked glycosylation site of the SU subunit abrogated receptor binding as well as binding to an Env-specific monoclonal antibody, which inhibits receptor interaction while not influencing processing or virion incorporation of Env. This result has led to the suggestion that this specific carbohydrate modification is important for the correct folding of the receptor-binding domain(s) of Env (Delos et al. 2002). Clearly, detailed X-ray structural analysis of the envelope glycoprotein from ASLV subgroups A–E, complexed with their cognate receptors, will ultimately be required to establish the precise roles of hr1, hr2, vr3, and N-linked oligosaccharides of Env in receptor binding.

3
Host Factors Influencing Infection: ASLV Receptors

A seminal body of work on host cell susceptibility factors for different ASLV subgroups led to the description of putative ASLV receptor genes (denoted *tv* for tumor virus) (Rubin 1965; Piranio 1967; Crittenden 1968). Specifically, the sensitivity of cells to ASLV subgroups A–E was mapped to three autosomal chicken loci denoted *tva* (Crittenden et al. 1964; Crittenden et al. 1967), *tvb* (Rubin 1965; Payne and Biggs 1966; Crittenden et al. 1967), and *tvc* (Payne and Biggs 1970; Motta et al. 1973). ASLV susceptibility and resistance alleles are associated with each of these loci (e.g., *tva^s* and *tva^r*), and susceptibility is always dominant (Rubin 1965; Vogt and Ishizaki 1965; Payne and Biggs 1966; Payne and Pani 1971). The *tva* and *tvc* loci are closely linked (Payne and Pani 1971) and were predicted to encode receptors for viral subgroups A and C, respectively (Vogt and Ishizaki 1965; Motta et al. 1973). The *tvb* locus is more complex, consisting of at least two dominant alleles (tvb^{S1} and tvb^{S3}) that confer differing patterns of susceptibility to infection by ASLV subgroups B, D, and E. The S1 allele confers susceptibility to ASLV subgroups B, D, and E, and the S3 allele confers susceptibility to infection only by ASLV subgroups B and D (Hanafusa et al. 1970; Vogt and Fris 1971; Crittenden et al. 1974; Robinson and Lamoreux 1976). In addition, susceptibility of cells to ASLV-E infection is controlled by intact endogenous proviruses present in the chicken genome at a number of loci (termed ev loci for endogenous virus) (Smith 1986). Expression of ev genes can interfere with the function of ASLV-E receptors or, alternatively, cause an increased immune response against ASLV infection. At the time of writing, three chicken ASLV receptors have been identified that correspond to the gene products of the tva^s, tvb^{S1}, and tvb^{S3} alleles. The gene product(s) of the tvc loci are not yet known.

3.1
ASLV Receptors

3.1.1
Subgroup A Viral Receptors: TVA800 and TVA950

The tva gene was cloned by using a gene transfer approach in which chicken and quail genomic DNA were introduced into mammalian cells that are normally resistant to ASLV infection (Bates et al. 1993; Young et al. 1993). The cloned DNA mapped to the chicken tva locus (Bates et al. 1998) and encoded the subgroup A-specific viral receptor. Two differentially spliced mRNA products of the quail gene (designated as TVA800 and TVA950) have been described that resulted from a retroviral vector-based exon-trapping strategy (Bates et al. 1993). TVA950 is a type I transmembrane protein with an N-terminal signal peptide (residues 1–19), an extracellular domain (residues 20–102), a membrane-spanning region (residues 103–125), and a small cytoplasmic tail (residues 126–157) (Fig. 2a). The N-terminal amino acids of TVA800, including the signal peptide and extracellular domain, are identical to those of TVA950. However, TVA800 lacks a transmembrane domain and is attached to the membrane instead via a glycosyl phosphatidylinositol (GPI) membrane anchor (Fig. 2a). This difference in membrane attachment seems to explain why TVA800 resides in lipid raft microdomains at the plasma membrane, whereas TVA950does not (Narayan et al. 2003). Both iso-

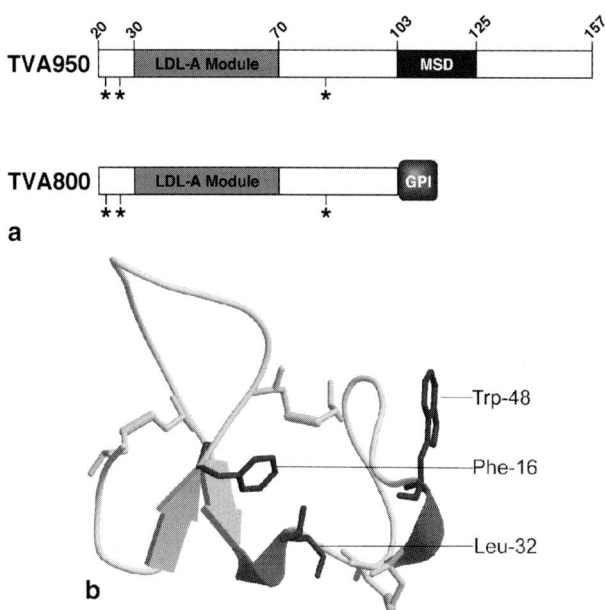

Fig. 2 a Schematic of TVA950 and TVA800. *MSD*, membrane-spanning domain. The *asterisks* indicate potential glycosylation sites. *Numbers* indicate amino acids in the precursor protein. The signal peptide is not shown. b Solution structure of the TVA LDL-A module. In this diagram residues Phe-16, Leu-34, and Trp-48, which form part of the hydrophobic patch, are indicated

forms of the TVA receptor are predicted to be modified at three sites of N-linked glycosylation (Fig. 2a) (Bates et al. 1993; Balliet et al. 1999).

ASLV-A Env specifically interacts with the extracellular domain of TVA (Connolly et al. 1994; Gilbert et al. 1994; Zingler and Young 1996; Balliet et al. 1999). The extracellular region of TVA contains a single cysteine-rich domain with a high degree of homology to the ligand-binding repeat of LDL receptors, termed the LDL-A module. As with LDL-A modules of other proteins (Blacklow and Kim 1996; Bieri et al. 1998), the six cysteine residues of the TVA LDL-A module form three intramolecular disulfide bonds arranged in a 1–3, 2–5, 4–6 configuration (Fig. 2b) (Belanger et al. 1995; Tonelli et al. 2001; Wang et al. 2002). Also, like many other LDL-A modules, TVA has a high affinity for calcium and coordination of a single calcium ion is required for correct protein folding (Bieri et al. 1998; Wang et al. 2001). Truncation of the extracellular domain of TVA revealed that the LDL-A module alone is sufficient to support viral entry (Rong and Bates 1995). ASLV Env has a high affinity for the ectodomain of TVA (K_D=0.3 nM) that remains relatively constant over a range of temperatures (Zingler and Young 1996; Balliet et al. 1999). This interaction is only slightly weakened by removal of N-linked sugars from TVA, suggesting that these oligosaccharides play a minor role in receptor-envelope binding (Balliet et al. 1999).

3.1.2
ASLV-A Envelope–Receptor Interactions

Extensive mutational analysis of the ectodomain of TVA identified three key amino acids, Asp-46, Glu-47, and Trp-48, that are necessary for viral receptor function (Zingler et al. 1995; Zingler and Young 1996; Rong et al. 1998b). Additional important amino acids were identified in a gain-of-function study, in which nonconserved residues of a human LDL-A module were replaced with the corresponding amino acids from the LDL-A module of TVA. This study revealed that residues Leu-34, His-38, and Gly-49 were also required for efficient ASLV-A entry (Rong et al. 1998a).

Analysis of the solution structure of the TVA LDL-A module demonstrated that the side chains of both Asp-46 and Glu-47, along with the carbonyl oxygens of Leu-34 and His-38, most likely directly participate in the coordination of the calcium ion (Tonelli et al. 2001). As mutation of Asp-46 and Glu-47 lead to a loss of calcium binding and a decrease in the overall stability of the protein (Wang et al. 2001), it is possible that mutation of His-38, Asp-46, or Glu-47 alters the overall structure of TVA and ultimately disrupts the Env binding site (Rong et al. 1998b; Tonelli et al. 2001). Trp-48 is exposed on the surface of TVA and lies flat against the backbone of Arg-45 (Fig. 2b) (Tonelli et al. 2001). As this large hydrophobic residue is not buried within the TVA molecule, it is unlikely that Trp-48 participates directly in the folding or overall stability of the protein but rather it is likely that it plays a direct role in the interaction with the viral envelope glycoprotein. Indeed, consistent with this hypothesis, substitution of Trp-48 with a hydrophilic or a small nonpolar residue results in a receptor that is unable to support infection (Zingler et al. 1995; Rong et al. 1998b). However, mutation of Trp-48 to a bulky hydrophobic amino acid, such as a tyrosine or phenylalanine, results in a receptor with almost wild-type activity (Zingler and Young 1996). Interestingly, although ASLV-A Env can interact with an altered TVA receptor, with residue Trp-48 replaced with an alanine (Zingler and Young 1996; Hernandez et al. 1997), this mutant receptor cannot support infection by ASLV-A (Zingler et al. 1995; Rong et al. 1998b) or induce the conformational changes in Env that are thought to occur during viral entry (Hernandez et al. 1997). Therefore, in addition to a role in ASLV-A Env binding, residue Trp-48 may also play a key part in activating the fusion potential of the viral envelope glycoprotein.

Residues Leu-34 and Gly-49 form part of a hydrophobic patch on the surface of the receptor (Fig. 2b) (Tonelli et al. 2001). This hydrophobic area is comprised of both Trp-48 and Gly-49 and extends into the N-domain of the LDL-A module to include Leu-34, Gln-31, and Phe-16 (Tonelli et al. 2001). As both Leu-34 and Gly-49 are required for association with ASLV-A Env and form part of a hydrophobic patch on the surface of TVA, it is possible that these amino acids play a direct role in establishing contacts with the envelope glycoprotein of ASLV-A (Tonelli et al. 2001). Despite the presence of the conserved amino acids Phe-16 and Gln-31 in the hydrophobic patch of TVA, a direct role for these residues in the association of ASLV-A Env remains to be demonstrated. It is interesting to speculate that the residues of the hydrophobic patch of TVA interact with a hydrophobic binding pocket of ASLV Env and help correctly orient Trp-48 to a specific interaction site of Env.

At present the natural ligand and function of TVA are unknown, and it is consequently not currently possible to determine whether ASLV-A Env interacts with its receptor in a manner similar to its natural ligand. However, many LDL-A module ligands possess clusters of basic residues that are required for receptor binding (Wilson et al. 1991). Sequence comparison of the envelope glycoproteins of many ASLV subgroups revealed a basic cluster of amino acids only in the hr2 region of ASLV-A Env (Rong et al. 1997). Alanine scanning analysis of these basic residues revealed that Arg-210, Arg-213, Arg-223, Arg-224, and Lys-227 are all required for efficient receptor interaction, indicating that ASLV-A Env potentially possesses properties similar to those of LDL-A ligands (Rong et al. 1997). Indeed, analysis of the surface charge of TVA reveals a cluster of negatively charged amino acids in the C-terminal region of the LDL-A module (Tonelli et al. 2001) that could interact with the basic residues of the subgroup A envelope glycoprotein, although many of these residues seem to be involved in coordinating the calcium ion.

In addition to the amino acid residues already described it is likely that additional residues of TVA are required for efficient interaction with ASLV-A Env. Analysis of ASLV-A Env mutants in binding studies with both chicken and quail TVA demonstrated that three mutations in the hr1 region of Env (E149K, Y142N and E149K/Y142N) abrogated binding to the quail, but not the chicken, TVA receptor (Holmen et al. 2001). As chicken and quail TVA differ only in the N-terminal regions, presumably there are amino acid determinants within these regions that can also impact receptor function.

From these data, it is possible to evoke a model by which ASLV-A Env interacts with TVA. In this model, the hr1 and hr2 domains of ASLV-A Env cooperate to form a receptor-binding site that recognizes specific structural elements of TVA that include surface acidic amino acids and the hydrophobic patch. It is possible that the hydrophobic patch of TVA aids in the orientation of Env with the receptor protein to allow a precise association of ASLV-A Env with Trp-48, perhaps via insertion into a hydrophobic pocket similar to that observed with other retroviral receptors. Indeed, residues Phe-43 of the HIV receptor CD4 and Tyr-235 of the ecotropic murine leukemia virus (MLV) receptor mCAT-1 make specific hydrophobic contacts with their respective envelopes and are essential for receptor activity (Moebius et al. 1992; Albritton et al. 1993; Malhotra et al. 1996; Kwong et al. 1998). This raises the possibility that retroviruses utilize a common recognition mechanism to promote efficient binding with their cognate receptors. The molecular mechanisms that control the association of TVA with ASLV-A Env and their homology to other LDL-A module–ligand interactions will be definitively solved after crystallization of the envelope glycoprotein in complex with TVA.

At present the nature of the defect in chicken tva^r has not been defined and sequence analysis of the LDL-A module of tva^r allele from chickens has revealed no significant differences from that of tva^s (Bates et al. 1998). As this allele is fully recessive to tva^s, it is possible that tva^r is a defective gene that does not give rise to a protein product or, alternatively, may encode a protein that either interacts weakly with, or does not interact at all with, ASLV-A Env. For example, it is possible that the tva^r gene encodes a protein containing alterations in residues that affect the general fold of the molecule in a manner similar to mutations of Asp-46.

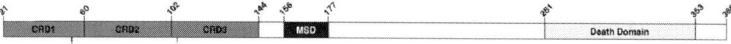

Fig. 3 Schematic of TVB. *CRD*, cysteine-rich domain; *MSD*, membrane-spanning domain. The *asterisks* indicate potential glycosylation sites. The *numbers* indicate amino acids in the precursor protein. The signal peptide is not shown

3.1.3
Subgroup B, D and E Viral Receptors: TVB^{S1} and TVB^{S3}

Two alleles of the *tvb* locus, *tvb^{S1}* and *tvb^{S3}* encode receptors for ASLV-B, -D, and -E and ASLV-B and -D, respectively. The *tvb^{S3}* gene was cloned by a gene transfer approach (Brojatsch et al. 1996; Smith et al. 1998). Analysis of its protein product revealed that like TVA, TVB^{S3} is a type I membrane protein consisting of a signal peptide (residues 1–21), a small extracellular domain (residues 22–155) anchored to the lipid bilayer via a C-terminal membrane-spanning domain (residues 156–177), and a cytoplasmic domain (residues 178–361) (Fig. 3). TVB^{S3} is a member of the tumor necrosis factor receptor (TNFR) family and contains three cysteine-rich domains (CRDs) in the extracellular domain and a cytoplasmic death domain (Fig. 3). The overall topology of TVB^{S3} suggests that it is the chicken homolog of the TNFR-related human death receptors [TNFR apoptosis-inducing ligand (TRAIL) receptors] TRAIL-R1 and TRAIL-R2 (Adkins et al. 2001). The finding that TVB^{S3} contains a cytoplasmic death domain is intriguing because the viruses that utilize this receptor for entry, ASLV-B and ASLV-D, are both cytopathic and may exert their cytopathic effect (CPE) via this domain during the acute phase of infection (Brojatsch et al. 1996).

The *tvb^{S1}* allele was isolated from a chicken cDNA library based on its homology to *tvb^{S3}* (Adkins et al. 2000), and the ectodomain of this receptor contains all of the viral interaction determinants (Adkins et al. 2001). A sequence comparison of TVB^{S1} and TVB^{S3} revealed that these two proteins are identical except for a single serine residue in the CRD2 domain of TVB^{S3} (Ser-62) that is altered to cysteine in TVB^{S1} (Cys-62) (Adkins et al. 2000). Interestingly, the TVB homolog from turkey cells (TVB^T), which allows entry of only ASLV-E, also contains a cysteine residue at position 62 (Adkins et al. 1997), indicating that Cys-62 is crucial for the interaction of ASLV-E with its receptors. Mutational analysis of the cysteine residues of TVB^{S1} has also indicated that ASLV-E binding may require a specific disulfide bond formed between residues Cys-46 and Cys-59 of the receptor, whereas an unpaired cysteine at position 62 or 77 may negatively impact this interaction (Adkins et al. 2000).

The tvb^r allele was recently identified and found to contain a premature stop codon so that it encodes only a 57-amino acid peptide of TVB that includes the 21-amino acid leader sequence of the receptor (Klucking et al. 2002). Thus the fully recessive nature of this allele is presumably explained by the severely truncated nature of its protein product.

3.1.4
ASLV-B Interaction with TVB^{S1}

Unlike in the case of ASLV-E Env, the interaction of ASLV-B Env with TVB^{S1} does not seem to require any specific disulfide bonding pattern in the receptor (Adkins et al. 2000). Indeed, the subgroup B Env-receptor interaction is maintained after deglycosylation or reduction and denaturation of the receptor, a result that led to the hypothesis that ASLV-B Env recognizes a linear subfragment of TVB (Adkins et al. 2001). Subsequent peptide scanning analysis of TVB confirmed this prediction and revealed that a 15-amino acid linear peptide derived from the N-terminal region of TVB^{S1} (residues 32–46) contains sufficient information to act as a minimal subgroup B-specific viral receptor: The peptide bound specifically to ASLV-B SU and supported subgroup B viral entry into receptor-negative cells (Knauss and Young 2002). Three residues within this peptide were essential for receptor activity (Leu-36, Gln-37, and Tyr-42) (Knauss and Young 2002). The presence of an essential aromatic amino acid in both TVA (residue Trp-48) and TVB (residue Tyr-42) suggests that the activation of these ASLV envelope glycoproteins could occur via a similar mechanism. However, a similar minimal binding peptide of TVA, which contained essential amino acids for interaction with ASLV-A Env including Trp-48, inhibited ASLV-A entry (Zingler et al. 1995). This suggests that additional residues are required to activate the fusogenic potential of ASLV-A Env in addition to those of the minimal TVA binding peptide.

The simple requirements of TVB for ASLV-B receptor function lend further credence to the concept that ASLV-B and ASLV-E interact with the TVB receptor in fundamentally different ways. However, direct experimental evidence for this hypothesis is currently lacking. Although

ASLV-B Env can be activated by the receptor-derived minimal peptide, it is still unclear how activated virions are able to infect cells that lack receptor. As it has been demonstrated that virions adsorb on both susceptible and nonsusceptible cells to similar levels (Piranio 1967) (see also Sect. 8.2 of the chapter by Tailor et al. and Sect. 2.2 of the chapter by Sandrin et al., this volume), the initial interactions of ASLV virions with cells could be independent of receptor.

3.1.5
Nonreciprocal Interference Pattern of TVB^{S1} with ASLV Subgroups B, D, and E

Although TVB^{S1} is a functional receptor for ASLV-B, ASLV-D, and ASLV-E, these viral subgroups exhibit a nonreciprocal interference pattern. When cells expressing TVB^{S1} are infected with ASLV-B or -D, they become resistant to superinfection by all three of these ASLV subgroups (-B, -D, and -E). This effect results from the formation of complexes between newly synthesized ASLV-B Env and the TVB receptor either during intracellular trafficking of both proteins or at the cell surface. The net effect of these interactions is that the cellular receptor cannot promote additional rounds of viral entry (Weiss 1993).

In contrast to cells infected with ASLV-B or ASLV-D, those infected with ASLV-E are resistant to superinfection only by other subgroup E-specific viruses. This nonreciprocal interference pattern is explained by the existence of two forms (types 1 and 2) of TVB^{S1} that presumably differ in their intrachain disulfide bonding patterns (Adkins et al. 2001). The type 1 form acts as a receptor for all three ASLV subgroups (-B, -D, and -E), whereas the type 2 form is a receptor specific for ASLV subgroups B and D (Adkins et al. 2001). Thus the superinfection resistance pattern is probably explained by ASLV-B and ASLV-D interfering with the activities of both types of receptor whereas ASLV-E infection interferes only with the activity of the type 1 receptor, leaving the type 2 receptor available at the cell surface to support further rounds of subgroup B and D virus entry (Adkins et al. 2001).

The finding that the envelope glycoprotein of ASLV-E interacts specifically with only one of the two forms of TVB^{S1} supports the idea that this virus recognizes structural elements, possibly dictated by the intrachain disulfide bonding pattern, within the general fold of the TVB receptor (see Sect. 3.3.1). Consistent with this idea, mutational analysis of TVB^{S1}

has revealed that residues in both the CRD1 and CDR2 regions of TVB[S1] are important for subgroup E-specific viral receptor function and several key amino acid residues in the CRD2 region of the receptor have been identified (Tyr-67, Asn-72, and Asp-73) (S. Klucking, and J.A.T. Young, manuscript in preparation).

4
Viral Entry Mechanisms

4.1
ASLV-Receptor Interactions: Receptor Priming and Low-pH Activation

After association with receptors at the cell surface, ASLV infection proceeds via a series of conformational changes in Env that ultimately result in fusion of viral and cellular membranes. For many viruses, such as Influenza A virus, the envelope glycoprotein is triggered by the low-pH environment of acidic intracellular organelles after internalization of the virus by receptor-mediated endocytosis. In contrast, the envelope glycoproteins of viruses that utilize a pH-independent entry mechanism, such as those of most retroviruses, are triggered by association with the cognate receptor, or in some cases also by coreceptors, often at the cell surface.

Recent analysis of ASLV entry has led to a model in which this virus utilizes a novel entry mechanism that combines aspects of both pH-independent and pH-dependent entry mechanisms (Mothes et al. 2000). ASLV infection is abolished in the presence of lysosomotropic reagents, such as bafilomycin, that neutralize the pH of intracellular organelles and inhibit low-pH-dependent cellular processes (Mothes et al. 2000). The requirement for low pH in ASLV entry maps solely to Env, as ASLV particles pseudotyped with the envelope glycoprotein of MLV (which mediates pH-independent entry) are resistant to the effect of the lysosomotropic reagent (Mothes et al. 2000). Conversely, MLV particles pseudotyped with ASLV Env entered cells in a strictly low-pH-dependent manner (Mothes et al. 2000). The low-pH-induced signal appears to activate ASLV Env directly, because the block to ASLV infection imposed by bafilomycin can be overcome after treatment of cell-associated virus with low pH, presumably by inducing fusion of virions at the plasma membrane (Mothes et al. 2000). Finally, efficient cell-cell fusion can be induced between cells expressing ASLV Env and cells expressing cognate receptors after treatment of the cells at low pH, but not at neutral pH (Gilbert et al. 1990; Mothes et al. 2000).

It appears that the internalization of ASLV virions is also required for infection, as ASLV entry is severely abrogated in cells expressing a dominant-negative form of dynamin that inhibits endocytosis from the cell surface (Mothes et al. 2000). More recently it was demonstrated that the uptake of ASLV-A virions from the cell surface, and their subsequent trafficking to intracellular acidic sites of fusion, can occur via two distinct pathways and differ because of the presence or absence of TVA in lipid raft microdomains (Narayan et al. 2003).

Collectively these data indicate that the ASLV envelope glycoprotein requires a low-pH activation step during infection, most likely after uptake of the virus and trafficking to an acidic intracellular compartment. However, several key differences seem to exist between the entry mechanism of ASLV and those used by other low-pH-dependent viruses. For example, low-pH treatment of Influenza A virus causes a dramatic loss of viral infectivity, most likely because of premature triggering of the envelope glycoprotein and the insertion of the hydrophobic fusion peptide into viral membranes (Stegmann et al. 1987; Puri et al. 1990). ASLV, on the other hand, is resistant to inactivation at low pH (Gilbert et al. 1990; Mothes et al. 2000). Instead, ASLV virions preloaded with a soluble form of their cognate receptor become highly sensitive to inactivation by low -pH treatment, an effect that seems to be correlated with oligomerization of the TM subunit of Env (Mothes et al. 2000) in a manner similar to that observed with other envelope glycoproteins during fusion activation (Weissenhorn et al. 1999; Mothes et al. 2000). Thus the sensitivity of ASLV Env to low-pH activation depends on its prior interaction with the cognate receptor (a step designated as receptor priming) (Fig. 4). Finally, ASLV differs from other low-pH-dependent viruses in that the virions can avoid cellular degradation and reside stably at an intracellular site of fusion when entry is blocked by incubating cells with lysosomotropic reagents (Mothes et al. 2000; Narayan et al. 2003). Therefore, it is possible that ASLV can access intracellular compartment(s) different from those involved in the intracellular trafficking of other low-pH-dependent viruses.

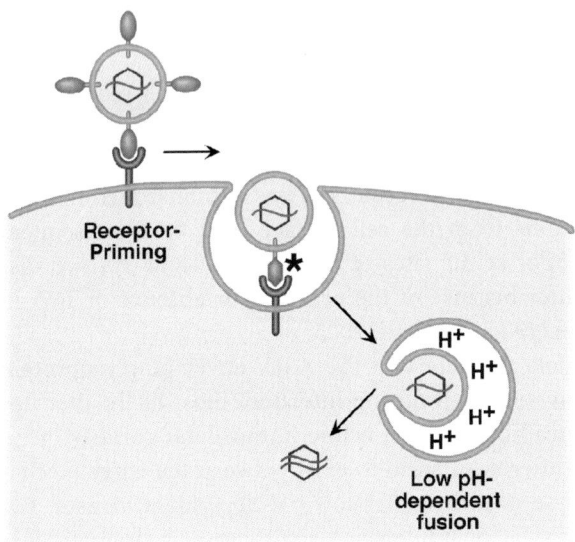

Fig. 4 Model for receptor-primed, low-pH-dependent entry of ASLV. The *asterisk* indicates the receptor-primed envelope glycoprotein

4.2
ASLV Env-Dependent Viral Fusion

For class I viral fusion proteins, such as influenza HA and HIV gp120/gp41, triggering of the envelope glycoprotein is thought to involve an initial extensive conformational change that leads to the exposure of the hydrophobic fusion peptide, normally sequestered from the aqueous solution within the protein, and its subsequent insertion into target membranes (Skehel and Wiley 2000; Eckert and Kim 2001). In this extended conformation, the envelope glycoprotein is proposed to span both viral and target membranes (Carr and Kim 1993; Bullough et al. 1994; Qiao et al. 1998). Further conformational changes are then proposed that reorient the fusion protein such that the fusion peptide and the membrane-spanning domain lie in close proximity at the same end of the protein (Skehel and Wiley 1998; Eckert and Kim 2001). In this conformation, the viral and target membranes are forced into contact, promoting the fusion of the contacting lipid bilayers, termed hemifusion (Chernomordik et al. 1995; Melikyan et al. 1995, 1997). After hemifusion, further conformational changes in the fusion protein are then proposed that include the association of N- and C-terminal heptad repeat domains to form a closely packed, thermostable, six-helix bundle(6HB) (Skehel and Wiley 1998; Weissenhorn et al. 1999; Eckert and Kim 2001). It is thought that the energy liberated during formation of the stable 6HB, and possibly from association of the fusion peptide and the membrane-spanning domain of the fusion protein, is used to bring the viral and cellular membranes closer together, thus promoting full fusion of the lipid bilayers (for detailed reviews on this topic, see Skehel and Wiley 2000; Eckert and Kim 2001). The fusion peptide of the Influenza A virus fusion protein is exposed and inserted into lipid bilayers after triggering of the HA at low pH (Stegmann et al. 1991; Tsurudome et al. 1992; Weber et al. 1994; Durrer et al. 1996). Similar association with target membranes has also been observed in the fusion proteins of other viruses, including Semliki Forest virus (Wahlberg et al. 1992; Bron et al. 1993; Klimjack et al. 1994), vesicular stomatitis virus, and rabies virus (Durrer et al. 1995), under conditions that trigger viral fusion. In contrast, analysis of the soluble ectodomain of ASLV-A Env after association with soluble TVA revealed that the hydrophobic fusion peptide is exposed at neutral pH (Gilbert et al. 1995), conditions under which ASLV fusion does not occur (Mothes et al. 2000). Furthermore, association with its cognate receptor led to the hydrophobic association of the soluble form of ASLV-A Env with artificial lipid bilayers via the TM subunit (Hernandez et al. 1997; Damico et al. 1999). More recently it was demonstrated that intact ASLV-B particles can associate with lipid bilayers in a hydrophobic manner at neutral pH after interaction with a soluble form of TVB^{S1}(R.J.O. Barnard and J.A.T. Young, manuscript in preparation).

Together, these data suggest that receptor association with ASLV Env at neutral pH induces a conformational change in the viral glycoprotein leading to exposure of the hydrophobic fusion peptideand its subsequent insertion into the target membrane. This conclusion contrasts with those obtained from studies of all other known viral fusion proteins, because insertion of the ASLV TM fusion peptide into the target membrane appears to occur before receipt of the physiological fusion-activating trigger (i.e., low pH). Consequently, unlike Influenza A virus, which exhibits a complete loss of viral infectivity at low pH [due to premature triggering of HA and insertion of its fusion peptide into the viral membrane (Stegmann et al. 1987; Puri et al. 1990)], no such inactivation is observed with soluble receptor-loaded ASLV virions, which can remain highly infectious for several hours at 37°C (Snitkovsky and Young 1998, 2002;

Boerger et al. 1999; Mothes et al. 2000; Snitkovsky et al. 2000, 2001; Knauss and Young 2002). The relative stability of the receptor-loaded ASLV virions suggests that exposure of the ASLV TM fusion peptide, in the absence of a target membrane, could be a reversible event. As both soluble (Hernandez et al. 1997; Damico et al. 1998) and virion-associated (R.J.O. Barnard and J.A.T. Young , manuscript in preparation) forms of ASLV Env associate stably with lipid bilayers after receptor priming, it is conceivable that the target membrane may trap the transiently exposed fusion peptide state of ASLV Env, thus stabilizing the membrane-associated conformation. As all of these conformational changes are predicted to occur in the absence of the low-pH-dependent trigger for ASLV Env-mediated fusion, this model predicts that viral fusion pauses after formation of the membrane-associated form of Env before low-pH-dependent triggering.

As lipid mixing, measured by the transfer of fluorescent lipids (R-18) from labeled ASLV virions with target membranes, was observed even under conditions where low-pH-dependent cellular processes are inhibited (Gilbert et al. 1990), it is possible that after formation of the membrane-associated intermediate ASLV Env-dependent fusion could progress to a lipid mixing stage before low-pH triggering. Indeed, such pre-6HB intermediates have been isolated with inhibitory peptides, which act by inhibiting the formation of the 6HB (Melikyan 2000), that permit lipid mixing but not content mixing in HIV (Munoz-Barroso et al. 1998) and in a paramyxovirus (Joshi et al. 1998). However, it remains to be established whether the intermediates isolated in these two studies were bona fide intermediates of viral fusion. An alternative explanation for the lipid mixing observed in R-18-labeled ASLV fusion experiments is that it occurred as a result of degradation of some labeled ASLV virions during incubation of cells with lysosomotropic reagents or, alternatively, was due to a nonspecific transfer of lipids between viral and cellular membranes.

It is interesting to speculate that, after receptor-priming, ASLV Env exists in an intermediate state between the extended conformation (fusion peptideinserted in the target membrane) and the final fusogenic state (6HB). Such a model would predict that after receptor priming and membrane association incubation at low pH will trigger ASLV Env to undergo additional conformational changes that ultimately complete the fusion reaction, most likely via formation of a 6HB. Further research will be required to fully test this model. For instance, it remains to be established whether the receptor-primed, membrane-associated form of ASLV is the pH-sensitive intermediate required for low-pH triggering of ASLV Env-dependent membrane fusion. In addition, many of the intermediates proposed by this model, such as formation of the 6HB, also remain to be established. It would be interesting to definitively ascertain whether lipid mixing occurs after receptor priming, as indicated by studies with R-18-labeled ASLV virions (Gilbert et al. 1990). Once the intermediates of ASLV Env-dependent fusion are better understood, they will undoubtedly provide new insights into the molecular mechanisms of membrane fusion by other class I viral fusion proteins.

5
GATE Proteins (General Adaptors for Targeted Virus Entry)

The knowledge gained from analysis of ASLV Env-receptor interactions has allowed for the development of a new retrovirus-based viral targeting system that is based on the use of GATEs (general adaptors for targeted virus entry). GATEs are soluble proteins comprised of the extracellular domains of either the TVA or TVB receptors fused to a ligand for a cell surface receptor or instead to a single-chain antibody. These reagents serve as molecular bridges between the ASLV envelope protein contained on the surface of a retroviral vector and a cell surface protein or marker located on the surface of a desired target cell type. As described in Sect. 4.2 of the chapter by Sandrin et al., this volume, these reagents support efficient and specific entry into cell types of interest presumably because they retain the capacity to prime the wild-type ASLV Env glycoprotein for subsequent low -pH-induced activation. By contrast, it has been difficult to achieve robust viral targeting by an alternative approach involving ligand insertion directly into retroviral envelope glycoproteins (see Sects. 6.1–6.4 of the chapter by Sandrin et al.). The use of GATEs holds much promise for approaches that involve retrovirus-mediated gene delivery to specific cell types, including those associated with gene therapy protocols).

6
Conclusions

ASLV Env-receptor interactions have provided a remarkably tractable system for understanding how retroviral Env glycoproteins mediate viral entry. Since the identification of the TVA and TVB receptors, a great deal of information has been obtained on the molecular requirements for their association with ASLV Env. However, the precise molecular contacts made between each ASLV envelope glycoprotein and its cognate receptor will ultimately only be solved when the three-dimensional structures of ASLV Env-receptor complexes are elucidated. As the ASLV subgroup A–E Env proteins share a high degree of sequence homology, with the exception of the variable regions mentioned in Sect. 2, it is likely that they all share a common overall structure. Therefore, it would be especially interesting to see how each ASLV subgroup has evolved to allow for its specific interaction with the cognate receptor. In addition, as aromatic amino acid residues of both the TVA and TVB receptors are required for viral entry (Zingler and Young 1996; Knauss and Young 2002), it would be interesting to see whether these residues are oriented in the same manner in the putative receptor-binding pockets created by the hr1 and hr2 regions. If so, this would indicate a common mechanism by which the fusion potential of ASLV Env is activated after receptor association.

Studies of ASLV-receptor interactions have led to the identification of a third type of viral entry mechanism that borrows features from the two major mechanisms of viral entry involving either receptor-dependent or low-pH-dependent triggering of the viral glycoprotein. In the case of ASLV, the viral glycoprotein is "primed" by receptor contact so that it becomes competent for subsequent low-pH-dependent fusion activation. Further research is required to fully understand the underlying molecular mechanisms of this two-step model of ASLV entry. For example, it is possible that after receptor priming and Env association with the target membrane further conformational changes can occur in Env at neutral pH that lead to a stable hemifusion state. If so, the elucidation of the nature of this state would be highly informative for understanding the process of virus-cell membrane fusion as such an intermediate has not been seen before. This model also predicts that ASLV infection occurs via acidic intracellular compartments, but the identity of these compartments is not yet known. Finally, it remains to be established whether ASLV is the only virus that can utilize a receptor-primed, low-pH-dependent mode of entry. In particular, it will be interesting to discern whether the Ebola virus, which also requires low pH for infection (Takada et al. 1997; Wool-Lewis R. and Bates 1998) and contains a fusion protein with significant homology to the TM subunit of ASLV, shares some commonality with ASLV entry. To establish the precise molecular events that lead to ASLV entry will require the union of several biological disciplines such as cell biology, electrophysiology, and in vitro biochemistry.

Note to be added in proof. A recent study by Earp et al., using pyrene-labeled virions, has provided stronger evidence that ASLV can reach a lipid-mixing stage of the fusion reaction at neutral pH during infection. (Earp LJ, Delos SE, Netter RC, Bates P, White JM (2003). The Avian Retrovirus Avian Sarcoma/Leukosis Virus Subtype A Reaches the Lipid Mixing Stage of Fusion at Neutral pH. J. Virol. 77:3058–3066)

Acknowledgements. We thank Jean Yves-Sgro for his help in the preparation of Fig. 2b. We thank Sara Klucking for her critical reading of this manuscript. This work was supported by NIH Grants CA-62000 and CA-70810 (to J.A.T.Y).

References

Adkins HB, Blacklow SC, Young JAT (2001) Two functionally distinct forms of a retroviral receptor explain the nonreciprocal receptor interference among Subgroup B, D and E avian leukosis viruses. J. Virol. 75:3520–3526

Adkins HB, Brojatsch J, Naughton J, Rolls MM, Pesola JM, Young JAT (1997) Identification of a cellular receptor for subgroup E avian leukosis virus. Proc Natl Acad Sci USA 94:11617–11622

Adkins HB, Brojatsch J, Young JAT (2000) Identification and characterization of a shared TNFR-related receptor for subgroup B, D, and E Avian leukosis viruses reveal cysteine residues required specifically for subgroup E entry. J. Virol. 74:3572–3578

Albritton LM, Kim JW, Tseng L, Cunningham JM (1993) Envelope-binding domain in the cationic amino acid transporter determines the host range of ecotropic murine retroviruses. J. Virol. 67:2091–2096

Balliet J, Grendron K, Bates P (2000) Mutational analysis of the subgroup A Avian Sarcoma and Leukosis Virus putative fusion peptide domain. J. Virol. 74:3731–3739

Balliet JW, Berson J, D'Cruz CM, Huang J, Crane J, Gilbert JM, Bates P (1999) Production and characterization of a soluble, active form of TVA, the subgroup A Avian Sarcoma and leukosis virus receptor. J. Virol. 73:3054–3061

Bates P, Rong L, Varmus HE, Young JAT, Crittenden LB (1998) Genetic mapping of the cloned subgroup A Avian Sarcoma and Leukosis virus receptor gene to the TVA locus. J. Virol. 71:2505–2508

Bates P, Young JAT, Varmus HE (1993) A receptor for Subgroup A Rous Sarcoma Virus is related to the low density lipoprotein receptor. Cell 74:1043–1051

Belanger C, Zingler K, Young JAT (1995) Importance of cysteines in the LDLR-related domain of the subgroup A Avian Leukosis and Sarcoma virus receptor for viral entry. J. Virol. 69:1019–1024

Bieri S, Adkins AR, Lee HT, Winzor DJ, Smith R, Kroom PA (1998) Folding, calcium binding, and structural characterization of a concatemer of the first and second ligand-binding modules of the low-density lipoprotein receptor. Biochemistry 37:10994–11002

Blacklow SC, Kim PS (1996) Protein folding and calcium binding defects arising from familial hypercholesterolemia mutations of the LDL receptor. Nat Struct Biol 3:758–562

Boerger AL, Snitkovsky S, Young JAT (1999) Retroviral vectors preloaded with a viral receptor-ligand bridge protein are targeted to specific cell types. Proc Natl Acad Sci U S A 96:9867–9872

Bova CA, Manfredi JP, Swanstrom R (1986) The env genes of avian retroviruses: Nucleotide sequence and molecular recombinants define host range determinants. Virology 152:343–354

Bova CA, Olsen JC, Swanstrom R (1988) The avian retrovirus env gene family: Molecular analysis of host range and antigenic variants. J. Virol. 62:75–83

Bova-Hill CA, Olsen JC, Swanstrom R (1991) Genetic analysis of the Rous sarcoma virus subgroup D env gene: Mammal tropism correlates with temperature sensitivity of gp85. J. Virol. 65:2073–2080

Brojatsch J, Naughton J, Rolls MM, Zingler K, Young JAT (1996) CAR1, a TNFR-related protein, is a cellular receptor for cytopathic Avian Leukosis-Sarcoma Viruses and mediates apoptosis. Cell 87:845–855

Bron R, Wahlberg JM, Garoff H, Wilschut J (1993) Membrane fusion of Semliki Forest virus in a model system: correlation between fusion kinetics and structural changes in envelope glycoprotein. EMBO J. 12:693–701

Buchhagen DL, Hanafusa H (1978) Intracellular precursors of the major glycoprotein of avian oncoviruses in chicken embryo fibroblasts. J. Virol. 25:845–851

Bullough PA, Hughson FM, Skehel JJ, Wiley DC (1994) Structure of influenza hemagglutinin at the pH of membrane fusion. Nature 371:19–20

Cao J, Sullican N, Desjardin E, Parolin C, Robinson J, Wyatt R, Sodroski J (1997) Replication and neutralization of human Immunodeficiency virus type 1 lacking the V1 and V2 variable loops of the gp120 envelope glycoprotein. J. Virol. 71:9808–9812

Carr CM, Kim PS (1993) A spring-loaded mechanism for the conformational change of influenza hemagglutinin. Cell 73:823–32

Chambers P, Pringle CR, Easton AJ (1991) Heptad repeat sequences are located adjacent to hydrophobic regions in several types of virus fusion glycoprotein. J. Gen. Virol. 71:3075–3080

Chernomordik L, Kozlov MM, Zimmerberg J (1995) Lipids in biological membrane fusion. J Membr Biol 146:1–14

Coffin JM, Champion M, Chabot F (1978) Nucleotide sequence relationships between the genomes of an exogenous and an endogenous avian tumour virus. J. Virol. 28:972–991

Connolly L, Zingler K, Young JAT (1994) A soluble form of a receptor for Subgroup A Avian Leukosis and Sarcoma Virus (ALSV-A) blocks infection and binds directly to ALSV-A. J. Virol. 68:

Crittenden LB (1968) Observations on the nature of a genetic cellular resistance to avian tumor viruses. J Natl Cancer Inst 41:145–153

Crittenden LB, Okazaki W, Reamer R (1964) Genetic resistance to Rous sarcoma virus in embryo cell culture and embryos. Natl. Cancer Inst. Monogr. 17:161–177

Crittenden LB, Smith EJ, Weiss RA, Sarma PS (1974) Host gene control of endogenous avian leukosis virus production. Virology 57:128–138

Crittenden LB, Stone HA, Reamer RH, Okazaki W (1967) Two loci controlling genetic cellular resistance to Avian Leukosis-Sarcoma Viruses. J. Virol. 1:898–904

Damico R, Rong L, Bates P (1999) Substitutions in the receptor-binding domain of the avian sarcoma and leukosis virus envelope uncouple receptor-triggered structural rearrangements in the surface and transmembrane subunits. J. Virol. 73:3087–3094

Damico RL, J. Crane, Bates P (1998) Receptor-triggered membrane association of a model retroviral glycoprotein. Proc Natl Acad Sci U S A 95:2580–2585

Delos SE, Burdick MJ, White JM (2002) A single glycosylation site within the receptor-binding domain of the avian sarcoma/leukosis virus glycoprotein is critical for receptor binding. Virology 294:354–363

Delos SE, Gilbert JM, White JM (2000) The central prolines of an internal viral fusion peptide serves two important roles. J. Virol. 74:1686–1693

Dong JY, Dubay JW, Perez LG, Hunter E (1990) Mutations within the proteolytic cleavage site of the Rous sarcoma virus glycoprotein define a requirement for dibasic residues for intracellular cleavage. J. Virol. 66:865–74

Dorner AJ, Coffin JM (1986) Determinants for receptor interaction and cell killing on the avian retrovirus glycoprotein gp85. Cell 45:365–374

Dorner AJ, Stoye JP, Coffin JM (1985) Molecular basis of host range variation in avian retroviruses. J. Virol. 53:32–39

Durrer P, Galli C, Hoenke S, Corti C, Gluck R (1996) H^+-induced membrane insertion of influenza virus hemagglutinin Involves the HA2 amino-terminal fusion peptide but not the coiled coil region. J. Biol. Chem. 271:13417–21

Durrer P, Gaudin Y, Ruigrok RW, Graf R, Brunner J (1995) Photolabeling identifies a putative fusion domain in the envelope glycoprotein of rabies and vesicular stomatitis viruses. J. Biol. Chem. 270:17575–17581

Eckert DM, Kim PS (2001) Mechanisms of viral membrane fusion and its inhibition. Annu Rev Biochem. 70:777–810

Einfeld D, Hunter E (1988) Oligomeric structure of a prototype retrovirus glycoprotein. Proc Natl Acad Sci U S A 85:8688–92

England JM, Bolognesi DP, Dietzschold B, Halpern MB (1977) Evidence that a precursor glycoprotein is cleaved to yield the major glycoprotein of Avian Tumor Virus. J. Virol. 21:810–814

Gallaher WR (1996) Similar structural models of the transmembrane proteins of Ebola and Avian Sarcoma Virus. Cell 85:477–478

Gilbert JM, Bates P, Varmus HE, White JM (1994) The receptor for the subgroup A avian leukosis-sarcoma viruses binds to subgroup A but not to subgroup C envelope glycoprotein. J. Virol. 68:5623–5628

Gilbert JM, Hernandez LD, Balliet JW, Bates P, White JM (1995) Receptor-induced conformational changes in the subgroup A avian leukosis and sarcoma virus envelope glycoprotein. J. Virol. 69:7410–5

Gilbert JM, Mason D, White JM (1990) Fusion of Rous Sarcoma Virus with host cells does not require exposure to low pH. J. Virol. 64:5106–5113

Hanafusa H (1965) Analysis of the defectiveness of Rous Sarcoma Virus III. Determining the influence of a new helper virus on the host range and susceptibility to interference of RSV. Virology 25:248-255

Hanafusa H, Miyamoto T, Hanafusa T (1970) A cell-associated factor essential for formation of an infectious form of Rous sarcoma virus. Proc Natl Acad Sci USA 66:314-321

Hara H, Tanaka A, Kaji A (1996) Presence of a hypervariable region within the hr2 domain of the host range determining sequences of the envelope glycoprotein gp85 (SU) of subgroup-A avian sarcoma-leukosis viruses. Virus Genes 12:37-46

Hernandez LD, Peters RJ, Delos SE, Young JAT, Agard DA, White JM (1997) Activation of a retroviral membrane fusion protein: Soluble receptor-induced liposome binding of the ALSV envelope glycoprotein. J. Cell Biol. 139:1455-1464

Hernandez LD, White JM (1998) Mutational analysis of the candidate internal fusion peptide of the Avian Leukosis and Sarcoma virus subgroup A envelope glycoprotein. J. Virol. 72:3259-3267

Holmen SL, Federspiel MJ (2000) Selection of a subgroup A Avian Leukosis Virus [ALV(A)] envelope resistant to soluble ALV(A) Surface glycoprotein. Virology 273:364-373

Holmen SL, Melder DC, Federspiel MJ (2001) Identification of key residues in Subgroup A Avian Leukosis Virus envelope determining receptor binding affinity and infectivity of cells expressing chicken or quail Tva receptor. J. Virol. 75:726-737

Holmen SL, Salter DW, Payne WS, Dodgson JB, Hughes SH, Federspiel MJ (1999) Soluble forms of the subgroup A Avian Leukosis Virus [ALV(A)] receptor Tva significantly inhibit ALV(A) infection in vitro and in vivo. J. Virol. 73:10051-10060

Hunter E, Hill E, Hardwick M, Bhown A, Schwartz DE, Tizard R (1983) Complete sequence of the Rous sarcoma virus env gene: Identification of structural and functional regions of its product. J. Virol. 46:920-936

Johnson WE, Desrosiers RC (2002) Viral Persistence: HIV's strategies of immune system evasion. Annu. Rev. Med. 43:499-518

Joho RH, Billeter MA, Weissmann C (1975) Mapping of biological functions of RNA of avian tumor viruses : Location of regions required for transformation and determination of host range. Proc Natl Acad Sci U S A 73:4772-4776

Joshi SB, Dutch RE, Lamb RA (1998) A core trimer of the Paramyxovirus fusion protein: Parallels to Influenza virus hemagglutinin and HIV-1 gp-41. Virology 248:20-34

Klemenz R, Digglemann H (1978) The generation of the two envelope glycoproteins of Rous Sarcoma Virus from a common precursor polypeptide. Virology 85:63-74

Klimjack MR, Jeffery S, Kielian M (1994) Membrane and protein interactions of a soluble form of Semliki Forest virus fusion protein. J. Virol. 68:6940-6946

Klucking S, Adkins HA, Young JAT (2002) Resistance to infection by subgroups B, D, and E avian sarcoma and leukosis virus explained by a premature stop codon within a resistance allele of the tvb receptor gene. J. Virol. 76:7918-7921

Knauss DJ, Young JAT (2002) A fifteen-amino-acid TVB peptide serves as a minimal soluble receptor for Subgroup B Avian Leukosis and Sarcoma Viruses. J. Virol. 76:5404-5410

Kwong PD, Wyatt R, Robinson HL, Sweet RW, Sodroski J, Hendrickson WA (1998) Structure of an HIV gp120 envelope glycoprotein in complex with the CD4 receptor and a neutralizing human antibody. Nature 393:648–659

Lee JS, Varmus HE, Bishop JM (1979) Virus-specific messenger RNAs in permissive cells infected by Avian Sarcoma Virus. J. Biol. Chem. 254:8015–8022

Malhotra S, Scott A, Zavorotinskaya T, Albritton L (1996) Analysis of the murine ecotropic leukemia virus receptor reveals a common biochemical determinant on diverse cell surface receptors that is essential to retrovirus entry. J. Virol. 70:321–326

Melikyan GB, Brener SA, Ok DC, Cohen FS (1997) Inner but not outer membrane leaflets control the transition from glycosylphosphatidylinositol-anchored influenza hemagglutinin-induced hemifusion to full fusion. J Cell Biol 136:995–1005

Melikyan GB, R.M., Markosyan, H., Hemmati, M.K., Delmedico, D.M., Lambert, F.S., Cohen (2000) Evidence that the transition of HIV-1 gp41 into a six-helix bundle, not the bundle configuration, induces membrane fusion. J. Cell Biol. 151:413–424

Melikyan GB, White JM, Cohen FS (1995) GPI-anchored influenza hemagglutinin induces hemifusion to both red blood cell and planar bilayer membranes. J Cell Biol 131:679–91

Moebius U, Clayton L, Abraham S, Harrison S, Reinherz E (1992) The human immunodeficiency virus gp120 binding site on CD4: delineation by quantitative equilibrium and kinetic binding studies of mutants in conjunction with a high-resolution CD4 atomic structure. J. Exp. Med. 176:507–517

Moelling K, Hayami M (1977) Analysis of precursors to the envelope glycoproteins of avian RNA tumor viruses in chicken and quail cells. J. Virol. 22:598–607

Mothes W, Boerger AL, Narayan S, Cunningham JM, Young JAT (2000) Retroviral entry mediated by receptor priming and low pH triggering of an envelope glycoprotein. Cell 103:679–689

Motta JV, Crittenden LB, Pollard WO (1973) The inheritance of resistance to subgroup C leukosis-sarcoma viruses in New Hampshire chickens. Poult. Sci. 52:578–86

Munoz-Barroso I, Durell S, Sakaguchi K, Appella E, Blumenthal R (1998) Dilation of the human immunodeficiency virus-1 envelope glycoprotein fusion pore revealed by the inhibitory action of a synthetic peptide from gp31. J. Cell Biol. 140:315–323

Narayan S, Barnard RJO, Young JAT (2003) Two retroviral entry pathways distinguished by lipid raft association of the viral receptor and differences in viral infectivity. J. Virol. 77:

Payne IN, Biggs PM (1966) Genetic basis of cellular susceptibility to the Schmidt-Ruppin and Harris strains of Rous Sarcoma Virus. Virology 29:190–198

Payne LN, Biggs PM (1970) Genetic resistance of fowl to MH2 reticuloendothelioma virus. J. Gen. Virol. 7:177–85

Payne LN, Pani PK (1971) Evidence for linkage between genetic loci controlling response of fowl to subgroup A and subgroup C sarcoma viruses. J. Gen. Virol. 13:253–9

Perez LG, Hunter E (1987) Mutations within the proteolytic cleavage site of the Rous sarcoma virus glycoprotein that block processing to gp85 and gp37. J. Virol. 61:1609–14

Piranio F (1967) The mechanism of genetic resistance of chick embryo cells to infection by Rous sarcoma virus-Bryan strain (BS-SRV) Virology 32:700–707

Purchio AF, Jovanovich S, Erikson RL (1980) Sites of synthesis of viral proteins in avian sarcoma virus-infected chicken cells. J. Virol. 35:629–36

Puri A, Booy FP, Doms RW, White JM, Blumenthal R (1990) Conformational changes and fusion activity of influenza virus hemagglutinin of the H2 and H3 subtypes : effects of acid pretreatment. J. Virol. 64:3824–3832

Qiao H, Pelletier SL, Hoffman L, Hackert J, Armstrong RT, White JM (1998) Specific Single or double proline substitutions in the "spring-loaded" coiled-coil region of the influenza hemagglutinin impair or abolish membrane fusion activity. J. Cell Biol. 141:1335–47

Robinson HL, Lamoreux WF (1976) Expression of endogenous ALV antigens and susceptibility to subgroup E in three strains of chickens (endogenous C type virus) Virology 69:50–62

Rong L, Bates P (1995) Analysis of the subgroup A avian sarcoma and leukosis virus receptor: the 40-residue, cysteine rich, low density lipoprotein receptor repeat motif of Tva is sufficient to mediate viral entry. J. Virol. 69:4847–4853

Rong L, Edinger A, Bates P (1997) Role of basic residues in the subgroup-determining region of the subgroup A avian sarcoma and leukosis virus envelope in receptor binding and infection. J. Virol. 71:3458–3465

Rong L, Gendron K, Bates P (1998a) Conversion of a human low-density lipoprotein receptor ligand-binding repeat to a virus receptor: Identification of residues important for ligand specificity. Proc Natl Acad Sci USA 95:8467–8472

Rong L, Gendron K, Strohl B, Shenoy R, Wool-lewis RJ, Bates P (1998b) Characterization of determinants for envelope binding and infection in Tva, the subgroup A Avian Sarcoma and Leukosis Virus receptor. J. Virol. 72:4552–4559

Rubin H (1965) Genetic control of cellular susceptibility to pseudotypes of Rous Sarcoma Virus. Virology 26:270–276

Schneider-Schaulies J (2000) Cellular receptors for viruses: links to tropism and pathogenesis. J. Gen. Virol. 81:1413–1429

Schwarz DE, Tizard R, Gilbert W (1983) Nucleotide sequence of Rous Sarcoma Virus. Cell 32:853–869

Skehel JJ, Wiley DC (1998) Coiled coils in both intracellular vesicle and viral membrane fusion. Cell 95:871–874

Skehel JJ, Wiley DC (2000) Receptor binding and membrane fusion in virus entry: The Influenza Hemagglutinin. Annu Rev Biochem. 69:531–569

Smith EJ (1986) Endogenous Avian Leukemia Viruses. In: GF De Boer, (ed.) Vol 1. Avian Leukosis. Martinus Nijhoff Publishing, Boston, pp 101–130

Smith EJ, Brojatsch J, Naughton J, Young JAT (1998) The CAR1 gene encoding a cellular receptor specific for subgroup B and D avian leukosis viruses maps to the chicken *tvb* loci. J. Virol. 72:3501–3503

Snitkovsky S, Niederman TMJ, Carter RC, Mulligan BS, Young JAT (2000) A TVA-single-chain antibody fusion protein mediates specific targeting of a subgroup A avian leukosis virus vector to cells expressing a tumor-specific form of the epidermal growth factor receptor. J. Virol. 74:9540–9545

Snitkovsky S, Niederman TMJ, Mulligan RC, Young JAT (2001) Targeting avian leukosis virus subgroup A vectors by using a TVA-VEGF bridge protein. J. Virol. 75:1571–1575

Snitkovsky S, Young JAT (1998) Cell-specific viral targeting mediated by a soluble retroviral receptor-ligand fusion protein. Proc Natl Acad Sci U S A 95:7063–7068

Snitkovsky S, Young JAT (2002) Targeting retroviral vector infection to cells that express heregulin receptors using Tva-heregulin bridge protein. Virology 292:150–155

Stamatotos L, Cheng-Mayer C (1998) An envelope modification that renders a primary, neutralization-resistant clade B Human Immunodeficiency Virus Type 1 isolate highly susceptible to neutralization by sera from other clades. J. Virol. 72:7840–7845

Stegmann T, Booy FP, Wilschut J (1987) Effects of low pH on influenza virus. Activation and inactivation of the membrane fusion capacity of the hemagglutinin. J. Biol. Chem. 262:17744–17749

Stegmann T, Delfino JM, Richards FM, Helenius A (1991) The HA2 subunit of influenza hemagglutinin inserts into the target membrane prior to fusion. J. Biol. Chem. 266:18404–18410

Takada A, Robison C, Gotto H, Sanchez A, Murti KG, Whitt MA, Kawaoka Y (1997) A system for functional analysis of Ebola virus glycoprotein. Proc Natl Acad Sci U S A 94:14764–14769

Taplitz R, Coffin J (1997) Selection of an avian retrovirus mutant with extended receptor usage. J. Virol. 71:7814–7819

Tonelli M, Peters RJ, James TL, Agard DA (2001) The solution structure of the viral binding domain of Tva, the cellular receptor for subgroup A avian leucosis and sarcoma virus. FEBS Lett. 509:162–268

Tsichlis PN, Coffin JM (1980) Recombinants between endogenous and exogenous avian tumor viruses : Role of the C region and other portions of the genome in the control of replication and transformation. J. Virol. 33:238–249

Tsichlis PN, Conklin KF, Coffin JM (1980) Mutant and recombinant avian retroviruses with extended host range. Proc Natl Acad Sci USA 77:536–540

Tsurudome M, Gluck R, Graf R, Falchetto R, Schaller U (1992) Lipid Interactions of the hemagglutinin HA2 NH2-terminal segment during influenza virus-induced membrane fusion. J. Biol. Chem. 267:20225–32

Vogt PK (1965) A heterogeneity of Rous Sarcoma Virus revealed by selectively resistant chick embryo cells. Virology 25:237–247

Vogt PK, Fris RR (1971) An avian leukosis virus related to RSV (O): properties and evidence for helper activity. Virology 43:223–234

Vogt PK, Ishizaki R (1965) Reciprocal patterns of genetic resistance to avian tumor viruses in two lines of chickens. Virology 26:664–672

Volchkov VE, Blinov VM, Netesov SV (1992) The envelope glycoprotein of Ebola virus contains an immunosuppressive-like domain similar to oncogenic retroviruses. FEBS Lett. 305:181–184

Wahlberg JM, Bron R, Wilschut J, Garoff H (1992) Membrane fusion of Semliki Forest Virus involves homotrimers of the fusion protein. J. Virol. 66:7309–7318

Wang Q-Y, Dolmer K, Huang W, Gettins PGW, Rong L (2001) Role of calcium in protein folding and function of TVA, the receptor of subgroup A Avian Sarcoma and Leukosis Virus. J. Virol. 75:2051–2058

Wang Q-Y, Huang W, Dolmer K, Gettins PGW, Rong L (2002) Solution structure of the viral receptor domain of Tva and its implications for viral entry. J. Virol. 76:2848–2856

Weber T, Paesold G, Galli C, Mischler R, Semenza G (1994) Evidence for H^+-induced insertion of influenza hemagglutinin HA2 N- terminal segment into viral membrane. J. Biol. Chem. 269:18353–58

Weiss RA (1993) Cellular receptors and viral glycoproteins involved in retrovirus entry. In: JA Levy, (ed.) Vol 2. The Retroviridae. Plenum Press, New York, pp 1–108

Weissenhorn W, Dessen A, Calder LJ, Harrison SC, Skehel JJ, Wiley DC (1999) Structural basis for membrane fusion by enveloped viruses. Mol Membr Biol 16:3–9

Wilson C, Wardell MR, Weisgraber KH, Mahley RW, Agard DA (1991) Three-dimensional structure of the LDL receptor-binding domain of human apolipoprotein E. Science 252:1817–1822

Wool-Lewis. R., Bates P (1998) Characterization of Ebola virus entry by using pseudotyped viruses : Identification of receptor-deficient cell lines. J. Virol. 72:3155–3160

Young JAT, Bates P, Varmus HE (1993) Isolation of a chicken gene that confers susceptibility to infection by subgroup A Avian Leukosis and Sarcoma Viruses. J. Virol. 67:1811–1816

Zingler K, Belanger C, Peters RJ, Agard DA, Young JAT (1995) Identification and characterization of the viral interaction determinant of the subgroup A Avian Leukosis Virus receptor. J. Virol. 69:4261–4266

Zingler K, Young JAT (1996) Residue Trp-48 of Tva is critical for viral entry but not for high-affinity binding to the SU glycoprotein of Subgroup A Avian Leukosis and Sarcoma Virus. J. Virol. 70:7510–7516

Targeting Retroviral and Lentiviral Vectors

V. Sandrin[1] · S. J. Russell[2] · F.-L. Cosset[1]

[1] Laboratoire de Vectorologie Rétrovirale et Thérapie Génique,
  Unité de Virologie Humaine, INSERM U412, Ecole Normale Supérieure de Lyon,
  46 allée d'Italie, 69364 Lyon Cedex 07, France
  E-mail: flcosset@ens-lyon.fr
[2] Molecular Medicine Program, Guggenheim 18, Mayo Clinic, 200 First Street SW,
  Rochester, MN 55905, USA

1	Introduction	138
2	Early Events of Virus Entry: Keys for the Design of Retargeted Vectors	139
2.1	Overview of Fusion Activation of Viral Glycoproteins	140
2.2	Non-specific Factors of Virus-Cell Attachment	143
3	Exploiting the Natural Tropism of Glycoproteins from Enveloped Viruses	144
3.1	Mechanisms of Pseudotype Formation	145
3.2	Engineering of Pseudotype Formation	146
3.3	Properties of Pseudotyped Vectors	147
4	Targeting with Adaptor Molecules	148
4.1	Early Approaches	148
4.2	Fusogenic Adaptors	149
5	Engineering of Viral Glycoprotein	150
5.1	Retroviral Glycoproteins	150
5.2	Glycoproteins from Other Enveloped Viruses	151
6	Direct Targeting: Targeting by Host Range Extension	152
6.1	Concepts	152
6.2	Loss of Binding-Fusion Coupling	152
6.3	Receptor-Mediated Virus Sequestration	153
6.4	Implications for Direct Targeting Strategies	154
6.5	Direct Targeting Strategies Using pH-Dependent Viral Glycoproteins	155
7	Selective Targeting: Escorting Viral Entry	157
8	Indirect Targeting: Targeting by Host Range Restriction	159
8.1	Concepts	159
8.2	Inverse Targeting	159
8.3	Protease Targeting	161
8.4	Non-receptor-specific Blocking Domains	161

8.5 Retargeting Gene Transfer by Two-Step Targeting Strategies 162
9   Concluding Remarks. 164
9.1 Conclusions. 164
9.2 Clinical Utility of Retroviral Targeting 165

References. 166

Abstract Retroviral vectors capable of efficient in vivo gene delivery to specific target cell types or to specific locations of disease pathology would greatly facilitate many gene therapy applications. The surface glycoproteins of membrane-enveloped viruses stand among the choice candidates to control the target cell receptor recognition and host range of retroviral vectors onto which they are incorporated. This can be achieved in many ways, such as the exchange of glycoprotein by pseudotyping, their biochemical modifications, their conjugation with virus–cell bridging agents or their structural modifications. Understanding the fundamental properties of the viral glycoproteins and the molecular mechanism of virus entry into cells has been instrumental in the functional alteration of their tropism. Here we briefly review the current state of our understanding of the structure and function of viral envelope glycoproteins and we discuss the emerging targeting strategies based on retroviral and lentiviral vector systems.

1
Introduction

For a decade and a half, the gene therapy research community has been captivated by the appealing concept of a targetable, injectable vector which will seek out and transduce a particular chosen target cell population after intravenous administration. This so-far elusive dream has driven many scientists to join the rapidly growing field of retroviral vector targeting research, which we have attempted to summarize in this review article. A strong underlying theme is that the development of viable targeting strategies has been possible only in the context of parallel advances in basic scientific understanding of the molecular details of retroviral entry from initial contact between virus and target cell through specific Env receptor interactions to triggering of membrane fusion. Indeed, much of our current understanding of these processes had a direct consequence in retroviral targeting studies.

From a purely structural perspective, several Env glycoproteins have been exhaustively studied to determine their structural plasticity including their ability to tolerate amino acid deletions, insertions, extensions, substitutions and non-covalent adaptations (e.g. through the use of bi-functional cross-linking agents). The surprising conclusion of these studies is that retroviral Env glycoproteins can tolerate innumerable structural modifications, and a great deal of progress has been made in analysing the effects of these changes on virus assembly, stability, attachment and entry. Indeed, analysis of these engineered Env, and of the biology of viruses into which they are incorporated, has significantly contributed to advances in our understanding of the early steps in virus entry (e.g. adhesion, receptor engagement and fusion triggering) and how each of these steps relates to specific details of Env structure.

With respect to the goal of retargeting virus entry, naïve optimism has been replaced by a more realistic appreciation of the structural and biological factors that constrain receptor choice, and this has led to the development of realistically viable targeting strategies. Also, there is now an appreciation that retargeted viruses are usually sub-optimal in their entry efficiency, and considerable emphasis is now given to optimisation of retargeted Env. Finally, attention is now gradually shifting from the study of retargeted Env in ex vivo tissue culture systems to the more complex and challenging questions associated with in vivo studies.

2
Early Events of Virus Entry: Keys for the Design of Retargeted Vectors

Enveloped viruses penetrate the host cells by a process of fusion between the viral and cell membranes (Hunter 1997). This process is catalysed by a fusogenic activity harboured by viral surface glycoproteins. A characteristic feature of the fusion glycoproteins of many membrane-enveloped viruses is that they are synthesised as inactive precursors which undergo several post-translational modifications in order to be displayed on virions in metastable forms (Carr et al. 1997). Metastable protein conformations are energy loaded and are considered as biologically active, that is, fusion competent in the case of the viral glycoproteins, which can be activated to trigger their function. After their activation, the fusion subunits of glycoproteins from several membrane-enveloped viruses undergo a dramatic refolding of their structure and the energy released by this conformational rearrangement is thought to be necessary for the fusion process.

2.1
Overview of Fusion Activation of Viral Glycoproteins

The surface of retroviruses consists of an array of membrane-anchored glycoproteins of both cellular and viral origins. The retroviral glycoproteins are expressed as trimers of two subunits, the SU (surface) and TM (transmembrane) proteins derived from a single protein precursor. The SU subunit harbours the determinants of interaction with the cell surface receptor, whereas the functions of the TM subunit include anchorage of the trimer complex in the viral membrane and achievement of membrane fusion (Fig. 1). The retroviral TM proteins share many similarities with the fusion subunits of other enveloped viruses such as filoviruses, paramyxoviruses and orthomyxoviruses (Kobe et al. 1999). The structure of the most stable conformations of these proteins has been determined and is thought to represent the fusion-active conformation of the proteins after their fusogenicity has been activated. The C-terminal region from each TM subunit packs into grooves on the outside of the triple-stranded coiled-coil, forming a six-helix bundle with the fusion peptide and transmembrane domain of TM being positioned at the same end of the molecule. This folding therefore brings the viral

Fig. 1A, B Schematic representation of chimeric retroviral envelope glycoproteins. **A** Domain organisation of the MLV envelope glycoprotein precursor. *SP*, signal peptide. The surface subunit (*SU*, in *orange*) consists of the receptor binding domain (*RBD*), the proline-rich region (*PRR*) and the carboxy-terminal domain (*C*). The transmembrane subunit (*TM, multi-coloured*) consists of an ectodomain comprising the fusion peptide (*FP,* in *red*) and an heptad repeat region (*HR,* in *blue*) followed by a transmembrane domain (*tmd*), a cytoplasmic tail (*cyt,* in *blue*) and the R peptide. The positions of some envelope glycoprotein subdomains are shown: *VRA* and *VRB*, variable regions A and B. The *bold arrows* mark the positions of cleavage of the envelope precursor. The *red arrows* show positions of the MLV glycoprotein which accommodate insertion/substitutions of peptides and/or polypeptides. **B** Examples of retargeted glycoproteins whose host range has been modified by using (a) bifunctional protein adaptors, (b) domain substitution (e.g., RBD), (c) insertion of small ligand peptides and (d) addition of large polypeptide ligands (see text for details)

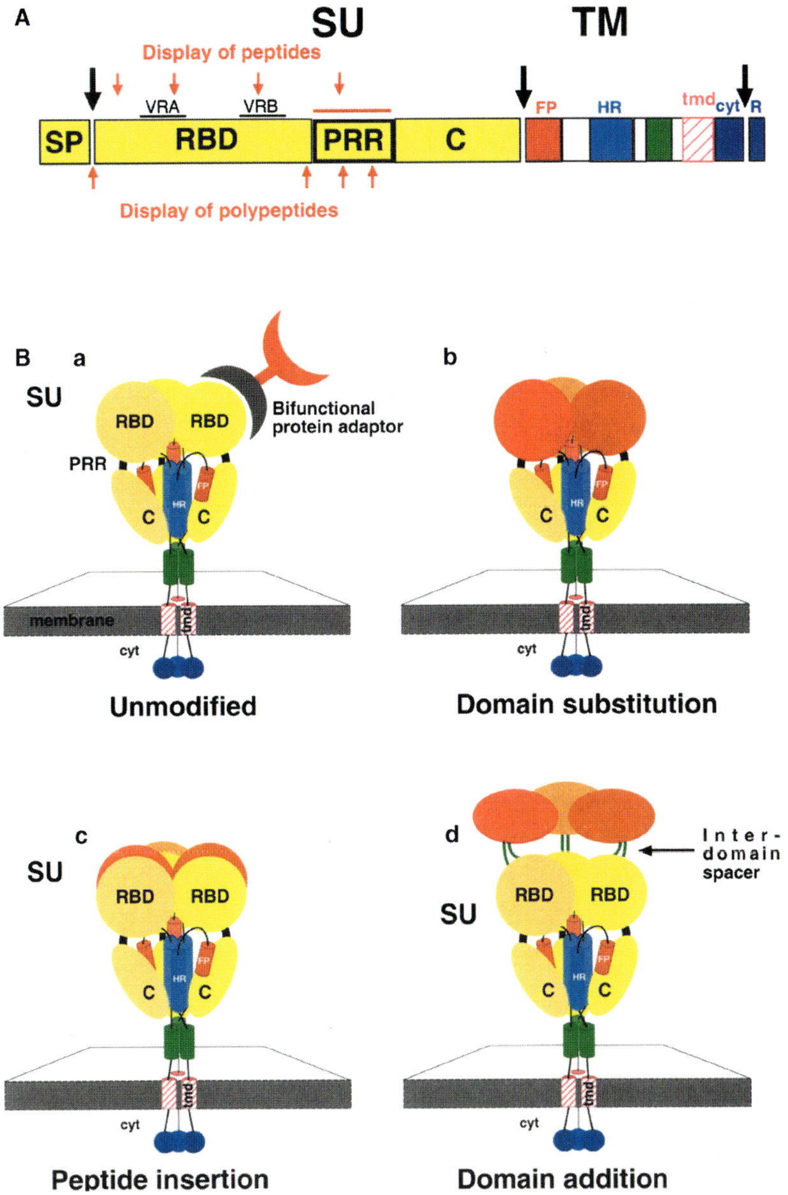

Targeting Retroviral and Lentiviral Vectors

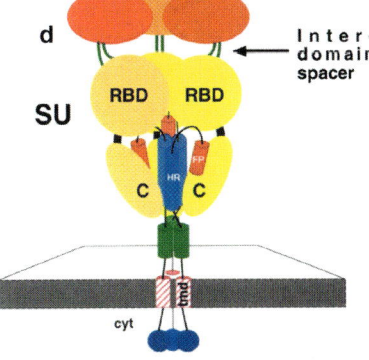

membrane close to the cell membrane and hence initiates the merging of the lipid bilayers and the formation of fusion pores.

Acquisition of metastability of the viral glycoproteins must be a highly precisely controlled process because their fusogenicity should not be activated inappropriately or prematurely, that is, before the virions have reached the target cell surface. Retroviruses have adopted several solutions in order to control acquisition and maintenance of metastability. First, Env glycoproteins are expressed as fusion-inactive protein precursors that can sequester their receptors inside cells at an early stage of their synthesis. The glycoproteins are then proteolytically matured, later in the cell secretory pathway, hence preventing untimely fusion activation (Hunter 1997). Second, interaction between subdomains of the glycoprotein maintains a fusion-inhibitory conformation (Barnett and Cunningham 2001; Lavillette et al. 1998, 2002). Additionally, the processed SU and TM Env subunits are held together via a labile disulfide bond whose isomerisation and disruption might provide more metastability to the Env complex and increased instability of the SU subunit (Pinter et al. 1997; Sanders 2000). Finally, for type C and D mammalian retroviruses, ultimate acquisition of fusion competency will only occur after virion budding and may be promoted by modification of the structure of Env complex through viral protease-mediated cleavage of the Env cytoplasmic tail (Bobkova et al. 2002; Brody et al. 1994; Ragheb and Anderson 1994; Rein et al. 1994).

The fusion process, that is, disruption of the metastable conformation, involves the activation of the viral fusion proteins and their subsequent refolding into fusion-active conformations (Hughson 1997). Two distinct pathways of fusion activation have been described. Fusogenicity of pH-dependent viruses, such as orthomyxoviruses, is activated by the acid pH found in endosomal vesicles into which the virions are routed after receptor binding (Skehel and Wiley 2000). In contrast, the fusion activation of pH-independent membrane-enveloped viruses, such as paramyxoviruses (Lamb 1993) and most retroviruses (McClure et al. 1990), is induced by interaction of their glycoproteins with their receptors and is thought to occur at neutral pH. A hybrid pathway, whereby initial receptor interaction primes the glycoprotein for subsequent low-pH triggering, has been described for retroviruses of the avian leukosis virus group (Mothes et al. 2000). The attachment subunits of the viral glycoproteins play an essential role in fusion activation as they contain residues that can activate the fusion subunits (Chen et al. 1998; Lavillette et al. 1998, 2000; Morrison 2001). For orthomyxoviruses, ionisation of residues that belong to both the attachment and fusion subunits is thought to induce the structural rearrangements of the glycoprotein (Chen et al. 1998). In contrast, activation of the fusion proteins of paramyxoviruses and retroviruses involves interactions between the attachment and fusion subunits and is necessarily coupled to receptor binding. Consistently, in addition to determinants that specify binding to the cell surface receptor, the attachment proteins from these viruses contain determinants that are involved in molecular dialogues with their respective fusion subunits. Optimal recruitment of these determinants is the key problem in targeting strategies using altered glycoproteins derived from viruses that are receptor dependent for fusion activation.

2.2
Non-specific Factors of Virus-Cell Attachment

Engineering viral tropism should not be limited to considering the role of the viral receptors and their interaction with the attachment subunits of the viral glycoproteins. Several other factors strongly influence the early events of infection. Recent studies have indicated that, despite the absence of receptors for their Env glycoproteins, retroviruses can nevertheless efficiently adsorb to the surface of adherent target cells (Abe et al. 1998; Pizzato et al. 1999, 2001; Sharma et al. 2000). The kinetics of virion attachment to the cell surface is similar in the presence and absence of specific receptor-env interaction (Pizzato et al. 1999). Such attachment is mediated by components on virus and cell surfaces which can be different from the viral Env and its cognate receptor (Fortin et al. 1997; Pizzato et al. 1999; Ugolini et al. 1999). Intercellular adhesion/communication molecules or proteins of the extra-cellular matrix, such as heparan sulfate proteoglycans, for example, play a major role in these initial steps of infection (Bounou et al. 2002; Fortin et al. 2000; Mondor et al. 1998) and perhaps are more important to mediate virus-cell attachment than the viral receptors themselves. Additionally, binding and subsequent internalisation of virions into cells lacking the viral receptor has also been described (Cosset et al. 1995; Marechal et al. 1998, 2001; Mondor et al. 1998). Moreover, under specific experimental conditions which can promote Env-independent membrane fusion, such receptor-independent virion-cell attachment may lead to efficient infection (Abe et al. 1998; Innes et al. 1990; Pizzato et al. 1999, 2001; Porter 2002; Porter et al. 1998; Sharma et al. 1997, 2000; Walker et al. 2002). Finally, for some mutant viral glycoproteins, nearly-wild-type levels of infectivity can be obtained in the absence of receptors for the viral SU (Barnett and Cunningham 2001; Lavillette et al. 2002; Wensel et al. 2003). This indicates that the most important function of the viral receptor, at least in cell culture, is not to allow attachment of the viral particles but rather to trigger fusion activation of the viral glycoprotein. A similar conclusion was also indirectly reached while characterising retroviruses coated with chimeric viral glycoproteins lacking the receptor binding domain of the SU or displaying heterologous binding domains (Barnett and Cunningham 2001; Barnett et al. 2001; Lavillette et al. 2001b; Pizzato et al. 2001; Porter 2002). Non-receptor-specific adsorption of the virus to the cell may play an important role by helping virions to reach the specific receptor and subsequently enter the cell. Therefore, because Env/receptor-independent binding precedes the recognition of the cognate receptors by virus particles, the concept of retargeting of retroviral vectors is challenged. They call into question the potential utility of modifying the viral tropism for systemic delivery. As discussed below, they stress the notion that the specific receptor-Env interactions that lead to triggering of the fusion functions of the viral Env glycoproteins, in addition to their binding properties, should be engineered in a cell type-specific manner to retarget infection. In fact, although non-specific adhesion may possibly lead to wastage of vector particles on non-target cells after inoculation in vivo, it is clear that it does not result in productive infection. Indeed, one of the best examples of a cell type-specific virus, HIV-1, is known to adhere to a variety of cell surface molecules on different non-target cells. Yet this does not prevent specific interaction and infection with the specific target cells.

3
Exploiting the Natural Tropism of Glycoproteins from Enveloped Viruses

Vectors derived from retroviruses offer particularly flexible properties in gene transfer applications given the numerous possible associations of various viral surface glycoproteins (determining cell tropism) with different types of viral cores (determining genome replication and integration) (Nègre et al. 2002). For example, association of the VSV-G glycoprotein with viral cores derived from lentiviruses results in vector pseudotypes which have broad tropism and can integrate into non-proliferating target cells (Naldini et al. 1996). Some in vivo gene transfer applications will require vectors that are targeted for specific cell entry and/or gene expression after systemic administration (Peng et al. 2001). Because of the wide distribution of its receptor, a lipid component of the plasma membrane (Seganti et al. 1986), VSV-G pseudotypes may bind to the surface of all cells encountered after inoculation before reaching the target cells. Moreover, VSV-G-pseudotyped vectors are rapidly inactivated by human serum (DePolo et al. 2000), and this might impose a limitation on the use of VSV-G as a glycoprotein to pseudotype vectors for systemic gene delivery. More selective tropisms could be achieved by taking advantage of the natural tropisms of glycoproteins from some membrane-enveloped viruses.

3.1
Mechanisms of Pseudotype Formation

Protein incorporation on retroviruses is not specific to the homologous viral glycoproteins. Over 40 host cell-derived proteins have been identified on the exterior of HIV-1 viral particles, including major histocompatibility complex class I (MHC-I) and MHC-II molecules, adhesion molecules, co-stimulation molecules and complement control proteins (Ott 1997). Additionally, many heterologous viral glycoproteins can be incorporated into retrovirus particles and mediate infectivity (Swanstrom and Wills 1997). This process—called pseudotyping—allows retroviral vectors to transduce a broader range of cells and tissues. Glycoproteins derived from most retroviruses and from many families of enveloped viruses have been found to allow pseudotype formation with retroviral and lentiviral vectors. Non-retroviral glycoproteins include those derived from vesiculoviruses (Burns et al. 1993; Naldini et al. 1996), lyssaviruses (Desmaris et al. 2001; Mochizuki et al. 1998), arenaviruses (Beyer et al. 2002; Miletic et al. 1999), hepadnaviridae (Sung and Lai 2002), paramyxoviridae (Hatziioannou et al. 2000; Kobayoshi et al. 2003; Kobinger et al. 2001; Spiegel et al. 1998), orthomyxoviruses (Dong et al. 1992; Hatziioannou et al. 1998; Sandrin et al. 2002), filoviruses (Kobinger et al. 2001; Wool-Lewis and Bates 1998), Flaviviridae (Bartosch et al. 2003) and alphaviruses (Morizono et al. 2001; Sharkey et al. 2001; Suomalainen and Garoff 1994). However, co-expression of a given glycoprotein with a heterologous viral core will not necessarily give rise to highly infectious viral particles. There are specific examples of restriction of pseudotype formation, notably between glycoproteins and viral cores derived from different retrovirus families (Christodoulopoulos and Cannon 2001; Lindemann et al. 1997; Mammano et al. 1997; Salmon et al. 2000; Sandrin et al. 2002; Schnierle et al. 1997; Stitz et al. 2000; Takeuchi et al. 1992a). Actually, functional associations between viral glycoproteins and viral cores are unpredictable, in large part because of our insufficient knowledge of the mechanisms which dictate assembly of retroviral particles. It is currently admitted that at least two types of mechanisms lead to assembly of homologous and heterologous, viral or cellular, glycoproteins on viral particles. The passive model of Env incorporation implies non-obligatory interactions between the pseudotyping glycoprotein and the viral core, provided that the former is sufficiently abundant at the site of virus budding (Pickl et al. 2001) and that its cytoplasmic tail does not bear determinants which are sterically incompatible with viral assembly or virion morphology (Swanstrom and Wills 1997). In this respect, heterologous glycoproteins harbouring short cytoplasmic tails are likely to be incorporated on lentiviral particles via a passive mechanism. On the other hand, in the active model of Env glycoprotein incorporation, interactions between the cytoplasmic tail of the pseudotyping glycoprotein and components of the virion core dictate assembly of viral particles. There is ample evidence in the literature to support the critical role of such interactions in viral assembly (reviewed in Freed 1998; Swanstrom and Wills 1997), at least for lentiviruses (Cosson 1996; Murakami and Freed 2000; Vincent et al. 1999; Wyma et al. 2000).

3.2
Engineering of Pseudotype Formation

The HIV-1 glycoprotein cannot pseudotype retroviral vectors derived from MLVs (Wilson et al. 1989). However, truncation of its long cytoplasmic tail enables pseudotype formation (Mammano et al. 1997; Schnierle et al. 1997) and allows specific gene transfer in $CD4^+$ cells (Lodge et al. 1998; Thaler and Schnierle 2001). This suggests that steric incompatibilities may prevent incorporation of the wild-type glycoproteins into retroviral particles. Likewise, the glycoproteins of type C and D mammalian retroviruses, like the GALV, the RD114 and the MPMV viruses, have been shown to harbour in their cytoplasmic tail a determinant which restricts incorporation on lentiviral cores (Christodoulopoulos and Cannon 2001; Salmon et al. 2000; Sandrin et al. 2002; Stitz et al. 2000; Takeuchi et al. 1992a). The relatively short cytoplasmic tails of type C/D mammalian retrovirus Env, about 30–40 amino acids long, harbour a 15- to 20-amino acid-long carboxy-terminal peptide—named R for MLVs—whose cleavage by the homologous viral core protease is required to activate the fusion potential of the glycoprotein (Bobkova et al. 2002; Brody et al. 1994; Ragheb and Anderson 1994; Rein et al. 1994). For pseudotype formation with homologous type C/D viral cores, lack of cleavage of the R peptide by the viral protease alters infectivity of pseudotyped virions but not Env incorporation (Brody et al. 1994; Rein et al. 1994). The cytoplasmic tail of MLV contains all the elements required for optimal pseudotyping of lentiviral cores (Christodoulopoulos and Cannon 2001; Salmon et al. 2000; Sandrin et al. 2002; Stitz et al. 2000). Based on these observations, efficient lentiviral vectors pseudotyped with chimeric glycoproteins derived from GALV and RD114 have been generated. These mutant Env harbour the cytoplasmic tail of the MLV-A Env whose cleavage site is compatible with the lentiviral proteases (Christodoulopoulos and Cannon 2001; Salmon et al. 2000; Sandrin et al. 2002; Stitz et al. 2000). It is likely because of its features that they are efficiently incorporated on lentiviral particles. The resulting chimeric glycoproteins preserve the host range of the initial glycoproteins and confer 25-fold-increased titres to lentiviral vectors.

3.3
Properties of Pseudotyped Vectors

There is considerable interest in exploring the properties of retroviral vectors pseudotyped with heterologous viral glycoproteins. This parameter is likely to modulate the physico-chemical properties of the vectors, their interaction with the host immune system and their host range. Importantly, vector pseudotypes might not always retain the host range of the parental viruses from which the pseudotyping glycoproteins were derived. For example, although the glycoprotein of the Mokola virus, a neurotropic lyssavirus, efficiently pseudotypes HIV-1 vectors (Mochizuki et al. 1998), the pseudotyped vectors do not reproduce the specific neurotropism of the parental virus (Desmaris et al. 2001). Nevertheless, even though the only case of a viral glycoprotein directing virus infection to a specific cell type is that of HIV-1 (Lodge et al. 1998; Thaler and Schnierle

2001), several studies have shown that the transduction efficiency of a given target cell type is directly dependent on the type of glycoprotein used to coat retroviral vectors. For instance, the use of surface glycoproteins derived from viruses which cause lung infection and infect via the airway epithelia, like Ebola virus or influenza virus, may prove useful for gene therapy of the human airway (Kobinger et al. 2001). There are many examples of preferential transduction of particular cell types. A recent study of lentiviral vectors pseudotyped with glycoproteins derived from a set of enveloped viruses indicated that exclusive transduction of retinal pigmented epithelium could be obtained after subretinal inoculations of some vector pseudotypes in rat eyes (Duisit et al. 2002). Lentiviral vectors pseudotyped with the glycoproteins from Ross River virus show superiority over vectors pseudotyped with VSV-G for in vivo gene delivery to the liver of mice (Kang et al. 2002). Likewise, screening of a large panel of pseudotyped vectors established the superiority of the GALV and RD114 glycoproteins for transduction of progenitor and differentiated haematopoietic cells (Hanawa et al. 2002; Kelly et al. 2000; Marandin et al. 1998; Movassagh et al. 1998; Porter et al. 1996; Sandrin et al. 2002). Finally, owing to the capacity of the influenza virus, Sindbis virus, MLV and GALV glycoproteins, among others, to pseudotype MLV and lentiviral vectors (Morizono et al. 2001; Nègre et al. 2000; Sandrin et al. 2002), several approaches can be undertaken to modify their tropism in order to modify the host range of vectors (see below).

4
Targeting with Adaptor Molecules

4.1
Early Approaches

Retroviruses recognise a relatively limited number of cell surface proteins as entry receptors (Overbaugh et al. 2001). Several retroviral glycoproteins (e.g. those of ecotropic MLV strains) do not recognise a receptor on human cells. Therefore, initial attempts to retarget retroviral tropism have consisted in cross-linking ecotropic vector particles and target cell surface molecules by using, for example, ligand-conjugated antibodies against the viral glycoprotein. The earliest experiments to test this approach employed a streptavidin bridging approach in which viruses were coated with biotinylated antibodies against the retroviral envelope (Etienne-Julan et al. 1992; Goud et al. 1988; Roux et al. 1989). Cells were coated with receptor-specific biotinylated antibodies (or ligands), and the streptavidin was used to cross-link the virus and cell-associated antibodies. With this relatively crude molecular bridging strategy, ecotropic retroviruses could be retargeted to human cells. Transduction of the targeted cells was very inefficient, and some of the cell surface molecules that were targeted could not function as surrogate receptors for the ecotropic vectors (Etienne-Julan et al. 1992; Roux et al. 1989).

4.2
Fusogenic Adaptors

Despite the relative inefficiency of these early results, interest in these strategies was recently revived with the development of more sophisticated adaptor molecules which can simultaneously retarget virion binding and trigger conformational changes in the glycoprotein of retroviruses which belong to the group of avian leukosis viruses (ALVs) (Snitkovsky and Young 1998). Such "intelligent" protein adaptors consist of recombinant polypeptides in which ligands are fused to soluble forms of the receptors for ALVs, which are single-spanning transmembrane molecules (Overbaugh et al. 2001). Thus these bifunctional bridge proteins bind virions to specific cell surface molecules and the retroviral receptor moiety activates viral entry into target cells. Proof of principle for this elegant targeting strategy, which does not require molecular engineering of the viral glycoprotein, has been established in vitro for adaptor molecules which carry EGF receptor binding determinants such as the EGF itself or an anti-EGF receptor single-chain antibody (Snitkovsky et al. 2000). Other cell surface receptors targeted with such adaptor molecules include the vascular endothelium growth factor and the heregulin receptor (Snitkovsky et al. 2001; Snitkovsky and Young 2002). The bridge proteins could be either pre-loaded on target cells before gene transfer or, interestingly, pre-loaded on ALV vector particles (Boerger et al. 1999). Thus the rather restricted host range of these avian retroviral vectors could be expanded to mammalian cells.

5
Engineering of Viral Glycoprotein

5.1
Retroviral Glycoproteins

Retroviral envelope glycoproteins can tolerate a variety of genetically encoded modifications. Initial attempts to engineer retroviral tropism consisted of the insertion of various ligand types, namely, growth factors, hormones, peptides or single-chain antibodies, in several locations on the viral surface glycoproteins so as to modify their host range by allowing them to bind human cell surface molecules different from the parent virus receptor. In some cases (Battini et al. 1998; Lorimer and Lavictoire 2000), the choice for insertion of heterologous polypeptides was rationalised by the structural information available for the MLV receptor binding domain (Fass et al. 1997; Linder et al. 1992, 1994). In most cases however, positions for polypeptide display were determined empirically, sometimes after screening for a large pool of insertion mutants of the MLV glycoprotein (Rothenberg et al. 2001). Examples of insertion sites in type C mammalian retrovirus glycoproteins—mainly the ecotropic and amphotropic MLV glycoproteins—which have been characterised and found to be functional, at least for retargeted binding, are shown in Fig. 1A. They include modifications of the glycoprotein such as (a) domain replacement (Barnett et al. 1999, 2001; Han et al. 1995; Kasahara et al. 1994; Matano et al. 1995), (b) peptide insertion in pre-folded domains (Ager et al. 1996; Battini et al. 1998; Bupp and Roth 2002; Gollan and Green 2002ab; Gordon et al. 2001a; Hall et al. 1997, 2000; Liu et al. 2000; Rothenberg et al. 2001; Valsesia-Wittmann et al. 1994; Wu et al. 1998, 2000) and (c) display of polypeptides as additional folded domains (Ager et al. 1996; Benedict et al. 1999; Buchholz et al. 1998; Chadwick et al. 1999; Chowdhury et al. 2002; Cosset et al. 1995; Erlwein et al. 2003, 2002; Fielding et al. 1998, 2000; Katane et al. 2002; Kayman et al. 1999; Khare et al. 2001; Konishi et al. 1998; Lorimer and Lavictoire 2000; Marin et al. 1996; Martin et al. 1998, 1999, 2002; Maurice et al. 1999, 2002; Merten et al. 2003; Morling et al. 1997; Nilson et al. 1996; Peng et al. 1997, 1999, 1998, 2001; Russell et al. 1993; Somia et al. 1995; Valsesia-Wittmann et al. 1996, 1997, 2001; Yajima et al. 1998; Zhao et al. 1999). Also, protease cleavage sites can be engineered into the anchoring linkers of N-terminally displayed polypeptides so that they can later be cleaved from the surface of the vector particles (Buchholz et al. 1998; Nilson et al. 1996; Peng et al. 1997) (Fig. 1).

Many of these chimeric glycoproteins fold correctly, are stably incorporated on virions, are susceptible to cleavage of the inserted protease substrate and allow efficient retargeted virion binding to the expected cell surface molecules. Large, foreign polypeptides have also been fused directly to all or part of TM (Chu and Dornburg 1995; Chu et al. 1994; Engelstadter et al. 2000; Jiang et al. 1998; Matano et al. 1995; Nguyen et al. 1998). However, for most N-terminally substituted chimeric envelope glycoproteins which have been studied to date, the efficiency of viral incorporation has been low, or undetected, possibly as a consequence of suboptimal folding, assembly or transport to the cell surface. Co-expression of such chimeras with unmodified glycoproteins appears to enhance their incorporation (Chu et al. 1994; Kasahara et al. 1994; Matano et al. 1995), suggesting that they need to be chaperoned for correct processing, transport to the cell surface and incorporation into vector particles as hetero oligomeric complexes.

5.2
Glycoproteins from Other Enveloped Viruses

As discussed above, retroviruses can be pseudotyped with several non-retroviral glycoproteins. Functional display of polypeptides in such glycoproteins has been established for the E2 surface glycoprotein of Sindbis virus (Morizono et al. 2001; Ohno et al. 1997) and for the influenza virus HA glycoprotein (haemagglutinin) (Hatziioannou et al. 1999; Patterson et al. 1999). Recombinant HA or E2 glycoproteins which displayed the polypeptides were correctly expressed and processed and stably incorporated on retroviral particles and could specifically retarget the binding of the virions (Hatziioannou et al. 1999; Morizono et al. 2001), indicating that insertion of large polypeptides did not alter the conformation of the chimeras.

6
Direct Targeting: Targeting by Host Range Extension

6.1
Concepts

Retroviral particles incorporating a number of different types of polypeptides capable of binding to a wide range of cell surface molecules have now been characterised. Direct targeting strategies rely on the simple idea that fusion activation of the chimeric envelope should be triggered by the interaction of the displayed ligand and the targeted cell surface molecule. In practise, this concept has met with limited success. Although the great majority of ligand-displaying envelope glycoproteins could specifically and efficiently bind the targeted cells, the infectivity of the corresponding viral particles was generally very poor, if not non-existent. Maximal infectious titres of 3,000 i.p./ml have been reported for the most successful approaches, namely, 4 logs lower than those obtained with wild-type glycoproteins. Such a low infectivity of retargeted retroviral vectors will clearly not be sufficient for most gene transfer applications. The poor infectivity of vectors for targeting by host range extension was due to two general properties of retargeted retroviral glycoproteins and their receptors: (a) their inability to induce membrane fusion and subsequent penetration of the viral core in the cytosol and (b) the sequestration of the targeted receptor-bound retroviral particles by some types of cell surface molecules, even when the target cells express the retroviral receptor.

6.2
Loss of Binding-Fusion Coupling

It is not always possible to predict the effect of the displayed polypeptides on the basic functions of the backbone envelope glycoprotein. Some ligands may affect the folding of the chimeric glycoprotein, transportation to the cell surface, its viral incorporation and its fusogenicity. However, even when the functionality of the binding and fusion domains of the chimeric glycoprotein has been optimised, by using interdomain spacers, for example (Ager et al. 1996; Valsesia-Wittmann et al. 1996, 1997), such retroviral vectors still give very low titres on target cells which only express the targeted cell surface molecules. In fact, lack of retargeted infection is not necessarily due to inactivation of the fusion machinery of the chimeric glycoproteins themselves, because several of these chimeras are fully functional for achieving membrane fusion, once they are allowed to bind cells expressing the natural retroviral receptors (Cosset et al. 1995). This confirms that, although the fusogenic potential of chimeric glycoproteins incorporated on the viral particles is intact, in the absence of the retroviral receptor the interaction of the displayed ligand with the targeted cell surface molecule is generally not able to activate the fusion functions of the chimeras. Infectivity of the recombinant retroviruses is therefore inhibited at a post-binding block (Benedict et al. 1999; Zhao et al. 1999). Thus the poor fusion activity of chimeric glycoproteins is attributed to the loss of coupling between retargeted binding and fusion activation. Closer examination of the molecular mechanism that couples binding to the natural retroviral receptors to fusion activation have in fact revealed the very sophisticated solution adopted by retroviruses to co-ordinate these two functions. As discussed above, this coupling involves complex inter-relations between the different subdomains of the glycoprotein complex (Barnett and Cunningham 2001; Barnett et al. 2001; Lavillette et al. 1998, 2000, 2001a, 2002; Zhao et al. 1997). Attempts to reconstitute this coupling via the interaction of a non-viral target receptor to a non-viral ligand have so far been unsuccessful, even with insertion into a fusion-competent retroviral glycoprotein (Russell and Cosset 1999).

6.3
Receptor-Mediated Virus Sequestration

The second essential feature of many targeted cell surface molecules is their ability to abolish infection, even when the retroviral receptor is present at the surface of targeted cells. For example, amphotropic retroviral envelope glycoproteins which display EGF have greatly impaired infectivity in human cells which express both EGF receptors and amphotropic receptors (Cosset et al. 1995; Nilson et al. 1996). Inhibition of infectivity is specifically caused by the interaction with the high-affinity EGF receptor, because competition with soluble EGF can restore infectivity via the amphotropic receptor. What allows some cell surface molecules to induce competitive virus sequestration is currently not known, although all tyrosine kinase receptors tested to date as targeted receptors induce competitive sequestration of bound viral particles, thus resulting in abrogation of their infectivity. Presumably, such receptors can sequester and/or traffic bound retroviruses to cell compartments which are not compatible with interaction with the amphotropic receptors. In the case of the EGF receptor, the EGF-displaying retroviral particles might mimic the natural ligand of this receptor and induce receptor dimerisation, endocytosis through clathrin-coated pits, a pathway which is not naturally adopted by MLVs (Lee et al. 1999), and, ultimately, routing to the lysosome. Treatment of target cells with chloroquine, an inhibitor of lysosomal degradation, yielded up to 100-fold increase of infectivity. Interestingly EGF-displaying retroviral vectors also fail to infect cells engineered to express mutant EGF receptors, lacking the cytoplasmic tail or the endocytosis signals, which are therefore unable to actively traffic receptor-bound particles to the degradation compartment (Cosset et al. 1995; Hatziioannou et al. 1998). Although such mutant receptors seem less potent to induce virus sequestration, it is possible that molecular events which precede active ligand-mediated endocytosis, for example, receptor dimerisation, may be responsible for such an effect.

6.4
Implications for Direct Targeting Strategies

There is obviously an additive effect between these two phenomena, that is, inability of targeted receptors to activate envelope fusogenicity and virus sequestration. >From a fundamental perspective, this strongly suggests that retroviruses have evolved and adapted to specific cell surface molecules to use them as entry ports not only because the latter can bind the viral particles but, above all, because they may exhibit specific determinants or may trigger essential cellular functions which allow both activation of envelope fusogenicity and cell entry on virus binding (Rodrigues and Heard 1999). It is anticipated that very few cell surface molecules may be able to exhibit the particular properties of retroviral receptors, as reflected both by the prominent number of targeted cell surface molecules which failed to allow retargeted virus entry and by the related topology and function of retroviral receptors for a given family of retroviruses (i.e. multitransmembrane symporters for type C mammalian retroviruses) (Overbaugh et al. 2001). More practically these two central issues have raised serious doubts as far as the ultimate goal of efficient retargeted gene delivery is concerned. A first question is related to the development of direct targeting strategies, that is, when the target cells do not express the retroviral receptor recognised by the backbone retroviral envelope and, therefore, when only the interaction between the displayed ligand and the targeted cell surface molecule should activate the fusogenicity of the envelope chimera. A second question concerns the possibility of circumventing the inability of most cell surface molecules to act as retroviral receptors and to develop targeting strategies that exploit—conditionally—retroviral receptors in a concomitant manner to assist retrovirus entry.

6.5
Direct Targeting Strategies Using pH-Dependent Viral Glycoproteins

The very specific fusion activation mechanism of retroviral glycoproteins precludes the development of direct targeting strategies using glycoproteins which are receptor dependent for fusion. In contrast, the ability of the glycoproteins of some membrane-enveloped viruses to fuse in low-pH endosomes associated with the high turnover rate of most cell surface molecules provides an alternative basis for targeting strategies. Examples of glycoproteins which use a pH-dependent fusion activation pathway, which are efficiently assembled on retroviral particles and which can be engineered for ligand-display are the E2 glycoprotein derived from Sindbis virus and the haemagglutinin (HA) of influenza virus (see above). The fusion mechanism of these glycoproteins has been extensively studied and does not appear to depend primarily on binding to their ubiquitous receptors (sialic acid for HA and laminin or heparan sulfate glycosaminoglycan for the Sindbis virus E2 glycoprotein) (Skehel and Wiley 2000; Smit et al. 1999). In fact, the activation of the fusion functions of these viral glycoproteins is achieved through acidification in the endosomes where the virions have been trafficked after binding to their receptors. Thus the physiologic signals that trigger the membrane fusion properties of these pH-dependent glycoproteins are much less specific than those of retroviral envelope glycoproteins and can activate their fusogenicity independently of their binding to receptors. Indeed, co-expression of fusion-defective MLV-based retargeted envelope glycoproteins with wild-type HA or with HAs which bear mutations that prevent sialic acid binding were shown to stimulate gene delivery in target cells (Hatziioannou et al. 1998; Lin et al. 2001). Therefore it is expected that, in contrast to retroviral envelope glycoproteins, the engineering of their host range via the insertion of ligands on these proteins is less likely to interfere with their fusion trigger.

As discussed above, several ligand types have been functionally displayed on HA or E2 glycoproteins, either as amino-terminal extensions of HA or by insertion into the HA or E2 structures themselves (Hatziioannou et al. 1999; Morizono et al. 2001; Patterson et al. 1999). As expected from the rather non-specific fusion-triggering properties of HA, virions generated with the HA chimeric glycoproteins had wild-type fusion activity when used to infect cells expressing the target surface molecules. Interestingly, in sharp contrast to retroviral chimeras, none of the targeted receptors abolished infectivity of retroviral vectors loaded with the HA chimeras on target receptor-positive cells. Retroviruses generated with EGF-HA chimeras were infectious on EGF receptor-positive cells and had titres similar to those of retroviral particles carrying wild-type HA proteins (Hatziioannou et al. 1999), consistent with the common endocytosis and trafficking properties of both molecules. The lack of receptor sequestration for retroviruses coated with chimeric HA glycoproteins is therefore very promising for the development of targeting strategies because it is anticipated that most retroviral chimeric glycoproteins fused to growth factors (Chadwick et al. 1999; Cosset et al. 1995; Fielding et al. 1998), or even to some single-chain antibodies (Benedict et al. 1999; Maurice et al. 2002; Pizzato et al. 2001; Zhao et al. 1999), will lead to virus sequestration. Moreover, the host range of retroviral vector particles coated with chimeric HA or E2 proteins could be selectively re-addressed to cells expressing the expected target cell surface molecules (Hatziioannou et al. 1999; Morizono et al. 2001; Patterson et al. 1999). Many types of receptor candidates for targeting can re-cycle from the cell surface and traffic into low-pH endosome (Mukherjee et al. 1997; Schwartz 1995). Therefore, it is likely that the fusogenicity of the pH-dependent chimeric glycoproteins bound to various targeted cell surface molecules will be activated during endocytosis and trafficking inside the cell, even if these chimeras are not attached to their wild-type receptors. In particular, an IgG-binding domain of protein A (domain ZZ), derived from *Staphylococcus aureus*, was inserted in the HA or E2 glycoproteins. Gene delivery by retroviral vectors carrying the chimeric glycoprotein could be retargeted in the presence of specific antibodies against the target cell surface molecules (Hatziioannou et al. 1999; Morizono et al. 2001). As both proteins can efficiently pseudotype primate lentiviral vectors (Christodoulopoulos and Cannon 2001;

Morizono et al. 2001; Sandrin et al. 2002), these results open the way to numerous in vivo applications in gene transfer areas.

7
Selective Targeting: Escorting Viral Entry

As discussed above, the signals which trigger fusion activation of the retroviral glycoproteins reside in intrinsic properties of the retroviral receptor. Therefore, it is anticipated that direct targeting strategies will not lead to useful retargeted retroviral vectors unless it is possible to (re)couple retargeted binding and activation of the envelope fusion machinery. Mutations that lower the activation threshold of envelope fusogenicity and thus facilitate the conversion of the pre-fusogenic native conformation of the retroviral envelope to its fusion active form (Fig. 1) have been characterised for different retroviral envelope glycoproteins in the SU (Lavillette et al. 1998, 2002) or in the TM (Reeves and Schulz 1997). The introduction of the former mutations into some chimeric envelope glycoproteins may enhance gene delivery by direct targeting. Other strategies have been explored to overcome the loss of binding-to-fusion coupling imposed by the stringent fusion properties of retroviral glycoproteins. Some of these approaches have consisted of the display of high-affinity ligands on glycoproteins which themselves recognise an ubiquitously expressed receptor, so as to exploit interaction between this receptor and the chimeric glycoprotein to assist viral entry. In essence, such approaches cannot give rise to highly specific targeting because cells lacking the targeted cell surface molecule should also be transduced because of the broad distribution of the (auxiliary) viral receptor. Strictly speaking, these strategies are called 'selective' targeting and they lead to preferential infection of target cells among other cell types. Several polypeptides have been displayed on retroviral glycoproteins which naturally recognise a receptor on the target cells (e.g. the amphotropic MLV glycoprotein). Thus, after a phase of interaction with the targeted cell surface molecule which, as discussed above, cannot activate fusion, cellular entry of retroviral vectors carrying such chimeric glycoproteins ultimately relies on the interaction with the natural retroviral receptor, which permits efficient membrane fusion. One such strategy consists of the inclusion of binding motifs on the amphotropic viral glycoprotein itself, in locations that do not affect their ability to promote binding to the natural receptor and subsequent membrane fusion (Fig. 1). Incorporation of a single-chain antibody against a melanoma antigen (HMWMAA) at the amino terminus of the amphotropic MLV glycoprotein resulted in preferential infection of HMWMAA-positive cells over HMWMAA-negative cells (Martin et al. 1998). Alternatively, the co-expression along with the wild-type glycoprotein of a second 'escorting' glycoprotein, which carries cell-specific binding determinants and which is usually defective for fusion, also permits the tethering of virion binding to tissues which abundantly express the target molecules. Recent examples of vector-escorting strategies focused on the incorporation on amphotropic MLV vector particles of matrix-targeting motifs (i.e. collagen binding peptides). This was shown to enhance retrovirus binding and transduction of human endothelial cells in vitro (Hall et al. 1997, 2000; Liu et al. 2000). Interestingly, such vectors could localise gene delivery to sites of vascular injury in vivo in rats (Gordon et al. 2001b; Hall et al. 2000) and in the angiogenic tumor vasculature in human cancer xenografts in nude mice (Gordon et al. 2001a).

Such a 'preferential' targeting cannot be highly specific in essence, and further experiments of vector bio-distribution will teach whether the increase of affinity, achieved through the addition of binding motifs, can be sufficient to consider non-significant the leak of infectivity to non-target cells. Nevertheless, in the case of vectors derived from the avian spleen necrosis virus (SNV), a more specific targeting can be envisaged through a similar approach (Chu and Dornburg 1995; Chu et al. 1994; Engelstadter et al. 2000, 2001; Jiang et al. 1998; Jiang and Dornburg 1999). Indeed, although SNV and simian D-type viruses belong to the same receptor interference group and appear to use the same receptor molecule (Overbaugh et al. 2001), the human allele of this receptor cannot mediate SNV entry into human cells, presumably because of its low affinity with the SNV glycoprotein (Engelstadter et al. 2000; Gautier et al. 1999; Jiang et al. 1998). However, in the context of cell surface-tethered virions that display both a wild-type glycoprotein and a chimeric glycoprotein with an engineered high-affinity binding motif, it is likely that the SNV glycoprotein could interact with the human receptor and may thus promote membrane fusion in a rather restricted manner (Engelstadter et al. 2000; Jiang and Dornburg 1999).

8
Indirect Targeting: Targeting by Host Range Restriction

8.1
Concepts

The retroviral vectors which are currently used for human clinical gene therapy applications can infect human target cells promiscuously. Strategies to restrict the host range properties of these vectors, focusing their infectivity on particular subsets of human target cells, are therefore being developed. The basis for host range restriction is the selective introduction of modifications into the retroviral envelope glycoproteins which destroy their ability to infect non-target cells. One important advantage of targeting by host range restriction is that because the natural virus entry pathway is exploited, fusion activation of the chimeric glycoproteins is more readily achieved. In addition, there potentially are safety advantages with this approach. Because the host range properties of the modified envelope are not expanded, there is no risk of generating a more highly pathogenic strain of the virus from which the vector is derived. Likewise, because infectivity is restricted to specific cell types, spreading of the vector particle is reduced.

At this point in time, two strategies have been developed for targeting retroviral vectors by host range restriction: inverse targeting and protease targeting. Inverse targeting involves the selective inhibition of infectivity on cells expressing the targeted receptor, whereas protease targeting involves the global suppression of infectivity with its selective reactivation on cells expressing a targeted protease.

8.2
Inverse Targeting

Several ligands displayed at the N-terminus of C-type retroviral envelope glycoproteins have been shown to inhibit infectivity on cells expressing the targeted receptor (Chadwick et al. 1999; Cosset et al. 1995; Fielding et al. 1998, 2000; Nilson et al. 1996). The original observation was that amphotropic vectors displaying EGF could efficiently bind to EGF receptor-positive target cells but could not infect them (Cosset et al. 1995). In contrast, these vectors could efficiently infect EGF receptor-negative target cells through the natural virus entry pathway. Thus interaction between the EGF-displaying vector and EGF receptors on the target cell led to specific neutralisation of virus infectivity. This phenomenon has been named 'receptor-mediated sequestration'. Sequestration has subsequently been observed for vectors displaying stem cell factor (SCF) (Fielding et al. 1998, 2000) or insulin-like growth factor (IGF-1) (Chadwick et al. 1999; Fielding et al. 2000) or displaying single-chain antibodies against EGF receptor CD33 (Zhao et al. 1999), the lymphocyte surface antigen CDw-52 and other tyrosine kinase or non-tyrosine kinase receptors (unpublished data). In-depth analysis of the sequestration of vectors displaying EGF or IGF-1 revealed that the efficiency of sequestration is dependent on the relative densities of two different receptor types on the target cell surface as well as on intrinsic biological properties of the receptors, such as their kinetics of internalisation (Chadwick et al. 1999). Thus high densities or rapid ligand-mediated internalisation of the targeted receptors leads to more efficient sequestration and reduction in virus titre, whereas high densities of the natural virus receptor or slow endocytosis of the targeted receptor leads to higher levels of infectivity. It appears that there is competition between these two receptor types (i.e. targeted receptor or viral receptor) for capture of virus particles which approach the cell surface. Those attaching to the natural virus receptors are able subsequently to mediate infection, whereas those attaching to the targeted receptors are neutralised, possibly as a consequence of rapid endocytosis and degradation in lysosomes.

Inverse targeting is the targeting strategy which exploits receptor-mediated virus neutralisation (Fielding et al. 1998). Thus retroviral vectors displaying EGF or SCF were shown to efficiently discriminate between haematopoietic and non-haematopoietic cell populations in tissue culture. The EGF-displaying vectors could efficiently infect EGF receptor-negative haematopoietic cells but were non-infectious for EGF receptor-positive epithelial carcinoma cells. Conversely, the SCF-displaying vectors failed to infect c-kit-positive haematopoietic cells but efficiently infected c-kit-negative epithelial carcinoma cells. Inverse targeting therefore has potential utility for the selective transduction of haematopoietic cells with therapeutic transgenes which confer resistance to cytotoxic drug therapy. The value of inverse targeting in this situation is that it can be used to minimise the risk of inadvertent transduction of contaminating cancer cells which express abundant EGF receptors.

The bio-distribution in vivo of inversely targeted vectors has been addressed after systemic inoculation in the tail vein of mice (Peng et al.

2001). Intravenous inoculation of non-targeted lentiviral vectors, carrying wild-type glycoproteins, leads to maximal reporter gene activity in liver and spleen with moderate or minimal expression in heart, skeletal muscle, lung, brain, kidney, ovaries and bone marrow. In contrast, EGF-displaying vectors inoculated intravenously are expressed maximally in spleen with very low-level expression detectable in EGF receptor-rich liver cells. Liver transduction by the EGF-displaying vector can be restored by pre-treating the animals with soluble EGF, suggesting that these vectors are inversely targeted to spleen cells.

8.3
Protease Targeting

On a parallel path, by capitalising on the sequestration properties of some cell surface molecules expressed on target cells, a specific gene delivery can also be envisaged (Chadwick et al. 1999; Martin et al. 1999, 2002; Peng et al. 1997, 1998, 1999). This depends on the definition of a molecular device which allows the virions to escape the sequestering receptor. This can be achieved by inserting, between the displayed virion-sequestrating ligand and the viral glycoprotein, peptide substrates cleaved by cell surface specific proteases (Fig. 1B). Infection therefore proceeds in two steps: in step one, the vector attaches to the cells via the displayed binding domain. In step two, the protease-sensitive linker which anchors the binding domain to the viral glycoprotein is cleaved by a specific protease. The underlying glycoprotein is then exposed and can subsequently interact with the natural viral receptor on the target cell and promote virus entry (Nilson et al. 1996). For example, EGF-displaying amphotropic retroviruses carrying a matrix metalloprotease (MMP) cleavage site could preferentially infect EGF receptor-positive MMP-rich target cells in vitro (Peng et al. 1997) and, moreover, could discriminate between MMP-rich and MMP-poor tumour xenografts implanted into nude mice (Peng et al. 1999).

8.4
Non-receptor-specific Blocking Domains

Although high-affinity ligands which lead to viral sequestration have been used for proof of principle studies (Nilson et al. 1996), they are not ideal for protease targeting because they only block virus infectivity on receptor-positive target cells (Chadwick et al. 1999; Cosset et al. 1995). Masking of the retroviral envelope functions can also be achieved in a very different and more general manner by using non-receptor-specific blocking domains such as, for example, trimerising cleavable (poly)peptides (Morling et al. 1997) or, alternatively, proline-rich spacers (Martin et al. 2003; Valsesia-Wittmann 2001; Valsesia-Wittmann et al. 1997). Such polypeptides can block infection in a way which is independent of the variable inclination of some displayed ligands to induce receptor-mediated virus sequestration. Binding assays have shown that these displayed homotrimers are able to block the interaction between the chimeric glycoprotein and the viral receptor, and it is assumed that the displayed trimerising polypeptides form a homotrimeric cap at the tip of the glycoprotein to which they are grafted, thereby masking its receptor binding sites. Relief of the block in infection can be achieved by inserting, between such virus entry-blocking domains and the viral glycoprotein, a protease cleavage site for which a—specific—cell surface protease is expressed on target cells (Morling et al. 1997). For example, display of homotrimeric leucine zipper peptides and globular domains which are capable of forming homotrimeric interactions, such as tumour necrosis factor or the trimerising extracellular domain of CD40 ligand (amino acids 116 to 261), on the amphotropic MLV glycoprotein, prevents infection (Morling et al. 1997). Full restoration of infectivity can be obtained after factor Xa protease treatment of the vectors, which display a factor Xa cleavage site after the trimerising blocking domains (Morling et al. 1997).

8.5
Retargeting Gene Transfer by Two-Step Targeting Strategies

The potential utility of the approach was subsequently demonstrated by generating vectors displaying chimeric glycoproteins which could be cleaved and activated by the plasminogen activator/plasmin system (Peng et al. 1998) or membrane-associated matrix metalloproteinases which are expressed on the surface of certain protease-rich tumours (Martin et al. 1999, 2002; Peng et al. 1997, 1999). These proteases are known to be important initiators of the proteolytic cascade which results in matrix degradation and plays a central part in cancer invasion metastasis and angiogenesis. In each case, the infectivity of the vectors which displayed the protease-cleavable chimeric glycoproteins was restored after exposure to the specific protease. Additionally, the MMP-activatable vectors were shown to be capable of discriminating between MMP-rich and MMP-poor cells in a heterogeneous cell population in vitro. Finally, the MMP-activatable vectors could selectively infect MMP-rich tumour xenografts implanted in mice (Martin et al. 2002; Peng et al. 1999), demonstrating the in vivo potential of the protease targeting strategy. Insertion of a single-chain antibody against a melanoma antigen at the amino terminus of the glycoprotein which displayed both the blocking domain and the MMP cleavage site resulted in specific transduction of melanoma xenografts with no spread of the vectors to spleen or liver (Martin et al. 2002). These results demonstrated the feasibility of using targeted retroviruses for in vivo gene delivery to tumours and highlighted the safety benefits of targeted retroviruses which do not infect other host tissues.

In addition to factor Xa, plasmin and the matrix metalloproteinases, there have been reports of retroviral vectors activatable by furin (Buchholz et al. 1998). A library of EGF-displaying replication-competent retroviruses was generated by inserting a randomised peptide linker between EGF and the MLV glycoprotein, thus offering potential cleavage sites for cellular proteases. This virus library was then propagated in EGF receptor-expressing selector cells which could not support EGF-displaying viruses. Most virus particles displayed a non-cleavable linker and were therefore sequestered by the EGF receptors and lost during selection. In contrast, some viruses encoded a linker cleaved by a cellular protease and were therefore able to enter and propagate in the selector cells by interacting with the natural viral receptor. The linker peptide sequences of the selected viruses contained arginine/lysine-rich motifs characteristic of the cleavage sites of proteases from the pro-protein convertase family, among which furin is ubiquitously expressed. The proof of principle was thereby established for the identification of cell surface-associated host proteases and for the selection of protease-activatable vectors from retroviral display libraries (Buchholz et al. 1998). A suitable cleavage signal for which there is a protease expressed at the target cell surface having been identified, it is also possible to further optimise the specificity and/or sensitivity of that signal by its subsequent randomisation and selection (Schneider et al. 2002).

These results have therefore raised the possibility that proteases of the cell surface, rather than receptors, could be used to target gene delivery, owing to the specific expression of many proteases at or close to the surface of tumour cells. In principle, any protease which does not degrade the envelope glycoprotein can be targeted using this strategy, provided a specific and sensitive cleavage signal has been identified.

9
Concluding Remarks

9.1
Conclusions

The most convenient and useful gene delivery vector should selectively transduce a particular chosen target cell population after intravenous administration. The quest for such an ideal vector has led the gene therapy research community to explore several strategies over the last few years. The initial concept that simply engineering the attachment of the viral envelope glycoproteins to the targeted cellular receptors would allow efficient virion penetration was revised and may appear as naïve in retrospect. Indeed, it has progressively become clearer that in addition to their role in viral attachment, viral receptors play a critical role in the activation of the fusogenicity of retroviral envelope glycoproteins and also may possibly trigger essential cellular functions to allow cell entry and subsequent integration of the viral genome into genomic cellular DNA. Likewise, the attachment subunits of retroviral glycoproteins not only contain determinants which specify binding to cell surface receptors but also contain essential determinants involved in complex intra- and inter-molecular dialogues which lead to the mobilisation of their fusogenic components. Recruitment of these determinants is a key problem in targeting strategies using engineered viral glycoproteins in all targeting strategies. The developing understanding of the complexity of the different steps which allow penetration of viruses into the cytoplasm of the infected cells after their initial interaction with the cell surface stimulated intense research in vectorology and led to emergence of highly sophisticated targeting strategies. Although advances are still expected in these areas and in our quest for ideal and powerful vectors, it is important to question the utility of retargeted viral vectors for in vivo gene delivery. Indeed, although targeting is a highly valid goal in gene therapy, it is important to recognize that a targeted vector may be completely ineffective if it cannot gain access to the appropriate target cell population in vivo. If one considers the ideal characteristics of a targetable, injectable vector carrying a therapeutic transgene for the treatment of disseminated malignancy, the issue of target cell accessibility is readily apparent. In this example, efficient gene delivery to the target cell population will be achieved only if the vector crosses the relatively impermeable tumour blood vessel and achieves a uniform distribution throughout the tumour parenchyma.

9.2
Clinical Utility of Retroviral Targeting

Perhaps the most important characteristics of retroviral vectors which distinguish them from other vector systems are the lack of vector sequences coding for immunogenic viral proteins in the vector genome and the ability to integrate efficiently into the host/cell genome such that the therapeutic transgene is transmitted to the future progeny of the targeted cell. Because of these properties, retroviral vectors are ideally suited for the transduction of stem cells and other proliferating target cell populations where the real targets for gene expression are the progeny of the initially transduced cells. Thus retroviral vectors are the logical choice for haematopoietic stem cell (HSC) transduction protocols seeking to correct genetic defects expressed in erythrocytes or white blood cells (lymphoid or myeloid) or in the megakaryocyte lineage. Indeed, the most successful application of gene therapy to date used retroviral vectors to transduce the HSCs of children afflicted with X-linked severe combined immune deficiency (SCID) (Cavazzana-Calvo et al. 2000). Moreover, proof of principle has been established in animal models for HSC gene therapy of sickle cell anaemia, thalassaemia, chronic granulomatous disease, lysosomal storage disorders, Fanconi's anaemia and many other diseases. However, for most of these diseases, unlike SCID, bone marrow reconstitution with genetically corrected HSCs cannot be achieved without using highly toxic myeloablative conditioning therapy to displace the defective HSCs. Thus, both for convenience (no need to manipulate HSCs ex vivo) and to circumvent the need for myeloablative conditioning therapy, targeted gene delivery to HSCs in vivo is a highly desirable goal. Also, with the recent recognition of the remarkable plasticity and diversity of circulating stem cells, it is possible to envisage numerous additional therapeutic scenarios involving stem cells which would be facilitated by the availability of targetable, injectable retroviral vectors.

T cell engineering is another burgeoning field of translational research in which genes are introduced into T cells to enhance their ability to home to tumour sites and to recognise and kill tumour cells (Chester et al. 2002). The current approach involving T cell isolation, ex vivo expansion and reinfusion would be greatly simplified by the availability of T cell-targeted, injectable retroviral vectors.

Vascular gene therapy also presents a variety of compelling scenarios in which targetable, injectable retroviral vectors could prove essential for the realisation of therapeutic goals. Examples include the delivery of genes to sites of angiogenesis for the treatment of cancer, diabetic retinopathy or rheumatoid arthritis; to sites of atherosclerotic plaque development for the treatment or prevention of ischaemic heart disease, stroke and peripheral vascular disease; and to the walls of small resistance vessels in the systemic or pulmonary circulations for the treatment of systemic or pulmonary hypertension.

More recently, because of their ability to transduce non-dividing cells, lentivirus vectors are being explored for direct in vivo gene transfer to non-dividing, terminally differentiated cells, for example, in brain and retina. However, in these instances, the argument for targeting is less compelling because the vectors are deposited precisely at the desired target site.

Acknowledgements. Our work is supported by the Agence Nationale pour la Recherche contre le SIDA (ANRS), the European Community (QLK3-1999-00859), Association Franco-Israélienne pour la Recherche Scientifique et Technologique (AFIRST), Association Française contre les Myopathies (AFM), Association pour la Recherche contre le Cancer (ARC), Centre National de la Recherche Scientifique (CNRS), and Institut National de la Santé et de la Recherche Médicale (INSERM).

References

Abe A, Chen ST, Miyanohara A, and Friedmann T (1998) In vitro cell-free conversion of noninfectious Moloney retrovirus particles to an infectious form by the addition of the vesicular stomatitis virus surrogate envelope G protein. J Virol 72:6356–61

Ager S, Nilson BHK, Morling FJ, Peng KW, Cosset F-L, and Russell SJ (1996) Retroviral display of antibody fragments; interdomain spacing strongly influences vector infectivity. Hum Gene Ther 7:2157–2164

Barnett AL, and Cunningham JM (2001) Receptor binding transforms the surface subunit of the mammalian C-type retrovirus envelope protein from an inhibitor to an activator of fusion. J Virol 75:9096–105

Barnett AL, Davey RA, and Cunningham JM (2001) Modular organization of the Friend murine leukemia virus envelope protein underlies the mechanism of infection. Proc Natl Acad Sci U S A 98:4113–8

Bartosch B, Dubuisson J, Cosset FL (2003) Infectious hepatitis C virus pseudo-particles containing functional E1–E2 envelope protein complexes. J Exp Med 197:633-42

Battini JL, Danos O, and Heard JM (1998) Definition of a 14-amino-acid peptide essential for the interaction between the murine leukemia virus amphotropic envelope glycoprotein and its receptor. J Virol 72:428–435

Benedict CA, Tun RY, Rubinstein DB, Guillaume T, Cannon PM, and Anderson WF (1999) Targeting retroviral vectors to CD34-expressing cells: binding to CD34 does not catalyze virus-cell fusion. Hum Gene Ther 10:545–557

Beyer WR, Westphal M, Ostertag W, and von Laer D (2002) Oncoretrovirus and lentivirus vectors pseudotyped with lymphocytic choriomeningitis virus glycoprotein: generation, concentration, and broad host range. J Virol 76:1488–95

Bobkova M, Stitz J, Engelstadter M, Cichutek K, and Buchholz CJ (2002) Identification of R-peptides in envelope proteins of C-type retroviruses. J Gen Virol 83:2241–6

Boerger AL, Snitkovsky S, and Young JA (1999) Retroviral vectors preloaded with a viral receptor-ligand bridge protein are targeted to specific cell types. Proc Natl Acad Sci U S A 96:9867–72

Bounou S, Leclerc JE, and Tremblay MJ (2002) Presence of host ICAM-1 in laboratory and clinical strains of human immunodeficiency virus type 1 increases virus infectivity and CD4(+)-T-cell depletion in human lymphoid tissue, a major site of replication in vivo. J Virol 76:1004–14

Brody BA, Rhee SS, and Hunter E (1994) Postassembly cleavage of a retroviral glycoprotein cytoplasmic domain removes a necessary incorporation signal and activates fusion activity. J Virol 68:4620–4627

Buchholz CJ, Peng K-W, Morling FJ, Zhang J, Cosset F-L, and Russell SJ (1998) In vivo selection of protease cleavage sites from retrovirus display libraries. Nat Biotechnol 16:951–954

Bupp K, and Roth MJ (2002) Altering retroviral tropism using a random-display envelope library. Mol Ther 5:329–35

Burns JC, Friedmann T, Driever W, Burrascano M, and Yee JK (1993) Vesicular stomatitis virus G glycoprotein pseudotyped retroviral vectors: concentration to very high titer and efficient gene transfer into mammalian and nonmammalian cells. Proc Natl Acad Sci U S A 90:8033–8037

Carr CM, Chaundhry C, and Kim PS (1997) Influenza hemagglutinin is spring-loaded by a metastable native conformation. Proc Natl Acad Sci USA 23:14306–14313

Cavazzana-Calvo M, Hacein-Bey S, Basile GdS, Gross F, Yvon E, Nusbaum P, Selz F, Hue C, Certain S, Casanova J, Bousso P, Deist F, and Fischer A (2000) Gene therapy of human severe combined immunodeficiency (SCID)-X1 disease. Science 288:669–672

Chadwick MP, Morling FJ, Cosset F-L, and Russell SJ (1999) Modification of retroviral tropism by display of IGF-I. J Mol Biol 285:485–494

Chen J, Lee KH, Steinhauer DA, Stevens DJ, Skehel JJ, and Wiley DC (1998) Structure of the hemagglutinin precursor cleavage site, a determinant of influenza pathogenicity and the origin of the labile conformation. Cell 95:409–417

Chester J, Ruchatz A, Gough M, Crittenden M, Chong H, Cosset F-L, Diaz RM, Harrington K, Alvarez-Vallina L, and Vile R (2002) Tumor antigen-specific induction of transcriptionally targeted retroviral vectors from chimeric immune receptor-modified T cells. Nat Biotechnol 20:256–263

Christodoulopoulos I, and Cannon P (2001) Sequences in the cytoplasmic tail of the gibbon ape leukemia virus envelope protein that prevent its incorporation into lentivirus vectors. J Virol 75:4129–38

Chu THT, and Dornburg R (1995) Retroviral vector particles displaying the antigen-binding site of an antibody enable cell-type-specific gene transfer. J. Virol. 69:2659–2663

Chu THT, Martinez I, Sheay WC, and Dornburg R (1994) Cell targeting with retroviral vector particles containing antibody-envelope fusion proteins. Gene Therapy 1:292–299

Cosset F-L, Morling FJ, Takeuchi Y, Weiss RA, Collins MKL, and Russell SJ (1995) Retroviral retargeting by envelopes expressing an N-terminal binding domain. J. Virol. 69:6314–6322

Cosson P (1996) Direct interaction between the envelope and matrix proteins of HIV-1. EMBO J. 15:5783–5788

DePolo NJ, Reed JD, Sheridan PL, Townsend K, Sauter SL, Jolly DJ, and Dubensky TW (2000) VSV-G pseudotyped lentiviral vector particles produced in human cells are inactivated by human serum. Mol Ther 2:218–22

Desmaris N, Bosch A, Salaun C, Petit C, Prevost MC, Tordo N, Perrin P, Schwartz O, deRocquigny H, and Heard JM (2001) Production and neurotropism of lentivirus vectors pseudotyped with lyssavirus envelope glycoproteins. Mol Ther 4:149–56

Dong J, Roth MG, and Hunter E (1992) A chimeric avian retrovirus containing the influenza virus hemagglutinin gene has an expanded host range. J Virol 66:7374–7382

Duisit G, Conrath H, Saleun S, Folliot S, Provost N, Cosset F-L, Sandrin V, Moullier P, and Rolling F (2002) Five recombinant SIV pseudotypes lead to exclusive transduction of retinal pigmented epithelium in rat. Mol Ther. In press

Engelstadter M, Bobkova M, Baier M, Stitz J, Holtkamp N, Chu TH, Kurth R, Dornburg R, Buchholz CJ, and Cichutek K (2000) Targeting human T cells by retroviral vectors displaying antibody domains selected from a phage display library. Hum Gene Ther 11:293–303

Engelstadter M, Buchholz CJ, Bobkova M, Steidl S, Merget-Millitzer H, Willemsen RA, Stitz J, and Cichutek K (2001) Targeted gene transfer to lymphocytes using murine leukaemia virus vectors pseudotyped with spleen necrosis virus envelope proteins. Gene Ther 8:1202–6

Etienne-Julan M, Roux P, Carillo S, Jeanteur P, and Piechaczyk M (1992) The efficiency of cell targeting by recombinant retroviruses depends on the nature of the receptor and the composition of the artificial cell-virus linker. J. Gen. Virol. 73:3251–3255

Erlwein O, Buchholz CJ, Schnierle BS (2003) The proline-rich region of the ecotropic Moloney murine leukaemia virus envelope protein tolerates the insertion of the green fluorescent protein and allows the generation of replication-competent virus. J Gen Virol 84:369–373

Erlwein O, Wels W, Schnierle BS (2002) Chimeric ecotropic MLV envelope proteins that carry EGF receptor-specific ligands and the Pseudomonas exotoxin A translocation domain to target gene transfer to human cancer cells. Virology 302:333–341

Fass D, Davey RA, Hamson CA, Kim PS, Cunningham JM, and Berger JM (1997) Structure of a murine leukemia virus receptor-binding glycoprotein at 2.0 angstrom resolution. Science 277:1662–1666

Fielding A, Chapel-Fernandes S, Chadwick M, Bullough F, Cosset F-L, and Russell S (2000) A hyperfusogenic gibbon ape leukemia virus envelope glycoprotein: targeting of a cytotoxic gene by ligand display. Hum Gene Ther 11:817–826

Fielding AK, Maurice M, Morling FJ, Cosset F-L, and Russell SJ (1998) Inverse targeting of retroviral vectors: selective gene transfer in a mixed population of hematopoietic and nonhematopoietic cells. Blood 91:1802–1809

Fortin JF, Cantin R, Bergeron MG, and Tremblay MJ (2000) Interaction between virion-bound host intercellular adhesion molecule-1 and the high-affinity state of lymphocyte function-associated antigen-1 on target cells renders R5 and X4 isolates of human immunodeficiency virus type 1 more refractory to neutralization. Virology 268:493–503

Fortin JF, Cantin R, Lamontagne G, and Tremblay M (1997) Host-derived ICAM-1 glycoproteins incorporated on human immunodeficiency virus type 1 are biologically active and enhance viral infectivity. J Virol 71:3588–3596

Freed EO (1998) HIV-1 gag proteins: diverse functions in the virus life cycle. Virology 251:1–15

Gautier R, Jiang A, Rousseau V, Dornburg R, and Jaffredo T (1999) Avian reticuloendotheliosis virus strain A and spleen necrosis virus do not infect human cells. J Virol 74:518–522

Gollan TJ, and Green MR (2002a) Redirecting retroviral tropism by insertion of short, nondisruptive peptide ligands into envelope. J Virol 76:3558–63

Gollan TJ, and Green MR (2002b) Selective targeting and inducible destruction of human cancer cells by retroviruses with envelope proteins bearing short peptide ligands. J Virol 76:3564–9

Gordon EM, Chen ZH, Liu L, Whitley M, Liu L, Wei D, Groshen S, Hinton DR, Anderson WF, Beart RW, and Hall FL (2001a) Systemic administration of a matrix-targeted retroviral vector is efficacious for cancer gene therapy in mice. Hum Gene Ther 12:193–204

Gordon EM, Zhu NL, Forney-Prescott M, Chen ZH, Anderson WF, and FL FLH (2001b) Lesion-targeted injectable vectors for vascular restenosis. Hum Gene Ther 12:1277–87

Goud B, Legrain P, and Buttin G (1988) Antibody-mediated binding of a murine ecotropic Moloney retroviral vector to human cells allows internalization but not the establishment of the proviral state. Virology 163:251–254

Hall FL, Gordon EM, Wu L, Zhu NL, Skotzko MJ, Starnes VA, and Anderson WF (1997) Targeting retroviral vectors to vascular lesions by genetic engineering of the MoMLV gp70 envelope protein. Hum Gene Ther 8:2183-2192

Hall FL, Liu L, Zhu NL, Stapfer M, Anderson WF, Beart RW, and Gordon EM (2000) Molecular engineering of matrix-targeted retroviral vectors incorporating a surveillance function inherent in von Willebrand factor. Hum Gene Ther 11:983-93

Han X, Kasahara N, and Kan YW (1995) Ligand-directed retroviral targeting of human breast cancer cells. Proc Natl Acad Sci USA 92:9747-9751

Hanawa H, Kelly PF, Nathwani AC, Persons DA, Vandergriff JA, Hargrove P, Vanin EF, and Nienhuis AW (2002) Comparison of various envelope proteins for their ability to pseudotype lentiviral vectors and transduce primitive hematopoietic cells from human blood. Mol Ther 5:242-51

Hatziioannou T, Delahaye E, Martin F, Russell SJ, and Cosset F-L (1999) Retroviral display of functional binding domains fused to the amino-terminus of influenza haemagglutinin. Hum Gene Ther 10:1533-1544

Hatziioannou T, Valsesia-Wittmann S, Russell S, and Cosset F-L (1998) Incorporation of fowl plague virus hemagglutinin into murine leukemia virus particles and analysis of the infectivity of the pseudotyped retroviruses. J Virol 72:5313 5317

Hatziioannou T, Russell SJ, and Cosset F-L (2000) Incorporation of simian virus 5 fusion protein into murine leukemia virus particles and its effect on the co-incorporation of retroviral envelope glycoproteins. Virology 267:49-57

Hughson FM (1997) Enveloped viruses: a common mode of membrane fusion? Curr Biol 7:R565-9

Hunter E (1997) Viral entry and receptors. In "Retroviruses" (J M Coffin, S H Hughes and H E Varmus, eds.), pp. 71-120. Cold Spring Harbor Laboratory Press, New York, USA

Innes CL, Smith PB, Langenbach R, Tindall KR, and Boone LR (1990) Cationic liposomes (Lipofectin) mediate retroviral infection in the absence of specific receptors. J Virol 64:957-61

Jiang A, Chu TH, Nocken F, Cichutek K, and Dornburg R (1998) Cell-type-specific gene transfer into human cells with retroviral vectors that display single-chain antibodies. J Virol 72:10148-10156

Jiang A, and Dornburg R (1999) In vivo cell type-specific gene delivery with retroviral vectors that display single chain antibodies. Gene Ther 6:1982-7

Kang Y, Stein CS, Heth JA, Sinn PL, Penisten AK, Staber PD, Ratliff KL, Shen H, Barker CK, Martins I, Sharkey CM, Sanders DA, McCray PB, Jr., and Davidson BL (2002) In vivo gene transfer using a nonprimate lentiviral vector pseudotyped with Ross River Virus glycoproteins. J Virol 76:9378-88

Katane M, Takao E, Kubo Y, Fujita R, Amanuma H (2002) Factors affecting the direct targeting of murine leukemia virus vectors containing peptide ligands in the envelope protein. EMBO Rep 3:899-904

Kasahara N, Dozy AM, and Kan YW (1994) Tissue-specific targeting of retroviral vectors through ligand-receptor interactions. Science 266:1373-1376

Kayman SC, Park H, Saxon M, and Pinter A (1999) The hypervariable domain of the murine leukemia virus surface protein tolerates large insertions and deletions, enabling development of a retroviral particle display system. J Virol 73:1802-1808

Kelly P, Vandergriff J, Nathwani A, Nienhuis A, and Vanin E (2000) Highly efficient gene transfer into cord blood nonobese diabetic/severe combined immunodeficiency repopulating cells by oncoretroviral vector particles pseudotyped with the feline endogenous retrovirus (RD114) envelope protein. Blood 96:1206–1214

Khare PD, Shao-Xi L, Kuroki M, Hirose Y, Arakawa F, Nakamura K, Tomita Y, and Kuroki M (2001) Specifically targeted killing of carcinoembryonic antigen (CEA)-expressing cells by a retroviral vector displaying single-chain variable fragmented antibody to CEA and carrying the gene for inducible nitric oxide synthase. Cancer Res 61:370–5

Kobe B, Center RJ, Kemp BE, and Poumbourios P (1999) Crystal structure of human T cell leukemia virus type 1 gp21 ectodomain crystallized as a maltose-binding protein chimera reveals structural evolution of retroviral transmembrane proteins. Proc Natl Acad Sci USA 96:4319–4324

Kobinger GP, Weiner DJ, Yu QC, and Wilson JM (2001) Filovirus-pseudotyped lentiviral vector can efficiently and stably transduce airway epithelia in vivo. Nat Biotechnol 19:225–30

Konishi H, Ochiya T, Chester KA, Begent RH, Muto T, Sugimura T, and Terada M (1998) Targeting strategy for gene delivery to carcinoembryonic antigen-producing cancer cells by retrovirus displaying a single-chain variable fragment antibody. Hum Gene Ther 9:235–248

Lamb RA (1993) Paramyxovirus fusion: A hypothesis for changes. Virology 197:1–11

Lavillette D, Boson B, Russell S, and Cosset F-L (2001a) Membrane fusion by murine leukemia viruses is activated in cis or in trans by interactions of the receptor-binding domain with a conserved disulfide loop at the carboxy-terminus of the surface glycoproteins. J Virol 75:3685–3695

Lavillette D, Maurice M, Roche C, Russell SJ, Sitbon M, and Cosset F-L (1998) A proline-rich motif downstream of the receptor binding domain modulates conformation and fusogenicity of murine retroviral envelopes. J Virol 72:9955–9965

Lavillette D, Ruggieri A, Boson B, Maurice M, and Cosset F-L (2002) Relationship between SU subdomains that regulate the receptor-mediated transition from the native (fusion-inhibited) and fusion-active conformations of the murine leukemia virus glycoprotein. J Virol 76:9685–2002

Lavillette D, Ruggieri A, Russell SJ, and Cosset F-L (2000) Activation of a cell entry pathway common to type C mammalian retroviruses by soluble envelope fragments. J Virol 74:295–304

Lavillette D, Russell SJ, and Cosset F-L (2001b) Retargeting gene delivery by surface-engineered retroviral vector particles. Curr Opin Biotechnol 12:461–466

Lee S, Zhao Y, and Anderson WF (1999) Receptor-mediated moloney murine leukemia virus entry can occur independently of the clathrin-coated-pit-mediated endocytic pathway. J Virol 73:5994–6005

Lin AH, Kasahara N, Wu W, Stripecke R, Empig CL, Anderson WF, and Cannon PM (2001) Receptor-specific targeting mediated by the coexpression of a targeted murine leukemia virus envelope protein and a binding-defective influenza hemagglutinin protein. Hum Gene Ther 12:323–32

Lindemann D, Bock M, Schweizer M, and Rethwilm A (1997) Efficient pseudotyping of murine leukemia virus particles with chimeric human foamy virus envelope proteins. J. Virol 71:4815–4820

Linder M, Linder D, Hahnen J, Schott HH, and Stirm S (1992) Localization of the intrachain disulfide bonds of the envelope glycoprotein 71 from Friend murine leukemia virus. Eur J Biochem 203:65–73

Linder M, Wenzel V, Linder D, and Stirm S (1994) Structural elements in glycoprotein 70 from polytropic Friend mink cell focus-inducing virus and glycoprotein 71 from ecotropic Friend murine leukemia virus, as defined by disulfide-bonding pattern and limited proteolysis. J Virol 68:5133–5141

Liu L, Anderson WF, Beart RW, Gordon EM, and Hall FL (2000) Incorporation of tumor vasculature targeting motifs into moloney murine leukemia virus env escort proteins enhances retrovirus binding and transduction of human endothelial cells. J Virol 74:5320–8

Lodge R, Subbramanian RA, Forget J, Lemay G, and Cohen EA (1998) MuLV-based vectors pseudotyped with truncated HIV glycoproteins mediate specific gene transfer in CD4+ peripheral blood lymphocytes. Gene Ther 5:655–64

Lorimer IA, and Lavictoire SJ (2000) Targeting retrovirus to cancer cells expressing a mutant EGF receptor by insertion of a single chain antibody variable domain in the envelope glycoprotein receptor binding lobe. J Immunol Methods 237:147–57

Mammano F, Salvatori F, Indraccolo S, de Rossi A, Chieco-Bianchi L, and Göttlinger HG (1997) Truncation of the human immunodeficiency virus type 1 envelope glycoprotein allows efficient pseudotyping of Moloney murine leukemia virus particles and gene transfer into CD4+ cells. J Virol 71:3341–3345

Marandin A, Dubart A, Pflumio F, Cosset F-L, Cordette V, Chapel-Fernandes S, Coulombel L, Vainchenker W, and Louache F (1998) Retroviral-mediated gene transfer into human CD34+/38− primitive cells capable of reconstituting long-term cultures in vitro and in nonobese diabetic-severe combined immunodeficiency mice in vivo. Human Gene Ther 9:1497–1511

Marechal V, Clavel F, Heard JM, and Schwartz O (1998) Cytosolic Gag p24 as an index of productive entry of human immunodeficiency virus type 1. J Virol 72: 2208–12

Marechal V, Prevost MC, Petit C, Perret E, Heard JM, and Schwartz O (2001) Human immunodeficiency virus type 1 entry into macrophages mediated by macropinocytosis. J Virol 75:11166–77

Marin M, Noël D, Valsesia-Wittmann S, Brockly F, Etienne-Julan M, Russell SJ, Cosset F-L, and Piechaczyk M (1996) Targeted infection of human cells via MHC class I molecules by MoMuLV-derived viruses displaying single-chain antibody fragment-envelope fusion proteins. J. Virol 70:2957–2962

Martin F, Chowdhury S, Neil S, Phillipps N, and Collins MK (2002) Envelope-targeted retrovirus vectors transduce melanoma xenografts but not spleen or liver. Mol Ther 5:269–74

Martin F, Kupsch J, Takeuchi Y, Russell S, Cosset F-L, and Collins M (1998) Retroviral vector targeting to melanoma cells by single-chain antibody incorporation in envelope. Hum Gene Ther 9:737–746

Martin F, Neil S, Kupsch J, Maurice M, Cosset F-L, and Collins M (1999) Retrovirus targeting by tropism restriction to melanoma cells. J Virol 73:6923–6929

Martin F, Chowdhury S, Neil SJ, Chester KA, Cosset F-L, and Collins MK (2003) Targeted retroviral infection of tumor cells by receptor cooperation. J Virol 77:2753–2756

Matano T, Odawara T, Iwamoto A, and Yoshikura H (1995) Targeted infection of a retrovirus bearing a CD4-Env chimera into human cells expressing human immunodeficiency virus type 1. J. Gen. Virol. 76:3165–3169

Maurice M, Mazur S, Bullough FJ, Salvetti A, Collins MKL, Russell SJ, and Cosset F-L (1999) Efficient gene delivery to quiescent IL2-dependent cells by murine leukemia virus-derived vectors harboring IL2 chimeric envelope glycoproteins. Blood 94:401–410

Maurice M, Verhoeyen E, Salmon P, Trono D, Russell SJ, and Cosset F-L (2002) Efficient gene transfer into human primary blood lymphocytes by surface-engineered lentiviral vectors that display a T cell-activating polypeptide. Blood 99:2342–50

McClure MO, Sommerfelt MA, Marsh M, and Weiss RA (1990) The pH independence of mammalian retrovirus infection. J. Gen. Virol. 71:767–773

Merten CA, Engelstaedter M, Buchholz CJ, Cichutek K (2003) Displaying epidermal growth factor on spleen necrosis virus-derived targeting vectors. Virology 305:106–114

Miletic H, Bruns M, Tsiakas K, Vogt B, Rezal R, Baum C, Kühlke K, Cosset F-L, Ostertag W, Lother H, and Laer DV (1999) Retroviral vectors pseudotyped with lymphocytic choriomeningitis virus. J Virol 73:6114–6116

Mochizuki H, Schwartz JP, Tanaka K, Brady RO, and Reiser J (1998) High-titer human immunodeficiency virus type 1-based vector systems for gene delivery into nondividing cells. J. Virol. 72:8873–8883

Mondor I, Ugolini S, and Sattentau QJ (1998) Human immunodeficiency virus type 1 attachment to HeLa CD4 cells is CD4 independent and gp120 dependent and requires cell surface heparans. J Virol 1998:3623–34

Morizono K, Bristol G, Xie Y-M, Kung SK-P, and Chen ISC (2001) Antibody-directed targeting of retroviral vectors via cell surface antigens. J Virol 75:8016–8020

Morling FJ, Peng K-W, Cosset F-L, and Russell SJ (1997) Masking of retroviral envelope functions by oligomerizing peptide adaptors. Virology 234:51–61

Morrison TG (2001) The three faces of paramyxovirus attachment proteins. Trends Microbiol 9:103–5

Mothes W, Boerger AL, Narayan S, Cunningham JM, and Young JA (2000) Retroviral entry mediated by receptor priming and low pH triggering of an envelope glycoprotein. Cell 103:679–89

Movassagh M, Desmyter C, Baillou C, Chapel-Fernandes S, Guigon M, Klatzmann D, and Lemoine FM (1998) High-level gene transfer to cord blood progenitors using gibbon ape leukemia virus pseudotyped retroviral vectors and an improved clinically applicable protocol. Hum Gene Ther 9:225–234

Mukherjee S, Ghosh RN, and Maxfield FR (1997) Endocytosis. Physiol Rev 77:759–803

Murakami T, and Freed EO (2000) Genetic evidence for an interaction between human immunodeficiency virus type 1 matrix and alpha-helix 2 of the gp41 cytoplasmic tail. J Virol 74:3548–54

Naldini L, Blömer U, Gallay P, Ory D, Mulligan R, Gage FH, Verma IM, and Trono D (1996) In vivo gene delivery and stable transduction of nondividing cells by a lentiviral vector. Science 272:263–267

Nègre D, Duisit G, Mangeot P-E, Moullier P, Darlix J-L, and Cosset F-L (2002) Lentiviral vectors derived from simian immunodeficiency virus (SIV). In "Current Topics in Microbiology and Immunology" (D Trono, ed.), pp. 53–74

Nègre D, Mangeot P, Duisit G, Blanchard S, Vidalain P, Leissner P, Winter A, Rabourdin-Combe C, Mehtali M, Moullier P, Darlix J-L, and Cosset F-L (2000) Characterization of novel safe lentiviral vectors derived from simian immunodeficiency virus (SIVmac251) that efficiently transduce mature human dendritic cells. Gene Ther 7:1613–1623

Nguyen T, Pages J-C, Farge D, Briand P, and Weber A (1998) Amphotropic retroviral vectors displaying hepatocyte growth factor-envelope fusion proteins improve transduction efficiency of primary hepatocytes. Hum Gene Ther 9:2469–2479

Nilson BHK, Morling FJ, Cosset F-L, and Russell SJ (1996) Targeting of retroviral vectors through protease-substrate interactions. Gene Ther. 3:280–286

Ohno K, Sawai K, Iijima Y, Levin B, and Meruelo D (1997) Cell-specific targeting of Sindbis virus vectors displaying IgG-binding domains of protein A. Nat Biotechnol 15:763–767

Ott DE (1997) Cellular proteins in HIV virions. Rev Med Virol 7:167–180

Overbaugh J, Miller AD, and Eiden MV (2001) Receptors and entry cofactors for retroviruses include single and multiple transmembrane-spanning proteins as well as newly described glycophosphatidylinositol-anchored and secreted proteins. Microbiol Mol Biol Rev 65:371–89

Patterson SM, Swainsbury R, and Routledge EG (1999) Antigen-specific membrane fusion mediated by the haemagglutinin protein of influenza A virus: separation of attachment and fusion functions on different molecules. Gene Ther 6:694–702

Peng K-W, Vile RG, Cosset F-L, and Russell SJ (1999) Selective transduction of protease-rich tumors by matrix-metalloproteinase-targeted retroviral vectors. Gene Ther 6:1552–1557

Peng KW, F.J. Morling, Cosset F-L, Murphy G, and Russell SJ (1997) A gene delivery system activatable by disease-associated matrix metalloproteinases. Hum Gene Ther 8:729–738

Peng KW, Morling FJ, Cosset F-L, and Russell SJ (1998) A retroviral gene delivery system activatable by plasmin. Tumor Targeting 3:112–120

Peng KW, Pham L, Ye H, Zufferey R, Trono D, Cosset F-L, and Russell SJ (2001) Organ distribution of gene expression after intravenous infusion of targeted and untargeted lentiviral vectors. Gene Ther 8:1456–63

Pickl WF, Pimentel-Muinos FX, and Seed B (2001) Lipid rafts and pseudotyping. J Virol 75:7175–83

Pinter A, Kopelman R, Li Z, Kayman SC, and Sanders DA (1997) Localization of the labile disulfide bond between SU and TM of the murine leukemia virus envelope protein complex to a highly conserved CWLC motif in SU that resembles the active-site sequence of thiol-disulfide exchange enzymes. J Virol 71:8073–8077

Pizzato M, Blair ED, Fling M, Kopf J, Tomassetti A, Weiss RA, and Takeuchi Y (2001) Evidence for non-specific adsorption of targeted retrovirus vector particles to cells. Gene Ther 8:1088–96

Pizzato M, Marlow SA, Blair ED, and Takeuchi Y (1999) Initial binding of murine leukemia virus particles to cells does not require specific Env-receptor interaction. J Virol 73:8599–611

Porter CD (2002) Cationic liposomes for envelope-independent retroviral transduction and enhancement of fusion-deficient targeted viruses. Gene Ther. in press

Porter CD, Collins MKL, Tailor CS, Parker MH, Cosset F-L, Weiss RA, and Takeuchi Y (1996) Comparison of efficiency of infection of human gene therapy target cells via four different retroviral receptors. Hum Gene Ther 7:913–919

Porter CD, Lukacs KV, Box G, Takeuchi Y, and Collins MK (1998) Cationic liposomes enhance the rate of transduction by a recombinant retroviral vector in vitro and in vivo. J Virol 72:4832–40

Ragheb JA, and Anderson WF (1994) pH-independent murine leukemia virus ecotropic envelope-mediated cell fusion: Implications for the role of the R peptide and p12E TM in viral entry. J Virol 68:3220–3231

Reeves JD, and Schulz TF (1997) The CD4-independent tropism of human immunodeficiency virus type 2 involves several regions of the envelope protein and correlates with a reduced activation threshold for envelope-mediated fusion. J Virol 71:1453–1465

Rein A, Mirro J, Haynes JG, Ernst SM, and Nagashima K (1994) Function of the cytoplasmic domain of a retroviral transmembrane protein: p15E-p2E cleavage activates the membrane fusion capability of the murine leukemia virus env protein. J Virol 68:1773–1781

Rodrigues P, and Heard JM (1999) Modulation of phosphate uptake and amphotropic murine leukemia virus entry by posttranslational modifications of PIT-2. J. Virol.:3789–3799

Rothenberg SM, Olsen MN, Laurent LC, Crowley RA, and Brown PO (2001) Comprehensive mutational analysis of the Moloney murine leukemia virus envelope protein. J Virol 75:11851–62

Roux P, Jeanteur P, and Piechaczyk M (1989) A versatile approach to the targeting of specific cell types by retroviruses. Proc Natl Acad Sci USA 86:9079–9083

Russell SJ, and Cosset F-L (1999) Modifying the host range properties of retroviral vectors. J Gene Med 1:300–311

Russell SJ, Hawkins RE, and Winter G (1993) Retroviral vectors displaying functional antibody fragments. Nucl Acids Res 21:1081–1085

Salmon P, Nègre D, Trono D, and Cosset F-L (2000) A chimeric GALV-derived envelope glycoprotein harboring the cytoplasmic tail of MLV envelope efficiently pseudotypes HIV-1 vectors. J Gen Med 2 (suppl):23

Sanders DA (2000) Sulfhydryl involvement in fusion mechanisms. In "Fusion of biological membranes and related problems" (Hilderson and Fuller, eds.), pp. 483–514. Kluwer Academic/Plenum Publishers, New York

Sandrin V, Boson B, Salmon P, Gay W, Nègre D, Grand RL, Trono D, and Cosset F-L (2002) Lentiviral vectors pseudotyped with a modified RD114 envelope glycoprotein show increased stability in sera and augmented transduction of primary lymphocytes and CD34+ cells derived from human and non-human primates. Blood 100:823–832

Schneider RM, Medvedovska Y, Voelker B, Chadwick MP, Russell SJ, Cichutek K, and Buchholz CJ (2002) Matrix metalloprotease substrates selected in living human cells using retroviral peptide libraries. in press

Schnierle BS, Stitz J, Bosch V, Nocken F, Merget-Millitzer H, Engelstadter M, Kurth R, Groner B, and Cichutek K (1997) Pseudotyping of murine leukemia virus with the envelope glycoproteins of HIV generates a retroviral vector with specificity of infection for CD4-expressing cells. Proc Natl Acad Sci USA 94:8640–8645

Schwartz AL (1995) Receptor cell biology: receptor-mediated endocytosis. Pediatr Res 38:835–843

Seganti L, Superti F, Girmenia C, Melucci L, and Orsi N (1986) Study of receptors for vesicular stomatitis virus in vertebrate and invertebrate cells. Microbiologica 9:259–67

Sharkey CM, North CL, Kuhn RJ, and Sanders DA (2001) Ross River virus glycoprotein-pseudotyped retroviruses and stable cell lines for their production. J Virol 75:2653–9

Sharma S, Miyanohara A, and Friedmann T (2000) Separable mechanisms of attachment and cell uptake during retrovirus infection. J Virol 74:10790–5

Sharma S, Murai F, Miyanohara A, and Friedmann T (1997) Noninfectious virus-like particles produced by Moloney murine leukemia virus-based retrovirus packaging cells deficient in viral envelope become infectious in the presence of lipofection reagents. Proc Natl Acad Sci U S A 94:10803–8

Skehel JJ, and Wiley DC (2000) Receptor binding and membrane fusion in virus entry: the influenza hemagglutinin. Annu. Rev. Biochem. 69:531 69

Smit JM, Bittman R, and Wilschut J (1999) Low-pH-dependent fusion of Sindbis virus with receptor-free cholesterol- and sphingolipid-containing liposomes. J. Virol. 73:8476–8484

Snitkovsky S, Niederman T, Mulligan R, and Young J (2001) Targeting avian leukosis virus subgroup A vectors by using a TVA-VEGF bridge protein. J Virol 75:1571–5

Snitkovsky S, Niederman TM, Carter BS, Mulligan RC, and Young JA (2000) A TVA-single-chain antibody fusion protein mediates specific targeting of a subgroup A avian leukosis virus vector to cells expressing a tumor-specific form of epidermal growth factor receptor. J Virol 74:9540–5

Snitkovsky S, and Young JA (1998) Cell-specific viral targeting mediated by a soluble retroviral receptor-ligand fusion protein. Proc Natl Acad Sci USA 95:7063–7068

Snitkovsky S, and Young JA (2002) Targeting Retroviral Vector Infection to Cells That Express Heregulin Receptors Using a TVA-Heregulin Bridge Protein. Virology 292:150–5

Somia NV, Zoppé M, and Verma IM (1995) Generation of targeted retroviral vectors by using single-chain variable fragment: an approach to in vivo gene delivery. Proc Natl Acad Sci USA 92:7570–7574

Spiegel M, Bitzer M, Schenk A, Rossmann H, Neubert WJ, Seidler U, Gregor M, and Lauer U (1998) Pseudotype formation of Moloney Murine leukemia virus with Sendai virus glycoprotein F. J Virol 72:5269–5302

Stitz J, Buchholz C, Engelstadter M, Uckert W, Bloemer U, Schmitt I, and Cichutek K (2000) Lentiviral vectors pseudotyped with envelope glycoproteins derived from gibbon ape leukemia virus and murine leukemia virus 10A1. Virology 273:16–20

Sung VM, and Lai MM (2002) Murine retroviral pseudotype virus containing hepatitis B virus large and small surface antigens confers specific tropism for primary human hepatocytes: a potential liver-specific targeting system. J Virol 76:912–7

Suomalainen M, and Garoff H (1994) Incorporation of homologous and heterologous proteins into the envelope of Moloney murine leukemia virus. J Virol 68:4879–4889

Swanstrom R, and Wills JW (1997) Synthesis, assembly, and processing of viral proteins. In "Retroviruses" (J M Coffin, S H Hughes and H E Varmus, eds.), pp. 263–334. Cold Spring Harbor Laboratory Press, New York, USA

Takeuchi Y, Simpson G, Vile R, Weiss R, and Collins M (1992a) Retroviral pseudotypes produced by rescue of moloney murine leukemia virus vector by C-type, but not D-type, retroviruses. Virology 186:792–794

Thaler S, and Schnierle BS (2001) A packaging cell line generating CD4-specific retroviral vectors for efficient gene transfer into primary human T-helper lymphocytes. Mol Ther 4:273–9

Ugolini S, Mondo I, and Sattentau QJ (1999) HIV-1 attachment: another look. Trends Microbiol 7:144–9

Valsesia-Wittmann S (2001) Role of chimeric murine leukemia virus env beta-turn polyproline spacers in receptor cooperation. J Virol 75:8478–86

Valsesia-Wittmann S, Drynda A, Deleage G, Aumailley M, Heard J-M, Danos O, Verdier G, and Cosset F-L (1994) Modifications in the binding domain of avian retrovirus envelope protein to redirect the host range of retroviral vectors. J. Virol. 68:4609–4619

Valsesia-Wittmann S, Morling FJ, Hatziioannou T, Russell SJ, and Cosset F-L (1997) Receptor co-operation in retrovirus entry: recruitment of an auxilliary entry mechanism after retargeted binding. EMBO J 16:1214–1223

Valsesia-Wittmann S, Morling FJ, Nilson BHK, Takeuchi Y, Russell SJ, and Cosset F-L (1996) Improvement of retroviral retargeting by using amino acid spacers between an additional binding domain and the N terminus of Moloney murine leukemia virus SU. J. Virol. 70:2059–2064

Vincent MJ, Melsen LR, Martin AS, and Compans RW (1999) Intracellular interaction of simian immunodeficiency virus Gag and Env proteins. J Virol 73:8138–44

Walker SJ, Pizzato M, Takeuchi Y, Devereux S (2002) Heparin binds to murine leukemia virus and inhibits Env-independent attachment and infection. J Virol 76:6909–18

Wensel DL, Li W, Cunningham JM (2003) A virus-virus interaction circumvents the virus receptor requirement for infection by pathogenic retroviruses. Virol 77:3460-9

Wilson C, Reitz MS, Okayama H, and Eiden MV (1989) Formation of infectious hybrid virions with gibbon ape leukemia virus and human T-cell leukemia virus retroviral envelope glycoproteins and the gag and pol proteins of Moloney murine leukemia virus. J Virol 63:2374–8

Wool-Lewis RJ, and Bates P (1998) Characterization of Ebola virus entry by using pseudotyped viruses: identification of receptor-deficient cell lines. J Virol 72:3155–3160

Wu BW, Cannon PM, Gordon EM, Hall FL, and Anderson WF (1998) Characterization of the proline-rich region of murine leukemia virus envelope protein. J Virol 72:5383–5391

Wu BW, Lu J, Gallaher TK, Anderson WF, and Cannon PM (2000) Identification of regions in the Moloney murine leukemia virus SU protein that tolerate the insertion of an integrin-binding peptide. Virology 269:7–17

Wyma DJ, Kotov A, and Aiken C (2000) Evidence for a stable interaction of gp41 with Pr55(Gag) in immature human immunodeficiency virus type 1 particles. J Virol 74:9381–7

Yajima T, Kanda T, Yoshiike K, and Kitamura Y (1998) Retroviral vector targeting human cells via c-Kit-stem cell factor interaction. Hum Gene Ther 10:779–787

Zhao Y, Lee S, and Anderson WF (1997) Functional interactions between monomers of the retroviral envelope protein complex. J Virol 71:6967–6972

Zhao Y, Zhu L, Lee S, Li L, Chang E, Soong NW, Douer D, and Anderson WF (1999) Identification of the block in targeted retroviral-mediated gene transfer. Proc Natl Acad Sci U S A 96:4005–4010

Intracellular Trafficking of HIV-1 Cores: Journey to the Center of the Cell

J. D. Dvorin[1] · M. H. Malim[2]

[1] Department of Microbiology and Cell and Molecular Biology Graduate Group, University of Pennsylvania School of Medicine, Philadelphia, PA 19104-6148, USA

[2] Department of Infectious Diseases, Guy's, King's and St. Thomas' School of Medicine, King's College London, London, SE1 9RT, UK
E-mail: michael.malim@kcl.ac.uk

1	HIV-1 Infection and Preintegration Hurdles	180
1.1	HIV-1 Infection of Nondividing Cells	180
1.2	Brief Overview of Cytoplasmic Transport Machinery	181
1.3	Brief Overview of Nuclear Import Machinery	183
2	Uncoating and Cytoplasmic Transport of HIV-1	187
2.1	Bioactivity of Incoming Virions	187
2.2	Uncoating	188
2.3	Role of Actin Filaments for Cytoplasmic Transport	191
2.4	Role of Microtubules for Cytoplasmic Transport	192
2.5	Interaction with Virion-Associated Nuclear Shuttling Protein	193
3	Nuclear Import of the HIV-1 PIC	193
3.1	The HIV-1 PIC: Size and Components	193
3.2	The Role of MA in PIC Nuclear Import	194
3.3	The Role of Vpr in PIC Nuclear Import	196
3.4	The Role of IN in PIC Nuclear Import	197
3.5	Role of the DNA flap in PIC import	198
4	Conclusions	199
	References	202

Abstract After entry into the cytoplasm, many diverse viruses, including both RNA and DNA viruses, require import into the nucleus and access to the cellular nuclear machinery for productive replication to proceed. Because diffusion through the crowded cytoplasmic environment is greatly restricted, most (if not all) of these viruses must first be actively transported from the site of cytoplasmic entry to the nuclear periphery (Luby-Phelps 2000; Lukacs et al. 2000; Sodeik 2000). Having reached the nucleus, viruses have evolved assorted methods to overcome the formidable physical barrier that is presented by the nuclear envelope. This review examines how these issues relate to human immunodeficiency virus type-1 (HIV-1) infection. Specifically, HIV-1 uncoating, cytoplasmic transport, and nuclear entry are addressed.

1
HIV-1 Infection and Preintegration Hurdles

1.1
HIV-1 Infection of Nondividing Cells

HIV-1 and other lentiviruses are able to infect nondividing cells productively (Lewis et al. 1992; Sellon et al. 1992; Weinberg et al. 1991). This important property distinguishes the lentiviral subfamily of retroviruses from other retroviruses [for example, murine leukemia virus (MLV)] that cannot efficiently infect nondividing cells (Lewis and Emerman 1994; Roe et al. 1993). Infection of certain nonproliferating cell populations is important for viral transmission, disease pathogenesis, and, potentially, the establishment of persistent viral reservoirs. Specifically, postmitotic tissue macrophages and mucosal dendritic cells, as well as nondividing T cells, have been shown to be among the first cells infected after inoculation with HIV-1 or SIVmac (Hu et al. 2000; Schacker et al. 2001; Zhang et al. 1999). This particular attribute of lentivirus biology has been exploited in the development of lentiviral vector systems for the genetic manipulation of nondividing cell populations (Follenzi et al. 2000).

The long-standing dogma in retrovirus research has been that lentiviruses are unique among retroviruses in their ability to infect nondividing cells. The simple retrovirus MLV clearly does not infect nondividing cells and requires mitosis (most plausibly because of nuclear envelope breakdown) to gain access to the host cell genome (Lewis and Emerman 1994; Roe et al. 1993). Notably, insertion of a heterologous nuclear targeting signal into the MLV genome was not found to restore infectivity in nondividing cells (Lieber et al. 2000). The prevailing view was challenged by a recent study of Rous sarcoma virus (RSV), in which significant infection was reported in challenges of pharmacologically arrested cells (reported infectivity was tenfold lower than HIV-1 but tenfold higher than MLV) (Hatziioannou and Goff 2001; Katz et al. 2002).

The biological significance of this level of RSV infection of nondividing cells remains unresolved.

After entry of HIV-1 into the host cell cytoplasm, a multicomponent nucleoprotein complex is formed: the HIV-1 preintegration complex (PIC) or reverse transcription complex (RTC). The ability of HIV-1 to infect nondividing cells efficiently and to transit across an intact nuclear envelope has been attributed to karyophilic signals within the HIV-1 PIC that facilitate active transport through the nuclear pore complex (NPC) (Bukrinsky et al. 1992). It is also important to bear in mind that active nuclear import may also be critical for efficient infection of dividing cells. This could be because transit of PICs through NPCs constitutes a required step in replication or, more simply, because the tempo of replication would be accelerated.

1.2
Brief Overview of Cytoplasmic Transport Machinery

The size and shape of a cell is largely governed by the complicated organization of the cytoskeleton. The three major protein structures that form the cytoskeleton are actin filaments, microtubules (MTs), and intermediate filaments (see Table 1). The cytoskeleton is a dynamic structure that changes in reaction to both internal and external signals. The most inert of the three major structures are the intermediate filaments, 8- to 10-nm-diameter nonpolarized fibers that are polymers of a family of related proteins including keratins, lamins, and vimentin. No intermediate filament-associated motor proteins have been identified. Hence, intermediate filaments are not believed to contribute to the active, directional transport of cellular or viral proteins (Alberts et al. 1994).

Actin filaments (or microfilaments) are thinner than intermediate filaments, approximately 8 nm in diameter. These helical filaments are formed from repeated, uniformly oriented actin monomers. Thus actin filaments are polarized with a rapidly polymerizing plus (or barbed) end and a more slowly polymerizing minus (or pointed) end. The filaments are dynamic, and often the fibers undergo a process known as "treadmilling" in which the rate of new monomer binding to the plus end is equilibrated with the rate of depolymerization at the minus end. The actin cytoskeleton is intimately involved with many cellular processes including signaling, locomotion, and polarization (Alberts et al. 1994). Proteins in the myosin superfamily act as small ATPase motors

Table 1 Cytoskeleton and cytoplasmic transport (adapted from Sodeik 2000)

	Intermediate filaments	Actin microfilaments	Microtubules
Monomer	Keratins, lamins, vimentin (and several others)	Actin	α-Tubulin and β-tubulin
Filament polarity	No	Yes	Yes
Filament diameter	10 nm	5–9 nm	25 nm
Example of pharmacological inhibitor	–	Cytochalasin D	Nocodazole
Motor proteins (direction of motion)	None	Myosin family (plus end) Myosin VI (minus end)	Kinesin family (plus end) Dynein family (minus end) Unconventional kinesins (minus end)
Example of virus transport	–	Vaccinia virus	HSV-1 and adenovirus

that bind and move along actin filaments (usually toward the plus end) with energy generated from ATP hydrolysis. By binding to myosin motors, various cargoes achieve energy-dependent directional movement within the cytoplasm (Kamal and Goldstein 2002; Mermall et al. 1998; Vale and Milligan 2000).

The third major cytoskeletal structure is the microtubule. These hollow 25-nm filaments are constructed from tubulin, a heterodimer formed from the closely related α-tubulin and β-tubulin. Microtubules, like actin filaments, are polarized structures with a rapidly growing, highly dynamic plus end and a more slowly changing minus end that is usually anchored in the microtubule-organizing center (MTOC) (Alberts et al. 1994; Kamal and Goldstein 2002). The molecular motors for microtubules are divided into two families, kinesins and dyneins (Goldstein and Philp 1999; Hirokawa 1998; Kamal and Goldstein 2002; Vale and Milligan 2000). The kinesins bind cargo, either directly or via an intermediate "receptor" protein, and move processively toward the plus end of microtubules utilizing energy liberated by ATP hydrolysis. The dynein family of proteins function analogously but in the reverse direction, allowing transport of cargo toward the minus end of microtubules. The "unconventional" kinesins are the exception to this rule—they transport cargo toward the minus end of microtubules (Goldstein and Philp 1999).

Although the mechanism of cytoplasmic transport for HIV-1 is not well characterized (see below), the transport pathways used by some other viruses have been successfully elucidated (see Table 1). For example, directed retrograde transport along microtubules has been shown for herpes simplex virus 1 (HSV-1). With biochemical, pharmacological, and microscopy techniques, incoming HSV-1 capsids were shown to colocalize with cellular dynein and move toward the minus end of microtubules (Sodeik et al. 1997). It has also been shown that adenovirus is transported along microtubules by dyneins after entry into the cytoplasm (Leopold et al. 2000).

Viruses such as SV40 and vesicular stomatitis virus (VSV) take advantage of the actin cortex to facilitate viral endocytosis and entry. Transport of endocytic vesicles (containing the incoming virus particles) and delivery to specialized intracellular environments may be critical for the life cycle of these viruses (Kasamatsu and Nakanishi 1998; Marsh 2000; Sodeik 2000; Whittaker 1996; Apodaca 2001; Pelkmans et al. 2002). The use of actin microfilaments for cytoplasmic transport appears to be less well characterized than microtubule-based transport. One notable example of actin microfilament-based transport occurs late in the life cycle of vaccinia virus. The cell-associated enveloped vaccinia virus (VV CEV) exploits rapid actin filament polymerisation close to the plasma membrane to propel viral particles away from infected cells and to facilitate aims spread (Reitdorf et al. 2001).

1.3
Brief Overview of Nuclear Import Machinery

The defining feature of all eukaryotic cells is the presence of the nucleus. The contents of the nucleus are physically separated from the cytoplasm by the nuclear envelope (NE). Formed by two distinct lipid membrane bilayers with a small internal lumen, the NE prevents unregulated mixing of nuclear and cytoplasmic contents. The outer layer and lumen of the NE are contiguous with the endoplasmic reticulum (ER). The inner layer is separate from the ER and distinct in composition. The primary gatekeepers for entry or exit of proteins and nucleic acids across the NE are the NPCs, large multiprotein structures that stud the NE. Reflecting the activity state of the cell, the exact number of NPCs in the nucleus is not fixed but ranges between 3,000 and 5,000 for a proliferating human cell (Görlich and Kutay 1999). The estimated size of the NPC is ~125 MDa; it is formed from multiple copies of ~50–100 different protein subunits (known as nucleoporins) (Reichelt et al. 1990). The structure of the NPC complex is well characterized with eightfold symmetry around the axis formed perpendicular to the plane of the NE (Hinshaw et al. 1992). Both the inner and outer faces of the NPC have an additional ring structure with long fibrils that extend into the nucleus and cytoplasm, respectively. The distal ends of the nuclear fibrils interact with an additional ring structure, known as the nuclear basket (Goldberg and Allen 1992). A single opening in the NPC complex allows both diffusion of small molecules and active transport of larger proteins. This new model of the NPC proposes that the central pore is lined with the hydrophobic, phenylalanine-rich faces of the nucleoporins forming a lipophilic mesh (Ribbeck and Görlich 2001).

Several excellent and detailed reviews on nucleocytoplasmic transport have been published (Bayliss et al. 2000; Görlich and Kutay 1999; Kasamatsu and Nakanishi 1998; Mattaj and Englmeier 1998; Nakielny and Dreyfuss 1999). Therefore, this introduction only briefly outlines the pathways of nuclear import. Proteins and nucleic acids may enter the nucleus via the NPC by one of two different known pathways. First, a molecule may enter the nucleus by passive diffusion. This method of nuclear import is possible for particles less than ~9 nm (approximately the size of a ~50- to 60-kDa globular protein). However, passive diffusion is only efficient for molecules much smaller (<20–30 kDa) than this upper limit (Görlich and Kutay 1999). This pathway of nuclear transport may be enhanced by a process termed facilitated diffusion whereby the molecule binds a "carrier" protein after transiting through the NPC, effectively removing it from the population of "free" molecules and maintaining a higher apparent concentration gradient.

The second method is signal-mediated transport and is more pertinent to viral import (see Fig. 1) (Fouchier and Malim 1999). Most imported proteins contain nuclear localization signals (NLSs), often characterized by a clustering of basic amino acids, that bind an import receptor. The import receptor, together with its cargo, interacts with the NPC and is transported into the nucleus. Once inside the nucleus, the import receptor dissociates from its cargo and is transported back through the NPC to the cytoplasm. The directionality of nuclear trans-

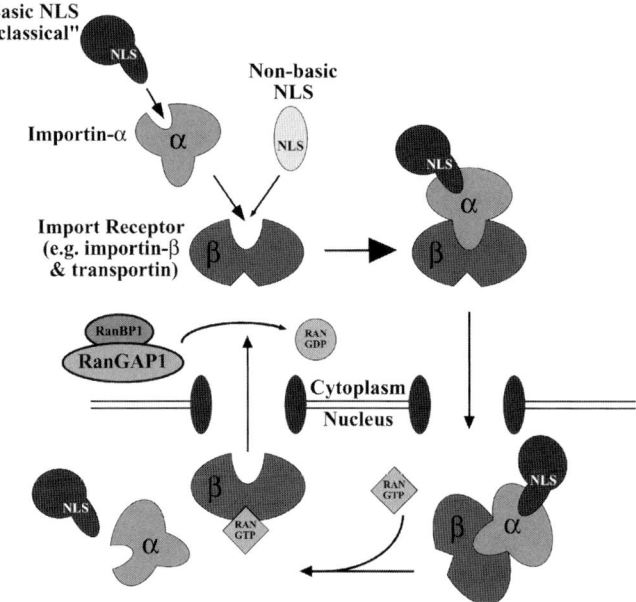

Fig. 1 Nuclear import pathway. In the cytoplasm, the import receptor binds NLS-containing proteins either directly or via the adapter protein, importin-α. The classic import pathway for basic NLSs requires importin-α. The binary or ternary complex is imported into the nucleus via the NPC. Once inside the nucleus, import receptor binding to Ran-GTP causes the complex to dissociate and release its cargo. The Ran-GTP/import receptor complex is exported through the NPC. In the cytoplasm again, RanGAP1 and RanBP1 activate Ran-GTP hydrolysis. The import receptor, after dissociation of Ran, is available for another round of import

port is provided by the Ran-GTP/Ran-GDP gradient. Import receptors release their cargo in the presence of Ran-GTP, and export receptors only bind their cargo in the presence of Ran-GTP. Ran, a small GTPase protein, is present in the cytoplasm and nucleus almost exclusively in the Ran-GDP and Ran-GTP forms, respectively. The intrinsic GTP-hydrolysis rate of Ran-GTP is very slow, and efficient hydrolysis only occurs in the presence of RanGAP, which increases enzymatic efficiency ~100,000-fold (Bischoff et al. 1994, 1995a; Klebe et al. 1995). Interaction with the Ran-binding protein RanBP1 increases this hydrolysis rate by an additional order of magnitude (Bischoff et al. 1995b). Both RanGAP1 and RanBP1 are located exclusively in the cytoplasm. Additionally, the intrinsic exchange rate of GTP for GDP is slow. However, the rate is increased nearly 100,000-fold by the exchange factor RCC1, which is located primarily inside the nucleus (Klebe et al. 1995). The differential localization of the exchange factors and GTPase-activating proteins maintains the Ran-GTP/Ran-GDP gradient, thus providing the energy to drive repeated active cycles of nuclear import and export (Görlich and Kutay 1999). Although the size limit for active nuclear transport was previously reported as ~26 nm, a recent study has suggested that the absolute size restriction for signal-mediated nuclear import of a rigid substrate (specifically, NLS-coated gold beads) is ~39 nm (Dworetzky and Feldherr 1988; Pante and Kann 2002).

Two examples of protein nuclear import are outlined to emphasize common themes. One, the NLS of the HIV-1 Rev protein, has been shown to bind directly to the importin-β import receptor (Henderson and Percipalle 1997; Truant and Cullen 1999). This binary complex then docks at the NPC via nucleoporin/importin-β interactions and is transported into the nucleus. Once inside the nucleus, importin-β binds to Ran-GTP and causes Rev to be released. The nuclear import of the SV40 large T antigen is similar but requires an additional factor, importin-α This pathway is used by many basic-type NLSs and is often termed the "classic pathway." Here, the NLS binds directly to importin-α, which, in turn, binds importin-β to form a trimeric complex that docks at the NPC and is transported into the nucleus. As above, the complex releases the SV40 large T antigen cargo after binding Ran-GTP inside the nucleus (Mattaj and Englmeier 1998).

Several published studies have attempted to identify the factors required for the nuclear import of the HIV-1 PIC. Although it is clear that the PIC must cross the intact NE in nondividing cells, and it is assumed that this passage occurs via the NPC, neither the mechanism nor the exact protein and nucleic acid requirements have been defined. The second half of this review focuses on the current status of research on HIV-1 PIC nuclear import.

2
Uncoating and Cytoplasmic Transport of HIV-1

2.1
Bioactivity of Incoming Virions

After entry into the cytoplasm, the incoming viral particle is not inert. Proteins packaged within the virion may have direct biological effects on the target cell (Poon et al. 1998; Subbramanian et al. 1998; Turelli et al. 2001; Wu and Marsh 2001). For instance, Vpr has been shown to arrest target cells at the G_2/M phase of the cell cycle, and it was reported that the amount of Vpr delivered into the cytoplasm by incoming virions can be sufficient to induce this effect (Poon et al. 1998). A recent study suggested that virion-delivered Vpr can also cause transient disruptions in the nuclear envelope and that this ability correlates with its cell cycle arrest activity (de Noronha et al. 2001). Additionally, cellular kinases have been identified within the virion, and it is possible that these kinases alter the activation state of the target cell (Jacqué et al. 1998; Sawai et al. 1994, 1996).

A second mechanism by which incoming virions may directly affect the target cell is by recruiting cellular proteins to the PIC. One protein reported to interact with the incoming HIV-1 PIC is the integrase-interacting protein Ini1 (Kalpana et al. 1994). This protein is a member of the Swi/Snf family of chromatin remodeling proteins and has been shown to shuttle in and out of the nucleus (i.e., it contains both a NLS and nuclear export signal) and to be packaged into HIV-1 virions (Craig et al. 2002; Yung et al. 2001). A recent study demonstrated a rapid and transient relocalization of Ini1 and another nuclear protein, PML, from the nucleus to the cytoplasm after HIV-1 infection (Turelli et al. 2001). Both Ini1 and PML were shown to colocalize with the incoming PIC. However, the authors suggested that this interaction was inhibitory for HIV-1 infection and therefore may not be acting to augment PIC transport. Whether Ini1 plays a role in the cytoplasmic transport or nuclear import of HIV-1 PICs is still unknown.

Unintegrated viral cDNAs provide a third mechanism for incoming virions to affect the target cell. These effects occur after uncoating and reverse transcription but before integration. For example, low-level expression of Nef from unintegrated viral cDNAs was shown to alter the activation state of resting $CD4^+$ T cells (Wu and Marsh 2001). Additionally, one study suggested that unintegrated viral cDNAs themselves can cause apoptosis (Li et al. 2001). Although the experiments in these studies were conducted with large inocula, it remains likely that the biological status of a cell changes shortly after challenge with HIV-1 virions (Corbeil et al. 2001).

2.2
Uncoating

The interaction of HIV-1 envelope proteins with the cognate receptors on target cells has been extensively studied (see Pierson and Doms, this volume; Berger et al. 1999). However, the events that occur immediately after membrane fusion and deposition of the HIV-1 core into the cytoplasm are not well understood. It is widely believed that the incoming viral core must partially disassemble to allow reverse transcription and cytoplasmic transport and that this uncoating process is critical for the successful completion of infection.

For this review, the term "uncoating" refers to the process of shedding viral or cellular proteins that are delivered into the cytoplasm by the incoming virion. Current evidence suggests that both viral and cellular proteins are involved in the process of uncoating and that uncoating may actually represent a continuum of steps as the PIC evolves into its final nuclear form (see Sect. 3.1). The Gag polyprotein (p55^{Gag}) that is assembled into progeny virions is processed during maturation by the viral protease, generating matrix (MA), capsid (CA), nucleocapsid (NC), p6, and other smaller peptides. MA associates with the inner face of the viral membrane, capsid (CA) forms the cone-shaped core surrounding the viral RNA, and NC interacts with the viral RNA (Freed 1998). Thus the same proteins that direct viral egress and budding must also facilitate uncoating and transport toward the nucleus during infection.

In addition to the early and organized dissociation of CA from the PIC (see Sect. 3.1 for a discussion of PIC composition), two viral accessory proteins may aid uncoating—Nef and Vif (Kotov et al. 1999; Ohagen and Gabuzda 2000). Although Nef is not absolutely required for viral replication in vitro, Δ*nef* viruses are attenuated in vivo (Fultz et al. 2001; Kestler et al. 1991; Kirchhoff et al. 1995; Piguet and Trono 1999). Nef is a 27-kDa myristoylated protein for which multiple functions, including downmodulation of a number of cell surface proteins and interaction with cellular signaling proteins, have been ascribed (Geyer et al.

2001; Piguet and Trono 1999). The infectivity defect observed with Δ*nef* viruses occurs after entry and before the completion of reverse transcription (Schwartz et al. 1995). The timing of this replicative inefficiency is suggestive of a defect in viral uncoating. Moreover, if the virus is manipulated to enter the cell via late endosomes (by pseudotyping with the envelope protein from vesicular stomatitis virus, VSV-G), wild-type infectivity is restored (Aiken 1997). This suggests that the environment of late endosomes may compensate for the absence of Nef-induced uncoating effects. As viruses with deletions in Nef still replicate, the role of Nef in virus uncoating can only be described as modulatory and not mandatory.

A second viral accessory protein that may be important for uncoating is Vif. Vif-deficient viruses fail to replicate and are debilitated in the synthesis and/or the accumulation of reverse transcripts in target cells (Courcoul et al. 1995; Simon and Malim 1996; von Schwedler et al. 1993). Although Vif evidently functions in virus-producing cells to suppress the activity of host cell antiviral genes e.g. CEM15/APOBEC3G (Sheehy et al. 2002), the deficiency of Δ*vif* virions in early postentry steps suggests that Vif's role is to ensure that viruses are assembled correctly and that they can uncoat and function properly in target cells. Consistent with this model, Vif has been shown to increase the stability of the viral core (Ohagen and Gabuzda 2000), and it remains possible that this reflects a "priming" event that facilitates proper uncoating within the target cell.

The most promising cellular factor identified thus far that may contribute to viral uncoating is cyclophilin A (CypA). CypA, a ubiquitous member of the cyclophilin family of peptidyl-prolyl isomerases, is the cellular binding protein for the potent immunosuppressive agent cyclosporin A (CsA) (Handschumacher et al. 1984). CypA is efficiently packaged into HIV-1 virions (approximately one copy of CypA per ten Gag molecules) through a direct interaction with the CA portion of Gag (Gamble et al. 1996; Luban et al. 1993). This interaction can be prevented by mutations in the CypA-binding site in CA, the glycine-proline dipeptide at codons 88 and 89, or by the presence of CsA during virus assembly (Braaten et al. 1996; Franke et al. 1994).

Somewhat reminiscent of Δ*nef* and Δ*vif* viruses, budding, Gag processing, RNA incorporation, and endogenous reverse transcription activity are normal for the CypA-deficient viruses, but infectivity and viral cDNA production are greatly reduced (Braaten et al. 1996). More recently, Luban and colleagues generated a CypA-null cell line by homologous recombination (Braaten and Luban 2001). As would be anticipated, replication of wild-type virus in this cell line was severely decreased, mutations that disrupted CypA binding had no additional deleterious effects on replication, and viruses with compensatory mutations in Gag that confer resistance to CsA replicated efficiently (Braaten and Luban 2001). Given its tight association with CA, a likely role for CypA in uncoating and CA removal is envisioned (Luban 1996). As is the case for Δnef viruses, utilization of the VSV-G envelope protein for viral entry restores the infectivity of virus produced in the presence of CsA to wild-type levels. However, VSV-G-mediated entry does not restore the infectivity of virus with a mutation at glycine 88 (which prevents CypA binding) (Aiken 1997), and an explanation for the discordance of these results is awaited. Of note, the role of CypA is fundamentally different from that of Vif because Δvif viruses are not rescued by CA mutations that confer CsA resistance (Yin et al. 1998).

Although one report has demonstrated that CypA is capable of catalyzing the *cis/trans* isomerization of the residue at amino acid 89 (Bosco et al. 2002), another study has shown that this isomerase activity does not appear to be required for the uncoating function (Saphire et al. 2002b). By utilizing fusion proteins between CypA (wild type or catalytic site mutant) and the HIV-1 accessory protein Vpr, it is possible to block the packaging of endogenous CypA by adding CsA and to package mutant (catalytically deficient) CypA *in trans* as a Vpr-fusion. By using this system, it was found that infectivity can be restored to CsA-treated virions but that the isomerase activity of CypA was not required.

Recent studies also invoke a role for CypA in virion assembly. Specifically, when CypA was added at a ratio of 1:10 (CypA:CA), it enhanced the ability of recombinant CA to form "tubes" in vitro. The same result was seen (at significantly higher concentrations of CypA) for tube assembly by one of the mutant forms of CA, G89W. The authors of this study suggest that the primary role of CypA-CA interactions is as a chaperone—preventing "nonproductive" CA-CA interactions (Grattinger et al. 1999). However, the uncoating and assembly models need not be mutually exclusive because correct assembly may allow correct "downstream" disassembly.

A few studies also suggested that CypA functions to enhance viral entry (Pushkarsky et al. 2001; Saphire et al. 1999; Sherry et al. 1998). One of these studies reported that CypA binding to the cellular surface receptor protein CD147 is the critical step mediated by CypA (Pushkarsky et al. 2001). Potentially reconciling these different proposed functions of CypA, one recent study demonstrated distinct roles for CypA during entry and postentry events in the viral life cycle (Saphire et al. 2002a). One final noteworthy point regarding CypA is that the Gag proteins from HIV-2 and SIVmac do not bind CypA and CsA does not inhibit their replication (Luban 1996). HIV-1 and HIV-2 are, however, different viruses, and it is plausible that the details of uncoating are different for each virus.

2.3
Role of Actin Filaments for Cytoplasmic Transport

The cytoplasmic transport of the HIV-1 PIC is one of the least-characterized steps of the viral life cycle. The bulk of research about interactions between the HIV-1 Gag polyprotein (or the Gag cleavage products--MA, CA, NC, and p6) and the cytoskeleton focuses on the role of these interactions as they pertain to viral egress and budding. Several groups have observed binding between Gag and actin filaments (Bukrinskaya et al. 1998; Ibarrondo et al. 2001; Liu et al. 1999; Wilk et al. 1999). Additionally, both actin and multiple actin-binding proteins were found to be packaged into virions (Ott et al. 2000; Ott et al. 1996).

Two studies have addressed the role of actin filaments during viral entry, uncoating, and cytoplasmic transport (Bukrinskaya et al. 1998; Iyengar et al. 1998). Stevenson and colleagues reported that the PIC tightly associates with the actin cytoskeleton after infection. Furthermore, the specificity and strength of this interaction is due to the binding of MA and actin filaments. When cytochalasin D (cyto D), an inhibitor of actin polymerization, was used to interfere with the MA-actin interaction during viral challenge, the accumulation of late viral cDNAs, but not early ones, was decreased 25-fold. This suggests an early role for interaction with the actin cytoskeleton during uncoating, perhaps as a means of facilitating penetration through the actin cortex. The finding that cyto D fails to block productive infection when added 1 h after challenge is consistent with such a model. Interestingly, the large infectivity defect observed in cyto D-treated cells could be overcome by VSV-G pseudotyping, suggesting that the microfilament requirement could be avoided by virions entering the cytoplasm via the endosome (Bukrinskaya et al. 1998).

Schwartz and colleagues reported that the virion output after challenge of peripheral blood mononuclear cells (PBMCs) pretreated with cyto D was reduced ~95% (Iyengar et al. 1998). Furthermore, this study reported that cyto D treatment prevents the actin-dependent colocalization of CD4 and CXCR4. This result may also help explain the restoration of wild-type infectivity observed with VSV-G-pseudotyped virions because such infections would not require actin-dependent receptor colocalization for entry (Bukrinskaya et al. 1998). In addition to receptor colocalization effects, it has also been proposed that depolymerization of actin filaments can prevent an intracellular signaling event that is required for productive infection (Iyengar et al. 1998).

2.4
Role of Microtubules for Cytoplasmic Transport

Several different classes of viruses are known to travel along microtubules during both the early and late stages of viral infection (Kasamatsu and Nakanishi 1998; Leopold et al. 2000; Tang et al. 1999; Tomishima et al. 2001; Whittaker et al. 2000). The proteins from these viruses interact directly, or via adapter proteins, with cellular kinesins or dyneins to facilitate active, directed transport along the intracellular "highway" system of microtubules. Alternatively, vesicles containing viruses, resulting from either endocytosis or budding into intracellular membranes, may be targeted for microtubule-dependent transport. The Gag proteins from several retroviruses, including HIV-1, have been shown to interact with the kinesin KIF-4 in yeast two-hybrid assays (Kim et al. 1998; Tang et al. 1999). Although the HIV-1 Gag-KIF-4 interaction was confirmed by coimmunoprecipitation from transfected cells, it has not yet been demonstrated in infected cells. Additionally, the functional consequences of the Gag-KIF-4 interaction await determination.

Recent elegant work from Hope and colleagues strongly implicated microtubule-mediated transport during the early stages of HIV-1 infection (McDonald et al. 2002). This group has combined a series of techniques to visualize simultaneously incoming viral particles, newly synthesized reverse transcripts, and different components of the cytoskeleton in real time. In this technique, assembling viral particles are labeled with Vpr-GFP, which then allows direct visualization of incoming virus (Schaeffer et al. 2001). Target cells are microinjected with fluorescently labeled dNTPs to allow the visualization of newly formed reverse transcripts. Finally, the cytoskeleton is labeled by microinjection with fluorescently labeled tubulin. After challenge with GFP-labeled HIV-1 virions, PICs, defined as viral complexes that colocalize with nascent cDNAs, were found to track along microtubules toward the nucleus (T. Hope, personal communication). Microtubules therefore appear to be the most promising candidate for HIV-1 PIC transport from the periphery of the cytoplasm to the region of the nuclear rim.

2.5
Interaction with Virion-Associated Nuclear Shuttling Protein

Using MA as bait for a yeast two-hybrid screen, an interaction with a virion-associated nuclear shuttling protein (VAN) was identified (Gupta et al. 2000). Bacterially expressed VAN was also shown to interact with MA fused to glutathione-S-transferase (GST-MA). The VAN protein was shown to contain both an NLS and a Crm1-dependent nuclear export signal (NES). Finally, VAN was found to be incorporated into HIV-1 virions, and the authors suggest a potential role for VAN in PIC transport and nuclear import (Gupta et al. 2000). The functional significance of this protein interaction is unclear, and role(s) in cytoplasmic transport and/or nuclear import are plausible.

3
Nuclear Import of the HIV-1 PIC

3.1
The HIV-1 PIC: Size and Components

The HIV-1 PIC is a dynamic entity that changes during uncoating, cytoplasmic transport, nuclear import, and transit to the final site of viral cDNA integration. Multiple groups have isolated and analyzed the composition of this large multicomponent complex (Bukrinsky et al. 1992; Farnet and Haseltine 1991; Fassati and Goff 2001; Gallay et al. 1996; Karageorgos et al. 1993; Li et al. 2001; Miller et al. 1997). The PICs isolated in these studies minimally contain the viral proteins MA, reverse transcriptase (RT), integrase (IN), Vpr and varying amounts of cellular proteins including HMG I(Y), importin-α, histones, and the nonhomologous end joining (NHEJ) proteins Ku70 and Ku90 . CA and NC are only observed in limited quantities within the PIC, and the apparent lack of

CA in the PIC sharply contrasts HIV-1 with what has been described for MLV (Bowerman et al. 1989; Miller et al. 1997). Importantly, the PICs also contain the viral nucleic acids—partially digested viral genomic RNA and newly synthesized cDNA (Fassati and Goff 2001). The estimated Stokes radius of the PIC is ~28 nm (Miller et al. 1997). Therefore, the PIC is too large to enter the nucleus by diffusion. Interestingly, the estimated 56-nm diameter of the PIC is larger than the 39-nm maximum dimension for signal-mediated nuclear import (Pante and Kann 2002). Thus a major conformational change or significant shedding of components must occur to reduce its dimensions before transport across the NPC. Supporting this hypothesis, the reported sedimentation velocities for nuclear-associated PICs (~80 S) were smaller than for cytoplasmic PICs (~100–300 S) (Fassati and Goff 2001). It is important to note that the bulk of studies characterizing PICs and their components have been done with cytoplasmic extracts isolated 1–8 h after infection. Because viral proteins have been observed in the nucleus very rapidly after infection (Bouyac-Bertoia et al. 2001; Bukrinskaya et al. 1996; Gallay et al. 1995a), it is not clear which experimental systems have identified bona fide PICs.

As stated above, the ability of HIV-1 to infect nondividing cells has been attributed to karyophilic signals within the PIC (Bukrinsky et al. 1992). Among the candidate viral proteins, MA, IN, and Vpr have all been identified as potential karyophiles (Bouyac-Bertoia et al. 2001; Bukrinsky et al. 1993; Depienne et al. 2000; Fouchier et al. 1998; Gallay et al. 1995a, 1997; Heinzinger et al. 1994; Jenkins et al. 1998; Pluymers et al. 1999; Vodicka et al. 1998). Additionally, the central single-stranded DNA flap generated during reverse transcription has also been implicated as a potential nuclear targeting signal (Zennou et al. 2000). The requirement for, and relative contribution to, nuclear import contributed by each of these signals continue to be controversial. This section of the review examines the evidence for and against each of these potential nuclear targeting signals within the HIV-1 PIC.

3.2
The Role of MA in PIC Nuclear Import

MA is a 17-kDa myristoylated protein that lines the inner side of the viral membrane and is derived from the amino terminus of the Gag polyprotein by cleavage during viral maturation (Freed 1998). MA was the first HIV-1 PIC protein to be assigned NLS activity. In an initial series of reports, disruption of the identified critical region of MA (^{25}GKKKYKLKH), which is similar to the canonical monopartite basic-type NLS, was shown to inhibit selectively viral replication and the nuclear accumulation of viral cDNA in nondividing cells but not in dividing cells (Bukrinsky et al. 1993; Gallay et al. 1995a; von Schwedler et al. 1994). Assignment of NLS activity to this region was reinforced by the observation that microinjected conjugates of bovine serum albumin (BSA) and a synthetic peptide spanning this region were specifically imported into the nucleus. Additionally, the import factor importin-α was shown to interact with MA as well as with the HIV-1 PIC (Gallay et al. 1996; Popov et al. 1998b).

The proposed mechanism that allows this MA-targeting dichotomy— to the plasma membrane during viral budding and to the nucleus during initial infection—is based on differential phosphorylation of MA (Bukrinskaya et al. 1996; Gallay et al. 1995a). According to this model, the MA component of Gag targets the polyprotein to the plasma membrane after translation. At a subsequent point, a portion of the MA molecules are phosphorylated (serine, threonine, and tyrosine phosphorylation have all been described), and this triggers a conformational switch allowing the retargeting of the protein to the nucleus (Bukrinskaya et al. 1996; Gallay et al. 1995a). Additionally, phosphorylation of the carboxy-terminal tyrosine residue has been reported to induce binding to IN and to facilitate infection of nondividing cells (Gallay et al. 1995b), although other groups did not see these effects (Bukrinskaya et al. 1996; Freed et al. 1997).

Additional studies have questioned the absolute requirement for MA for infection of nondividing cells (Fouchier et al. 1997; Freed et al. 1995; Reil et al. 1998). One study using multiple experimental approaches (transfection and microinjection) failed to detect a transferable NLS activity in the amino-terminal region of MA. Viruses with the ^{26}KK→TT mutations in MA were found to have a relatively modest and generalized replication defect in dividing and nondividing cells, as opposed to a defect that was exclusive to nondividing cells (Fouchier et al. 1997; Freed et al. 1995). A molecular basis for these results was suggested by the manifestation of a Gag-processing defect in the MA-mutant viruses (Fouchier et al. 1997). Finally, it was demonstrated not only that the basic region of MA was not required for infection of nondividing cells but that the entire globular domain of MA was dispensable (Reil et al. 1998).

3.3
The Role of Vpr in PIC Nuclear Import

The next protein from the HIV-1 PIC that was found to promote nuclear import was Vpr, a small accessory protein that is packaged into virions through a specific interaction with the p6 region of Gag (Checroune et al. 1995; Jenkins et al. 2001; Lu et al. 1995; Paxton et al. 1993). Viruses with disruptions in the *vpr* gene replicate less efficiently than wild-type viruses, and this defect is observed more profoundly in nondividing cells (Balliet et al. 1994; Connor et al. 1995; Eckstein et al. 2001; Fouchier et al. 1998; Freed et al. 1995; Heinzinger et al. 1994; Vodicka et al. 1998). When expressed in isolation, Vpr clearly accumulates in the nucleus (Fouchier et al. 1998). More importantly, heterologous fusion proteins of Vpr with maltose binding protein (MBP) or β-galactosidase (β-GAL) relocalize from the cytoplasm to the nucleus (Fouchier et al. 1998; Jenkins et al. 1998). Although not well defined, the mechanism of nuclear import of Vpr alone is somewhat unusual in that importin-α, importin-β, and the Ran system appear to be dispensable and Vpr itself interacts with nucleoporins (Fouchier et al. 1998; Jenkins et al. 1998; Popov et al. 1996, 1998a; Vodicka et al. 1998).

Although multiple studies have shown that Vpr contains a transferable NLS, the role of this activity in PIC nuclear import is less well defined. Viruses harboring disruptions in Vpr still infect nondividing cells (Balliet et al. 1994; Bouyac-Bertoia et al. 2001; Connor et al. 1995; Eckstein et al. 2001; Fouchier et al. 1998; Freed et al. 1995; Heinzinger et al. 1994; Vodicka et al. 1998). Therefore, the potential enhancement of PIC import imparted by Vpr, like MA, can only be modulatory and not required. It is important to note that viruses with combined disruptions in MA and Vpr still replicate in nondividing cells (Freed et al. 1995; Gallay et al. 1997). Furthermore, the delayed replication kinetics can be masked when target cells are infected at a high multiplicity of infection (MOI) (Gallay et al. 1997). Additionally, Vpr has been shown to possess other activities including cell cycle arrest and mild transactivation of transcription from the viral LTR (Felzien et al. 1998; Goh et al. 1998; Kino et al. 1999; Subbramanian et al. 1998; Wang et al. 1995). The relative contributions of each of these activities to the replicative defects observed for Δvpr viruses have yet to be segregated and defined.

3.4
The Role of IN in PIC Nuclear Import

The 32-kDa viral enzyme IN is absolutely required for efficient viral replication, catalyzing the enzymatic joining of the reverse-transcribed viral cDNA to the host cell genome (Brown 1997). Consequently, IN must be associated with the PIC during all steps leading up to and including integration. The IN protein also contributes to the efficiency of reverse transcription, most likely by serving a structural role to enhance the RT complex (Wu et al. 1999). Given that viruses with disruptions in both MA and Vpr can still replicate in nondividing cells, it has been presumed that additional karyophilic signals must exist in the PIC; IN has since been identified by several groups as a karyophilic protein (Depienne et al. 2000, 2001; Gallay et al. 1997; Pluymers et al. 1999).

The first study to identify the karyophilic properties of IN reported that two stretches of basic amino acids (^{186}KRK and ^{211}KELKQKQITK) were critical for interaction with importin-α and nuclear localization of the PIC (Gallay et al. 1997). Consistent with this finding, microinjection of a GST-IN fusion protein was found to localize to the nucleus. Furthermore, when cells were challenged with a triply mutated virus, lacking the basic domain of MA, Vpr, and IN, PIC components remained in the cytoplasm (Gallay et al. 1997). Although suggestive of an important role in PIC localization, the analysis of these mutations is complicated by their impact on other critical functions of IN. Specifically, disruption of these basic amino acid sequences alters the ability of IN to multimerize (Petit et al. 2000). One study reported that GFP-IN fusion proteins were primarily located in the nucleus of transfected cells and that disruption of the ^{186}KRK basic patch did not alter the nuclear localization of the fusion protein in this experimental system (Tsurutani et al. 2000).

Recent work from our laboratory identified a valine-arginine dipeptide motif at residues 165 and 166 of IN that is required for productive infection of dividing or nondividing cells (Bouyac-Bertoia et al. 2001). The stretch of amino acids from residues 161 to 173 was initially ascribed NLS activity. Although amino acid substitutions in the dipeptide motif alter the subcellular localization of virion-delivered IN during the early stages of infection, we now know that this region is not a transferable NLS (Dvorin et al. 2002). We demonstrated that V165A mutant viruses are blocked at a step in the life cycle after viral cDNA synthesis and before integration, with a modest decrease in the nuclear accumulation of viral cDNAs being observed (Limón et al. 2002a). Furthermore, the V165A IN protein, when supplied in *trans*, was able to restore infectivity to a virus harboring a catalytically dead IN protein, a finding that indicates that V165A IN has full catalytic function and is likely to be in the correct conformation. Possible explanations for why the V165A viral cDNA that reaches the nucleus fails to integrate (Bouyac-Bertoia et al. 2001) include this particular virus being defective for a postulated postnuclear entry trafficking step (see below for more discussion) or this IN protein being inactive in a manner that is not reflected in current assays.

The nuclear import pathway of IN, like that of Vpr, appears to be unusual (Depienne et al. 2001). Nuclear import of BSA conjugated to full-length IN did not require importin-α, importin-β, or GTP-hydrolysis by Ran and could not be competed with the NLSs of T antigen or hnRNP-A1; nuclear accumulation did, however, require ATP hydrolysis. Consistent with the notion that IN contains an NLS, recent work from the Muesing laboratory identified a potential NLS within the carboxy-terminal domain of IN. However, mutations that disrupt this putative NLS and decrease the nuclear accumulation of viral cDNAs also have deleterious effects on the early stages of reverse transcription (M. Muesing, personal communication).

3.5
Role of the DNA flap in PIC import

During HIV-1 reverse transcription, the synthesis of the positive cDNA strand occurs from two different primers. The upstream segment is initiated at the 3' poly-purine tract (PPT), and the downstream segment is initiated at the central poly-purine tract (cPPT). While displacing the downstream strand, synthesis of the upstream segment continues for 99 nucleotides after the cPPT until the viral RT complex stops at the central termination sequence (CTS). The resulting full-length viral cDNA therefore contains a central triple-stranded region of DNA, known as the DNA flap (Zennou et al. 2000). If the cPPT is disrupted, reverse transcription still occurs, but with the resulting cDNA containing a single, continuous, full-length positive strand.

Recent analyses of a virus carrying an inactivated cPPT (cPPT-D) reported a profound loss of infectivity and replication in both dividing and nondividing cells (Zennou et al. 2000). Viral cDNA synthesis occurred efficiently, but a substantial decrease in the nuclear forms of the viral cDNAs (LTR-circles) was observed suggesting a defect in nuclear import. Finally, fluorescence *in situ* hybridization (FISH) analysis of the viral cDNA confirmed the decrease in nuclear accumulation (Zennou et al. 2000). The contribution of the cPPT to efficient infection has been demonstrated for lentiviral vectors, where the presence of the cPPT increases transduction efficiency in nondividing cells (Dardalhon et al. 2001; Follenzi et al. 2000; Sirven et al. 2000; Zennou et al. 2000).

The critical requirement of the DNA flap for nuclear import has been challenged by recent work from both our and the Engelman laboratories (Dvorin et al. 2002; Limón et al. 2002b). We found that disruption of the cPPT in either the X4-tropic virus, HIV_{LA1}, or the R5-tropic virus, HIV_{YU-2}, had little effect on infection or replication in proliferating T cell lines or on the localization of the viral cDNA as measured by FISH. Although the HIV_{YU-2} cPPT-D virus was shown to replicate in PBMCs and monocyte-derived macrophages (MDMs) with modestly attenuated kinetics, the virus was still clearly infectious. It is possible that the increased replication efficiency of wild type viruses over cPPT-D viruses in primary cells may explain the improved transduction efficiency observed for cPPT-containing lentiviral vectors, though the molecular basis for this effect remains to be characterized. The basis for the inconsistencies over the importance of the cPPT to HIV-1 infection is not yet known.

4
Conclusions

The ability of HIV-1 to infect nondividing cells productively is presumed to be central to viral transmission and pathogenesis. After viral entry, the HIV-1 PIC must uncoat, move through the cytoplasm to the nucleus, enter the nucleus, and reach its final site of integration. Developing strategies to inhibit these steps of the HIV-1 life cycle may provide new therapeutic options for the treatment of HIV-1-infected individuals.

The early stages of the viral life cycle (after entry) have not been extensively studied, but some insightful reports do exist. CypA appears to be a critical factor for viral uncoating, and recent work from Hope and colleagues may provide new tools to understand both uncoating and cytoplasmic transport. It is interesting to note that viruses pseudotyped with VSV-G that enter the cell through the endosomal pathway are able to overcome Δ*nef* mutations as well as treatment with CsA or cyto D. These observations suggest that endosomal entry can act as a surrogate for the roles of Nef, CypA, and actin microfilaments and that each of these factors contributes to early events.

Although many published reports have examined the mechanism and requirements for PIC nuclear import, this aspect of the life cycle remains riddled with uncertainties and controversy. The apparent failure to identify a discrete, transferable NLS that is required for infection of nondividing cells, but is dispensable for infection of dividing cells, suggests that PIC nuclear import is complicated. One view is that the PIC contains multiple, potentially redundant, nuclear import signals that allow efficient movement of the PIC into the nucleus. Alternatively, nuclear targeting may be determined by a combination of multiple viral and cellular proteins (or factors) or by PIC proteins acting merely to recruit cellular proteins that contain the required localization signals. We also consider it possible that transport through the NPC constitutes a required step in the viral life cycle in both dividing and nondividing cells.

The findings of our laboratory suggest that there may be additional step(s) in replication between PIC nuclear import and integration. In particular, using methods that include FISH, we have observed that the viral cDNA from IN V165A mutant viruses reaches the nucleus in the presence of an apparently catalytically active IN protein but fails to integrate (Dvorin et al. 2002). Because this defect is complemented by a catalytically dead IN (D64A) IN protein, we suggested that the V165A IN protein may be deficient in conferring proper intranuclear localization to the PIC (Bouyac-Bertoia et al. 2001). In other words, this final targeting step could place the PIC in a permissive nuclear subenvironment for integration into the host cell genome. In this regard, it was recently established that HIV-1 displays a strong preference for integrating into transcriptionally active regions of the infected cell's genome (Schroder et al. 2002). We have also found that linear plasmid DNA is rapidly end-ligated (a commonly used surrogate marker for nuclear import) after transfection of cell cycle-arrested cells, a result that suggests linear DNAs can be rapidly imported into the nucleus in the absence of HIV-1 proteins or cell division (Dvorin et al. 2002). It is most likely that the nuclear import of such DNA occurs with the help of cellular NLS-bearing DNA binding proteins, although it is also possible that import may be direct (Salman et al. 2001; Wilson et al. 1999). A provocative interpretation of this result is that no viral sequences are needed for HIV-1 DNA

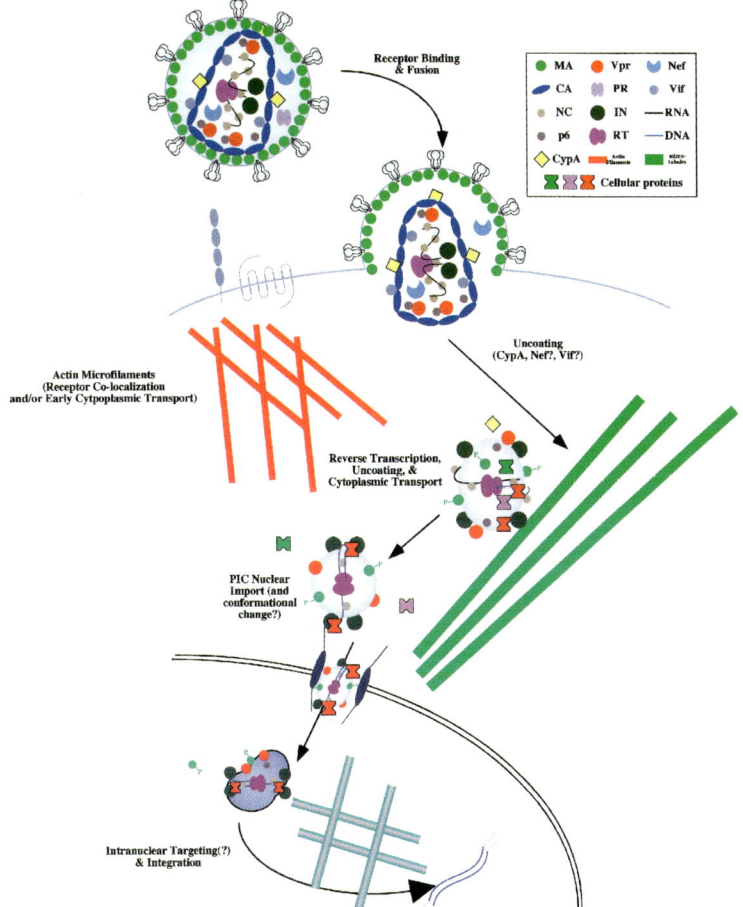

Fig. 2 Model for early steps in HIV-1 life cycle. After binding and membrane fusion, the viral core is released into the cytoplasm. A series of uncoating steps follow, involving actin microfilaments, Nef, and CypA, and lead to the removal of CA and preparation of the PIC for reverse transcription. During or after this step, the PIC is transported along microtubules toward the nucleus. The PIC, together with cellular proteins, interacts with the NPC, promoting active nuclear import, further uncoating or "trimming," and "priming" for integration. Finally, the PIC is selectively targeted to a permissive site where integration occurs, thus completing the first half of the viral life cycle

nuclear import other than the ability of PIC nucleic acids to associate "nonspecifically" with cellular karyophiles; the validity of such a model requires future testing. Should this hypothesis be borne out, an explanation for the restriction of productive MLV infection to proliferating cells would be required.

Synthesizing all of the information presented in this review, we propose the following model for the early steps of the viral life cycle (see Fig. 2). After entry of the viral core into the cytoplasm, a series of uncoating steps occur that appear to involve actin microfilaments, as well as the virion proteins Nef and CypA, and lead to the removal of CA and preparation of the PIC for reverse transcription. During or after this step, the PIC is transported along microtubules toward the nucleus. The PIC, together with cellular proteins, interacts with the NPC, promoting active nuclear import as well as possible further uncoating or "trimming" and "priming" for integration. Once inside the nucleus, the PIC is then selectively targeted to a permissive chromosomal site where appropriate integration occurs, thus completing the first half of the viral life cycle.

Acknowledgements. We thank Tom Hope, Mark Muesing, and Alan Engelman for generously discussing unpublished work from their laboratories and Seeta Badrinath for editorial assistance. Work in this laboratory is supported by NIH Research Grants and NIH Training Grants (GM-07170 and AI-07632). M.H.M. is an Elizabeth Glaser Scientist supported by the Elizabeth Glaser Pediatric AIDS Foundation.

References

Aiken, C. (1997). J Virol 71, 5871–5877
Alberts, B., Bray, D., Lewis, J., Raff, M., Roberts, K., and Watson, J. D. (1994). Molecular Biology of the Cell – Third Edition (R. Adams, ed.). Garland Publishing, Inc., New York
Balliet, J. W., Kolson, D. L., Eiger, G., Kim, F. M., McGann, K. A., Srinivasan, A., and Collman, R. (1994). Virology 200, 623–631
Bayliss, R., Corbett, A. H., and Stewart, M. (2000). Traffic 1, 448–456
Berger, E. A., Murphy, P. M., and Farber, J. M. (1999). Annu Rev Immunol 17, 657–700
Bischoff, F. R., Klebe, C., Kretschmer, J., Wittinghofer, A., and Ponstingl, H. (1994). Proc Natl Acad Sci USA 91, 2587–2591
Bischoff, F. R., Krebber, H., Kempf, T., Hermes, I., and Ponstingl, H. (1995a). Proc Natl Acad Sci USA 92, 1749–1753

Bischoff, F. R., Krebber, H., Smirnova, E., Dong, W., and Ponstingl, H. (1995b). EMBO J 14, 705-715

Bosco, D. A., Eisenmesser, E. Z., Pochapsky, S., Sundquist, W. I., and Kern, D. (2002). Proc Natl Acad Sci USA 99, 5247-5252

Bouyac-Bertoia, M., Dvorin, J. D., Fouchier, R. A., Jenkins, Y., Meyer, B. E., Wu, L. I., Emerman, M., and Malim, M. H. (2001). Mol Cell 7, 1025-1035

Bowerman, B., Brown, P. O., Bishop, J. M., and Varmus, H. E. (1989). Genes Dev 3, 469-478

Braaten, D., Franke, E. K., and Luban, J. (1996). J Virol 70, 3551-3560

Braaten, D., and Luban, J. (2001). EMBO J 20, 1300-1309

Brown, P. O. (1997). Integration. In "Retroviruses" (J. M. Coffin, S. H. Hughes and H. E. Varmus, eds.), pp. 161-203. Cold Spring Harbor Laboratory Press, Plainview, New York

Bukrinskaya, A., Brichacek, B., Mann, A., and Stevenson, M. (1998). J Exp Med 188, 2113-2125

Bukrinskaya, A. G., Ghorpade, A., Heinzinger, N. K., Smithgall, T. E., Lewis, R. E., and Stevenson, M. (1996). Proc Natl Acad Sci USA 93, 367-371

Bukrinsky, M. I., Haggerty, S., Dempsey, M. P., Sharova, N., Adzhubei, A., Spitz, L., Lewis, P., Goldfarb, D., Emerman, M., and Stevenson, M. (1993). Nature 365, 666-669

Bukrinsky, M. I., Sharova, N., Dempsey, M. P., Stanwick, T. L., Bukrinskaya, A. G., Haggerty, S., and Stevenson, M. (1992). Proc Natl Acad Sci USA 89, 6580-6584

Checroune, F., Yao, X. J., Gottlinger, H. G., Bergeron, D., and Cohen, E. A. (1995). J AIDS Hum Retrovirol 10, 1-7

Connor, R. I., Chen, B. K., Choe, S., and Landau, N. R. (1995). Virology 206, 935-944

Corbeil, J., Sheeter, D., Genini, D., Rought, S., Leoni, L., Du, P., Ferguson, M., Masys, D. R., Welsh, J. B., Fink, J. L., Sasik, R., Huang, D., Drenkow, J., Richman, D. D., and Gingeras, T. (2001). Genome Res 11, 1198-204

Courcoul, M., Patience, C., Rey, F., Blanc, D., Harmache, A., Sire, J., Vigne, R., and Spire, B. (1995). J.Virol 69 2068-2074

Craig, E., Zhang, Z. K., Davies, K. P., and Kalpana, G. V. (2002). EMBO J 21, 31-42

Dardalhon, V., Herpers, B., Noraz, N., Pflumio, F., Guetard, D., Leveau, C., Dubart-Kupperschmitt, A., Charneau, P., and Taylor, N. (2001). Gene Ther 8 190-198

De Noronha, C. M., Sherman, M. P., Lin, H. W., Cavrois, M. V., Moir, R. D., Goldman, R. D., and Greene, W. C. (2001). Science 294, 1105-8

Depienne, C., Mousnier, A., Leh, H., Le Rouzic, E., Dormont, D., Benichou, S., and Dargemont, C. (2001). J Biol Chem 276, 18102-7

Depienne, C., Roques, P., Creminon, C., Fritsch, L., Casseron, R., Dormont, D., Dargemont, C., and Benichou, S. (2000). Exp Cell Res 260, 387-395

Dvorin, J. D., Bell, P., Maul, G. G., Yamashita, M., Emerman, M., and Malim, M. H. (2002). J Virol 76, 12087-12096

Dworetzky, S. I., and Feldherr, C. M. (1988). J Cell Biol 106, 575-584

Eckstein, D. A., Sherman, M. P., Penn, M. L., Chin, P. S., De Noronha, C. M., Greene, W. C., and Goldsmith, M. A. (2001). J Exp Med 194, 1407-19

Farnet, C. M., and Haseltine, W. A. (1991). J.Virol 65 1910-1915

Fassati, A., and Goff, S. P. (2001). J Virol 75, 3626-3635

Felzien, L. K., Woffendin, C., Hottiger, M. O., Subbramanian, R. A., Cohen, E. A., and Nabel, G. J. (1998). Proc Natl Acad Sci USA 95, 5281–5286
Follenzi, A., Ailles, L. E., Bakovic, S., Geuna, M., and Naldini, L. (2000). Nat Genet 25, 217–222
Fouchier, R. A. M., and Malim, M. H. (1999). Adv Virus Res 52, 275–299
Fouchier, R. A. M., Meyer, B. E., Simon, J. H. M., Fischer, U., Albright, A. V., González-Scarano, F., and Malim, M. H. (1998). J. Virol 72, 6004–6013
Fouchier, R. A. M., Meyer, B. E., Simon, J. H. M., Fischer, U., and Malim, M. H. (1997). EMBO J. 16, 4531–4539
Franke, E. K., Yuan, H. E., and Luban, J. (1994). Nature 372, 359–362
Freed, E. O. (1998). Virology 251, 1–15
Freed, E. O., Englund, G., Maldarelli, F., and Martin, M. A. (1997). Cell 88, 171–174
Freed, E. O., Englund, G., and Martin, M. A. (1995). J Virol 69, 3949–3954
Fultz, P. N., Vance, P. J., Endres, M. J., Tao, B., Dvorin, J. D., Davis, I. C., Lifson, J. D., Montefiori, D. C., Marsh, M., Malim, M. H., and Hoxie, J. A. (2001). J Virol 75, 278–291
Gallay, P., Hope, T., Chin, D., and Trono, D. (1997). Proc Natl Acad Sci USA 94, 9825–9830
Gallay, P., Stitt, V., Mundy, C., Oettinger, M., and Trono, D. (1996). J.Virol 70, 1027–1032
Gallay, P., Swingler, S., Aiken, C., and Trono, D. (1995a). Cell 80, 379–388
Gallay, P., Swingler, S., Song, J., Bushman, F., and Trono, D. (1995b). Cell 83, 569–576
Gamble, T. R., Vajdos, F. F., Yoo, S., Worthylake, D. K., Houseweart, M., Sundquist, W. I., and Hill, C. P. (1996). Cell 87, 1285–1294
Geyer, M., Fackler, O. T., and Peterlin, B. M. (2001). EMBO Rep 2, 580–585
Goh, W. C., Rogel, M. E., Kinsey, C. M., Michael, S. F., Fultz, P. N., Nowak, M. A., Hahn, B. H., and Emerman, M. (1998). Nat Med 4, 65–71
Goldberg, M. W., and Allen, T. D. (1992). J Cell Biol 119, 1429–1440
Goldstein, L. S., and Philp, A. V. (1999). Annu Rev Cell Dev Biol 15, 141–183
Görlich, D., and Kutay, U. (1999). Annu Rev Cell Dev Biol 15, 607–660
Grattinger, M., Hohenberg, H., Thomas, D., Wilk, T., Muller, B., and Krausslich, H. G. (1999). Virology 257, 247–260
Gupta, K., Ott, D., Hope, T. J., Siliciano, R. F., and Boeke, J. D. (2000). J Virol 74, 11811–24
Handschumacher, R. E., Harding, M. W., Rice, J., Drugge, R. J., and Speicher, D. W. (1984). Science 226, 544–547
Hatziioannou, T., and Goff, S. P. (2001). J Virol 75, 9526–9531
Heinzinger, N. K., Bukrinsky, M. I., Haggerty, S. A., Ragland, A. M., Kewalramani, V., Lee, M.-A., Gendelman, H. E., Ratner, L., Stevenson, M., and Emerman, M. (1994). Proc Natl Acad Sci USA 91, 7311–7315
Henderson, B. R., and Percipalle, P. (1997). J Mol Biol 274, 693–707
Hinshaw, J. E., Carragher, B. O., and Milligan, R. A. (1992). Cell 69, 1133–1141
Hirokawa, N. (1998). Science 279, 519–526
Hu, J., Gardner, M. B., and Miller, C. J. (2000). J Virol 74, 6087–6095
Ibarrondo, F. J., Choi, R., Geng, Y. Z., Canon, J., Rey, O., Baldwin, G. C., and Krogstad, P. (2001). AIDS Res Hum Retroviruses 17, 1489–1500
Iyengar, S., Hildreth, J. E., and Schwartz, D. H. (1998). J Virol 72, 5251–5255

Jacqué, J.-M., Mann, A., Sharova, N., Brichacek, B., Enslen, H., Davis, R. J., and Stevenson, M. (1998). EMBO J 17, 2607–2618
Jenkins, Y., McEntee, M., Weis, K., and Greene, W. C. (1998). J Cell Biol 143, 875–885
Jenkins, Y., Pornillos, O., Rich, R. L., Myszka, D. G., Sundquist, W. I., and Malim, M. H. (2001). J Virol 75, 10537–10542
Kalpana, G. V., Marmon, S., Wang, W., Crabtree, G. R., and Goff, S. P. (1994). Science 266 2002–2006
Kamal, A., and Goldstein, L. S. (2002). Curr Opin Cell Biol 14, 63–68
Karageorgos, L., Li, P., and Burrell, C. (1993). AIDS Res Hum Retroviruses 9, 817–823
Kasamatsu, H., and Nakanishi, A. (1998). Annu Rev Microbiol 52, 627–686
Katz, R. A., Greger, J. G., Darby, K., Boimel, P., Rall, G. F., and Skalka, A. M. (2002). J Virol 76, 5422–5434
Kestler, I., H.W., Ringler, D. J., Mori, K., Panicall, D. L., Sehgal, P. K., Daniel, M. D., and Desrosiers, R. C. (1991). Cell 65, 651–662
Kim, W., Tang, Y., Okada, Y., Torrey, T. A., Chattopadhyay, S. K., Pfleiderer, M., Falkner, F. G., Dorner, F., Choi, W., Hirokawa, N., and Morse, H. C., 3rd. (1998). J Virol 72, 6898–6901
Kino, T., Gragerov, A., Kopp, J. B., Stauber, R. H., Pavlakis, G. N., and Chrousos, G. P. (1999). J Exp Med 189, 51–62
Kirchhoff, F., Greenough, T. C., Brettler, D. B., Sullivan, J. L., and Desrosiers, R. C. (1995). N Engl J Med 332, 228–232
Klebe, C., Bischoff, F. R., Ponstingl, H., and Wittinghofer, A. (1995). Biochemistry 34, 639–647
Kotov, A., Zhou, J., Flicker, P., and Aiken, C. (1999). J Virol 73, 8824–8830
Leopold, P. L., Kreitzer, G., Miyazawa, N., Rempel, S., Pfister, K. K., Rodriguez-Boulan, E., and Crystal, R. G. (2000). Hum Gene Ther 11, 151–165
Lewis, P., Hensel, M., and Emerman, M. (1992). EMBO J 11, 3053–3058
Lewis, P. F., and Emerman, M. (1994). J Virol 68, 510–516
Li, L., Olvera, J. M., Yoder, K. E., Mitchell, R. S., Butler, S. L., Lieber, M., Martin, S. L., and Bushman, F. D. (2001). EMBO J 20, 3272–3281
Lieber, A., Kay, M. A., and Li, Z. Y. (2000). J Virol 74, 721–734
Limón, A., Devroe, E., Lu, R., Ghory, H. Z., Silver, P. A., and Engelman, A. (2002a). J Virol 76, 10598–10607
Limón, A., Nakajima, N., Lu, R., Ghory, H. Z., and Engelman, A. (2002b). J Virol 76, 12078–12086
Liu, B., Dai, R., Tian, C. J., Dawson, L., Gorelick, R., and Yu, X. F. (1999). J Virol 73, 2901–2908
Lu, Y.-L., Bennett, R. P., Wills, J. W., Gorelick, R., and Ratner, L. (1995). J Virol 69, 6873–6879
Luban, J. (1996). Cell 87, 1157–1159
Luban, J., Bossolt, K. L., Franke, E. K., Kalpana, G. V., and Goff, S. P. (1993). Cell 73, 1067–1078
Luby-Phelps, K. (2000). Int Rev Cytol 192, 189–221
Lukacs, G. L., Haggie, P., Seksek, O., Lechardeur, D., Freedman, N., and Verkman, A. S. (2000). J Biol Chem 275, 1625–1629
Mattaj, I. W., and Englmeier, L. (1998). Annu Rev Biochem 67, 265–306

McDonald, D., Vodicka, M.A., Lucero, G., Svitkina, T.M., Borisy, G.G., Emerman, M., and Hope, T.J. (2002). J Cell Biol 159, 441–452
Mermall, V., Post, P. L., and Mosseker, M. S. (1998). Science 279, 527–533
Miller, M. D., Farnet, C. M., and Bushman, F. D. (1997). J Virol 71, 5382–5390
Nakielny, S., and Dreyfuss, G. (1999). Cell 99, 677–690
Ohagen, A., and Gabuzda, D. (2000). J Virol 74, 11055–11066
Ott, D. E., Coren, L. V., Johnson, D. G., Kane, B. P., Sowder, R. C., 2nd, Kim, Y. D., Fisher, R. J., Zhou, X. Z., Lu, K. P., and Henderson, L. E. (2000). Virology 266, 42–51
Ott, D. E., Coren, L. V., Kane, B. P., Busch, L. K., Johnson, D. G., Sowder, R. C., 2nd, Chertova, E. N., Arthur, L. O., and Henderson, L. E. (1996). J Virol 70, 7734–7743
Pante, N., and Kann, M. (2002). Mol Biol Cell 13, 425–434
Paxton, W., Connor, R. I., and Landau, N. R. (1993). J Virol 67, 7229–7237
Pelkmans, L., Puntener, D., and Helenius, A. (2002). Science 296, 535–539
Petit, C., Schwartz, O., and Mammano, F. (2000). J Virol 74, 7119–7126
Piguet, V., and Trono, D. (1999). Rev Med Virol 9, 111–120
Pluymers, W., Cherepanov, P., Schols, D., De Clercq, E., and Debyser, Z. (1999). Virology 258, 327–332
Poon, B., Grovit-Ferbas, K., Stewart, S. A., and Chen, I. S. Y. (1998). Science 281, 266–269
Popov, S., Dubrovsky, L., Lee, M.-A., Pennathur, S., Haffar, O., Al-Abed, Y., Tonge, P., Ulrich, P., Rexach, M., Blobel, G., Cerami, A., and Bukrinsky, M. (1996). Proc Natl Acad Sci USA 93, 11859–11864
Popov, S., Rexach, M., Ratner, L., Blobel, G., and Bukrinsky, M. (1998a). J Biol Chem 273, 13347–13352
Popov, S., Rexach, M., Zybarth, G., Reiling, N., Lee, M.-A., Ratner, L., Lane, C. M., Moore, M. S., Blobel, G., and Bukrinsky, M. (1998b). EMBO J 17, 909–917
Pushkarsky, T., Zybarth, G., Dubrovsky, L., Yurchenko, V., Tang, H., Guo, H., Toole, B., Sherry, B., and Bukrinsky, M. (2001). Proc Natl Acad Sci USA 98, 6360–6365
Reichelt, R., Holzenburg, A., Buhle, E. L., Jr., Jarnik, M., Engel, A., and Aebi, U. (1990). J Cell Biol 110, 883–894
Reil, H., Bukosvsky, A. A., Gelderblom, H. R., and Göttlinger, H. G. (1998). EMBO J 17, 2699–2708
Ribbeck, K., and Görlich, D. (2001). EMBO J 20, 1320–1330
Rietdorf, J., Ploubidou, A., Reckmann, I., Holmström, A., Frischknecht, F., Zettl, M., Zimmermann, T., and Way, M. (2001). Nat Cell Biol 3, 992–1000
Roe, T., Reynolds, T. C., Yu, G., and Brown, P. O. (1993). EMBO J 12 2099–2108
Salman, H., Zbaida, D., Rabin, Y., Chatenay, D., and Elbaum, M. (2001). Proc. Natl. Acad. Sci. USA 98, 7247–7252
Saphire, A. C., Bobardt, M. D., and Gallay, P. A. (1999). EMBO J 18, 6771–6785
Saphire, A. C., Bobardt, M. D., and Gallay, P. A. (2002a). J Virol 76, 4671–4677
Saphire, A. C., Bobardt, M. D., and Gallay, P. A. (2002b). J Virol 76, 2255–2562
Sawai, E. T., Baur, A., Struble, H., Peterlin, B. M., Levy, J. A., and Cheng-Mayer, C. (1994). Proc Natl Acad Sci USA 91, 1539–1543
Sawai, E. T., Khan, I. H., Montbriand, P. M., Peterlin, B. M., Cheng-Mayer, C., and Luciw, P. A. (1996). Curr Biol 6, 1519–1527

Schacker, T., Little, S., Connick, E., Gebhard, K., Zhang, Z. Q., Krieger, J., Pryor, J., Havlir, D., Wong, J. K., Schooley, R. T., Richman, D., Corey, L., and Haase, A. T. (2001). J Infect Dis 183, 555-562

Schaeffer, E., Geleziunas, R., and Greene, W. C. (2001). J Virol 75, 2993-3000

Schroder, A. R., Shinn, P., Chen, H., Berry, C., Ecker, J. R., and Bushman, F. (2002). Cell 110, 521-529

Schwartz, O., Marechal, V., Danos, O., and Heard, J. M. (1995). J Virol 69, 4053-409

Sellon, D. C., Perry, S. T., Coggins, L., and Fuller, F. J. (1992). J Virol 66, 5906-5913

Sheehy, A. M., Gaddis, N. C., Choi, J. D., and Malim, M. H. (2002). Nature 418, 646-450

Sherry, B., Zybarth, G., Alfano, M., Dubrovsky, L., Mitchell, R., Rich, D., Ulrich, P., Bucala, R., Cerami, A., and Bukrinsky, M. (1998). Proc Natl Acad Sci USA 95, 1758-1763

Simon, J. H. M., and Malim, M. H. (1996). J.Virol 70, 5297-5305

Sirven, A., Pflumio, F., Zennou, V., Titeux, M., Vainchenker, W., Coulombel, L., Dubart-Kupperschmitt, A., and Charneau, P. (2000). Blood 96, 4103-4110

Sodeik, B. (2000). Trends Microbiol 8, 465-472

Sodeik, B., Ebersold, M. W., and Helenius, A. (1997). J Cell Biol 136, 1007-21

Subbramanian, R. A., Kessous-Elbaz, A., Lodge, R., Forget, J., Yao, X. J., Bergeron, D., and Cohen, E. A. (1998). J Exp Med 187, 1103-1111

Tang, Y., Winkler, U., Freed, E. O., Torrey, T. A., Kim, W., Li, H., Goff, S. P., and Morse, H. C., 3rd. (1999). J Virol 73, 10508-10513

Tomishima, M. J., Smith, G. A., and Enquist, L. W. (2001). Traffic 2, 429-436

Truant, R., and Cullen, B. R. (1999). Mol Cell Biol 19, 1210-1217

Tsurutani, N., Kubo, M., Maeda, Y., Ohashi, T., Yamamoto, N., Kannagi, M., and Masuda, T. (2000). J Virol 74, 4795-4806

Turelli, P., Doucas, V., Craig, E., Mangeat, B., Klages, N., Evans, R., Kalpana, G., and Trono, D. (2001). Mol Cell 7, 1245-1254

Vale, R. D., and Milligan, R. A. (2000). Science 288, 88-95

Vodicka, M. A., Koepp, D. M., Silver, P. A., and Emerman, M. (1998). Genes Dev 12, 175-185

Von Schwedler, U., Kornbluth, R. S., and Trono, D. (1994). Proc Natl Acad Sci USA 91, 6992-6996

Von Schwedler, U., Song, J., Aiken, C., and Trono, D. (1993). J Virol 67, 4945-4955

Wang, L., Mukherjee, S., Jia, F., Narayan, O., and Zhao, L.-J. (1995). J Biol Chem 270, 25564-25569

Weinberg, J. B., Matthews, T. J., Cullen, B. R., and Malim, M. H. (1991). J Exp Med 174, 1477-1482

Whittaker, G. R., Kann, M., and Helenius, A. (2000). Annu Rev Cell Dev Biol 16, 627-651

Wilk, T., Gowen, B., and Fuller, S. D. (1999). J Virol 73 1931-1940

Wilson, G. L., Dean, B. S., Wang, G., and Dean, D. A. (1999). J Biol Chem 274, 22025-22032

Wu, X., Liu, H., Xiao, H., Conway, J. A., Hehl, E., Kalpana, G. V., Prasad, V., and Kappes, J. C. (1999). J Virol 73, 2126-2135

Wu, Y., and Marsh, J. W. (2001). Science 293, 1503-1506

Yin, L., Braaten, D., and Luban, J. (1998). J Virol 72, 6430-6436

Yung, E., Sorin, M., Pal, A., Craig, E., Morozov, A., Delattre, O., Kappes, J., Ott, D., and Kalpana, G. V. (2001). Nat Med 7, 920–926

Zennou, V., Petit, C., Guetard, D., Nerhbass, U., Montagnier, L., and Charneau, P. (2000). Cell 101, 173–185

Zhang, Z., Schuler, T., Zupancic, M., Wietgrefe, S., Staskus, K. A., Reimann, K. A., Reinhart, T. A., Rogan, M., Cavert, W., Miller, C. J., Veazey, R. S., Notermans, D., Little, S., Danner, S. A., Richman, D. D., Havlir, D., Wong, J., Jordan, H. L., Schacker, T. W., Racz, P., Tenner-Racz, K., Letvin, N. L., Wolinsky, S., and Haase, A. T. (1999). Science 286, 1353–1357

The Roles of Cellular Factors in Retroviral Integration

A. Engelman

Department of Cancer Immunology and AIDS, Dana Farber Cancer Institute,
44 Binney Street, Boston, MA 02115, USA
E-mail: alan_engelman@dfci.harvard.edu

1	Introduction	210
2	Mechanism of Retroviral Integration	210
3	Retroviral Integration Assays	211
3.1	Assays Using Preintegration Complexes	211
3.2	Assays with Purified Integrase Protein	213
3.2.1	Oligonucleotide-Based Assays	214
3.2.2	Assays with Mini-Viral Substrates	214
3.3	Assays for Integration In Vivo	215
4	Roles of Cellular Factors During 3′ Processing and DNA Strand Transfer	216
4.1	Reconstitution of Salt-Stripped PIC Activity	218
4.2	Stimulation of Purified Integrase Activity	219
4.3	Mechanism of Host Factor Function	221
5	The Roles of Cellular Factors During Gap Repair	223
5.1	Biochemical Assays Using Purified Components	223
5.2	Genetic Analyses of Gap Repair	225
6	Host Cell Factors Affecting Integration Target Site Selection	226
6.1	Genetic Analyses of Target Site Selection	227
6.2	In Vitro Assays Using Purified Integrase and PICs	227
6.3	Retrotransposons as Model Systems for Retroviral Target Site Selection	228
7	Future Directions	229
7.1	Inhibiting Retroviral Integration	230
	References	231

Abstract A key early step in the retroviral life cycle is the integration of reverse-transcribed viral cDNA into a chromosome of an infected cell. The key protein player in retroviral integration is the viral integrase, which enters the cell as part of the virus. Although purified integrase protein is necessary and sufficient to perform the basic catalytic DNA breakage and joining steps of retroviral integration, a variety of normal cellular proteins have been implicated as playing important roles in establishing the integrated provirus in cells. This chapter reviews the roles of host cell factors that function during integrase catalysis, during the repair of the resulting DNA recombination intermediate, and by potentially guiding viral preintegration complexes to their chromosomal locations for cDNA integration. The potential to interfere with proper integration by blocking either integrase catalysis or the function of cellular integration cofactors is also discussed.

1
Introduction

Retroviruses and their vectors must accomplish certain key steps early in the viral replication cycle to efficiently express genes in infected cells. These steps, which can be summarized as entry, uncoating, reverse transcription, nuclear localization, and integration, require the action of key viral proteins. In addition, each step likely requires the participation of essential host cell factors. Of all the early replication steps, host factor function is best understood for viral entry. In this case, viral envelope glycoproteins interact with specific cell surface proteins whose identities have been established for many retroviruses. The identities of the specific host factors involved in uncoating, reverse transcription, nuclear localization, and integration are less well defined than those involved in viral entry. This chapter reviews the roles of host proteins in integration. See Bushman (1999) for a previous review of host factor function in retroviral integration.

2
Mechanism of Retroviral Integration

After entry and uncoating viral reverse transcriptase copies viral RNA into linear double-stranded cDNA with long terminal repeats (LTRs), and this linear form is the substrate for integrase-mediated DNA recombination (Fujiwara and Mizuuchi 1988; Brown et al. 1989; Lee and Coffin 1991). The integrase interacts with short attachment (*att*) sites located at each end of the cDNA (reviewed in Katzman and Katz 1999; Engelman

1999). Because each LTR is comprised of U3, R, and U5 sequences, the upstream *att* site is U3 and the downstream site is U5.

Two integrase activities, 3' processing and DNA strand transfer, are required for integration. During the initial processing step, integrase cleaves a specific site near each 3' end of the viral cDNA, typically removing a dinucleotide (Fig. 1). This reaction can occur in the cytoplasm of cells infected with Moloney murine leukemia virus (MoMLV) (Fujiwara and Mizuuchi 1988; Brown et al. 1989; Roth et al. 1989), Rous sarcoma virus (RSV) (Lee and Coffin 1991), or human immunodeficiency virus type 1 (HIV-1) (Miller et al. 1997; Chen and Engelman 2000; 2001), indicating that 3' processing likely precedes nuclear localization in most instances. After nuclear entry, integrase transfers each cleaved viral end to the 5' phosphates of a double-stranded staggered cut in a cell chromosome. The product of DNA strand transfer, a gapped recombination intermediate with unjoined viral 5' ends, likely requires host cell enzymes for its repair (see Sect. 5.1 below). This yields the final integrated provirus (Fig. 1).

3
Retroviral Integration Assays

Retroviral integration can be measured with any of a number of different assay systems. These range from quantifying in vivo integration in infected cells to simplified in vitro assays using purified integrase protein and oligonucleotide DNA substrates. Before discussing the roles of cellular factors, it is important to review the different assays for measuring retroviral integration.

3.1
Assays Using Preintegration Complexes

Reverse transcription and integration take place in vivo in the context of large nucleoprotein complexes called reverse transcription complexes (RTCs) and preintegration complexes (PICs), respectively (reviewed in Goff 2001). In vitro integration was first demonstrated by Brown and colleagues using extracts of MoMLV-infected cells and purified bacteriophage lambda DNA as target (Brown et al. 1987). Subsequent physical analyses using indirect end-labeling and Southern blotting helped to define the PIC (Bowerman et al. 1989; Ellison et al. 1990; Farnet and

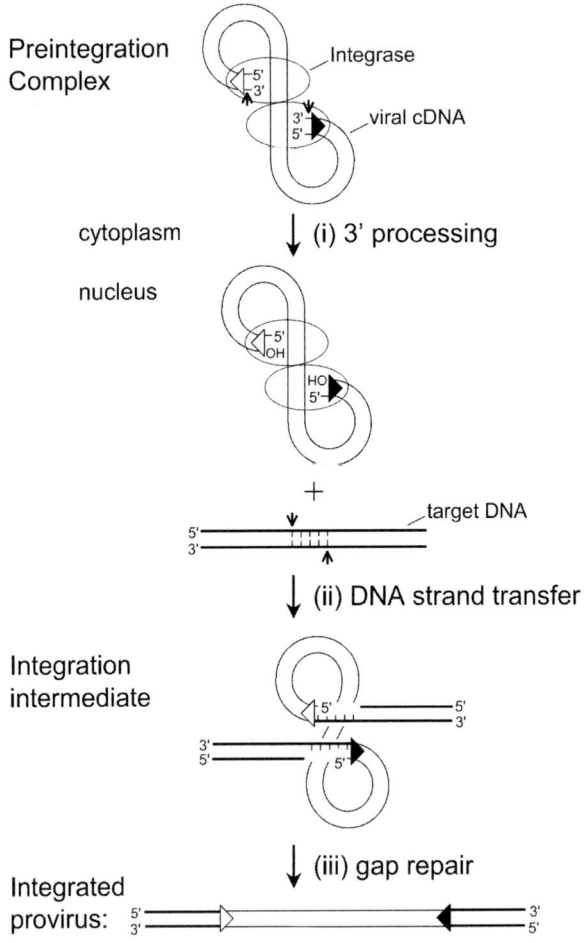

Fig. 1 Mechanism of retroviral integration. Integration proceeds via three steps, 3′ processing, DNA strand transfer, and gap repair. Whereas 3′ processing and DNA strand transfer are catalyzed by integrase, host cell enzymes likely participate in gap repair (see Sect. 5). After reverse transcription, a multimer of integrase is drawn holding the two ends of linear viral cDNA together. During 3′ processing, a dinucleotide is typically cleaved from each 3′ end (*vertical arrows*). After nuclear entry, integrase uses the recessed 3′-hydroxyl groups to make a double-stranded staggered cut in target DNA, which concomitantly joins the viral 3′ ends to the resulting 5′-phosphates. Although a 5-bp spacing in target DNA is shown, this varies from 4 to 6 bp depending on the virus. The viral 5′ ends remain unjoined in the resulting DNA recombination intermediate. Repair of this intermediate yields the integrated provirus. Although a dimer is drawn, the precise stoichiometry of the active integrase multimer is unknown. *Open triangle*, U3 *att* site; *filled triangle*, U5 *att* site

Haseltine 1990, 1991; Miller et al. 1997) and elucidate the mechanism of retroviral integration (Fujiwara and Mizuuchi 1988; Brown et al. 1989; Roth et al. 1989; Pauza, 1990; Lee and Coffin 1991). Quantification of in vitro PIC activity by Southern blotting is still in wide use. PICs are incubated with an excess of recombinant target DNA, which in many cases is linear 5.4-kb ΦX174. Because MoMLV cDNA is 8.8 kb, the integration product in this case is a 14.2-kb linear recombination intermediate (Fig. 1; Fujiwara and Mizuuchi 1988). More recent assays have used real-time quantitative PCR after integration into either immobilized (Hansen et al. 1999) or concatemerized (Brooun et al. 2001) target DNA to increase the sensitivity of detection of HIV-1 PIC activity.

Whereas the integrase enzyme and linear viral cDNA substrate are key components of all PICs, the identities of other viral components seem to differ among viruses. For example, certain antisera against the viral capsid protein quantitatively immunoprecipitated integration-competent MoMLV PICs, implying that capsid is associated with the majority of active MoMLV complexes (Bowerman et al. 1989). In contrast, HIV-1 matrix and reverse transcriptase proteins were readily detected in active PIC samples by Western blotting under conditions in which capsid was barely detected, suggesting that capsid is not a stoichiometric component of HIV-1 PICs (Miller et al. 1997). It is currently unclear whether these results represent real differences in PIC composition among viruses or whether different laboratory procedures and reagents might have also contributed to the findings.

3.2
Assays with Purified Integrase Protein

Retroviral integrase protein purified from any of a number of different sources displays 3' processing and DNA strand transfer activities using a variety of DNA substrates. These recombinant substrates tend to follow one of two different design strategies. Whereas synthetic double-stranded oligonucleotides generally contain just a single viral *att* site, longer restriction fragments incorporate *att* sites at both DNA ends. The longer substrates help to distinguish products that arose from the integration of just one viral DNA end versus normal two-ended integration (reviewed in Hindmarsh and Leis 1999).

3.2.1
Oligonucleotide-Based Assays

Simplified assays using short oligonucleotide substrates established that integrase is the only protein required for catalysis of 3' processing and DNA strand transfer (Katzman et al. 1989; Craigie et al. 1990; Katz et al. 1990; Sherman and Fyfe 1990; Bushman and Craigie 1991). Oligonucleotide substrates that contained a recessed 3' end and thus bypassed the requirement for 3' processing supported DNA strand transfer activity, demonstrating that *att* site cleavage is not a prerequisite for strand transfer activity (Craigie et al. 1990; Katz et al. 1990; Bushman and Craigie 1991; Lafemina et al. 1991).

3.2.2
Assays with Mini-Viral Substrates

Oligonucleotide-based assays were invaluable for deciphering basic aspects of integrase structure and function including protein domain structure, active site residues, and critical *att* site residues (reviewed in Brown 1997). One drawback of these simplified assays, however, was that integrase tended to integrate just one instead of two *att* sites into target DNA (Craigie et al. 1990; Bushman and Craigie 1991). Provirus formation requires the concerted integration of both U3 and U5 into both strands of target DNA (Fig. 1). If only one *att* site was joined instead of the usual two, the resulting Y-shaped recombination intermediate would likely resolve into its starting chromosomal and viral DNAs during gap repair, leading to virus excision and nonproductive infection. Thus mini-viral substrates, designed to detect the normal concerted integration of two *att* sites, assay a reaction pathway that is relevant to integration as it occurs in vivo.

In addition to containing an *att* site at each end, mini-viral substrates generally contain a genetic marker for selection in *Escherichia coli*. Although integration was initially scored after genetic selection (Fujiwara and Craigie 1989; Bushman and Craigie 1990; Bushman et al. 1990; Katz et al. 1990; Fitzgerald et al. 1992), direct visualization of radiolabeled products was subsequently demonstrated (Vora et al. 1994; Goodzari et al. 1995; Aiyar et al. 1996). Although designed to help quantify concerted integration, mini-viral substrates yielded significant levels of single-ended integration products (Vora and Grandgenett 1995; Aiyar et al. 1996;

Carteau et al. 1997, 1999; McCord et al. 1998; Goodzari et al. 1999; Hindmarsh et al. 1999). Despite this limitation, these systems helped establish that integrase is the only protein required to catalyze relatively efficient levels of concerted integration (Vora and Grandgenett 1995; McCord et al. 1998; Carteau et al. 1999; Goodzari et al. 1999; Sinha et al. 2002).

3.3
Assays for Integration In Vivo

Although local hot spots can be detected in vivo (Withers-Ward et al. 1994), retroviruses for the most part appear to integrate randomly throughout the animal cell genome (Withers-Ward et al. 1994; Carteau et al. 1998). Because of this, assay systems for quantitating integration in vivo must account for the relative randomness of retroviral integration. This has been approached in a couple of different ways. One is to cleave total cell DNA with a restriction enzyme that also cuts within the integrated provirus. This yields a heterogeneous population of virus-containing fragments whose sizes are defined by the distance between the viral cleavage site and the closest adjacent site in flanking genomic DNA. After intramolecular ligation, the frequency and distribution of in vivo integration can be assessed by inverse PCR and polyacrylamide gel electrophoresis (Lewis et al. 1992). Performing inverse PCR at limiting dilution afforded quantitative analysis of HIV-1 integration in different populations of CD4-positive cells (Chun et al. 1997).

A second strategy for measuring in vivo integration takes advantage of the highly repetitive nature of animal cell DNA. Human DNA, for example, contains $0.5–1.1 \times 10^6$ copies of *Alu* sequences, comprising 6%–13% of the genome (Mighell et al. 1997). Whereas integration was readily detected by PCR using *Alu* and HIV-specific primers (Benkirane et al. 1993; Courcoul et al. 1995; Sonza et al. 1996; Carteau et al. 1988), integration in the vicinity of other repetitive elements, for example, alphoid repeats, was disfavored (Carteau et al. 1988). A quantitative *Alu* PCR method, which incorporated a standard curve derived from a large sample of integrated proviruses, was recently described (Butler et al. 2001). The detection limit of this real-time PCR assay, about one integration per 100 cells, was well below the limits of more sensitive inverse (Chun et al. 1997) and ligation-mediated (Vandegraaff et al. 2001) PCR assays, which detected approximately one integration per 3×10^4 and 2×10^5 cells, respectively.

4
Roles of Cellular Factors During 3′ Processing and DNA Strand Transfer

Much of what is known concerning the roles of host cell factors during the initial 3′ processing and DNA strand transfer steps of retroviral integration came from analyses of PICs isolated from infected cells. PICs can be recovered from cells after lysis in buffers containing physiological or isotonic concentrations of salt (Brown et al. 1987; Ellison et al. 1990; Farnet and Haseltine 1990). MoMLV (Lee and Craigie 1994) and HIV-1 (Farnet and Bushman 1997; Chen and Engelman 1998) PICs purified by size after in vitro treatment with relatively high concentrations of salt lost their normal intermolecular DNA recombination activity (Fig. 2). For both viruses, extracts of uninfected cells restored normal integration, indicating that host cell proteins play essential roles in retroviral PIC function. Because virion lysates failed to restore activity to salt-stripped MoMLV (Lee and Craigie 1994) and HIV-1 (Farnet and Bushman 1997) PICs, the responsible cell factor(s) was apparently not packaged into virions. It is important to note that, unlike reactions with purified integrase, PICs isolated from infected cells rarely if ever integrate just a single viral *att* site in vitro (Chen and Engelman, 2001), and cell extracts apparently reconstituted this high rate of coupled integration activity (Lee and Craigie 1994; Farnet and Bushman 1997; Chen and Engelman 1998).

Salt-stripped MoMLV and HIV-1 PICs behaved somewhat differently in these in vitro reconstitution assays. Whereas salt-stripped HIV-1 PICs were apparently catalytically inactive (Farnet and Bushman 1997; Chen and Engelman 1998; Li et al. 1998), salt-stripped MoMLV PICs displayed robust autointegration activity (Lee and Craigie 1994; Li et al. 1998). Auto- or intramolecular integration refers to integration of the processed *att* sites into an internal part of the viral DNA itself instead of the normal intermolecular pathway into a separate target DNA molecule. Depending on the strand choice during integration, autointegration either severs the viral DNA into two nicked circles or forms one nicked circle with an inverted internal segment (Lee and Craigie 1994). Either of these outcomes is clearly detrimental to the virus. Thus, akin to relat-

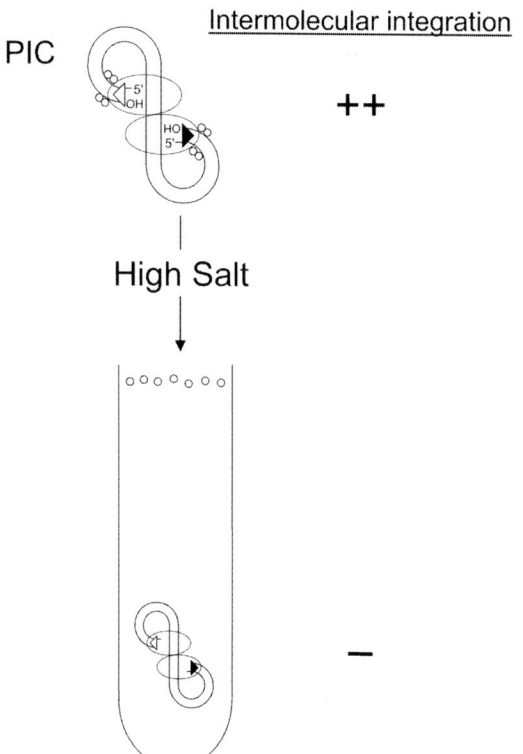

Fig. 2 High salt removes essential host cell cofactors from retroviral PICs. Host cell proteins (*small balls*) are drawn in association with the PIC. After treatment with high salt and size separation, host cell factors became dislodged from the PIC, rendering the starting integration-competent complex inactive for intermolecular DNA strand transfer activity (Lee and Craigie 1994; Farnet and Bushman 1997; Chen and Engelman 1998). Adding the top fraction from a sucrose gradient back to purified salt-stripped MoMLV complexes restored intermolecular strand transfer activity (Lee and Craigie 1994)

ed DNA transposition systems, retroviruses have apparently evolved a mechanism to protect themselves from self-destructive autointegration. In contrast to bacteriophage mu, which expresses its own protein to help suppress autointegration (Adzuma and Mizuuchi 1989), retroviruses have apparently usurped a normal cellular protein, the barrier-to-autointegration factor (BAF) (Lee and Craigie 1998), for protection from autointegration.

4.1
Reconstitution of Salt-Stripped PIC Activity

The finding that host cell extracts restored intermolecular integration activity to salt-stripped PICs defined in vitro biochemical assays for purifying the relevant factor(s). Whereas BAF was purified from mouse NIH/3T3 cells based on its ability to both suppress autointegration and restore intermolecular integration to salt-stripped MoMLV PICs (Lee and Craigie 1998), high mobility group (HMG) chromosomal protein A1 (formally HMG-I/Y; Bustin 2001) was purified from human Sup T1 T cells by its ability to restore integration activity to salt-stripped HIV-1 PICs (Farnet and Bushman 1997).

At approximately the same time these cellular proteins were purified, Craigie and coworkers devised a novel transposon-mediated DNA footprinting technique, called mu-mediated (MM)-PCR footprinting, to analyze the nucleoprotein structure associated with MoMLV PIC activity (Wei et al. 1997). MM-PCR footprinting revealed a bipartite structure at each cDNA end consisting of several hundred base pairs of protein protection together with smaller regions of enhanced transposition near each terminus (Wei et al. 1997). Whereas salt-stripping destroyed the so-called MoMLV intasome, uninfected cell extracts restored MoMLV PIC activity and intasome structure in parallel (Wei et al. 1997). Salt-stripping likewise destroyed the HIV-1 intasome, and adding back extracts of uninfected SupT1 cells restored HIV-1 PIC structure and function in parallel (Chen and Engelman 1998).

The independent identification of BAF and HMGA1 as essential cofactors for retroviral PIC function led to their side-by-side comparisons in functional reconstitution assays. For both MoMLV and HIV-1, BAF was approximately 500-fold more active than HMGA1 at restoring integration activity to salt-stripped PICs (Farnet and Bushman 1997; Chen and Engelman 1998; Li et al. 1998; Wei et al. 1998), and only BAF restored the native intasome structures (Chen and Engelman 1998; Wei et al. 1998). BAF apparently played an indirect role in restoring the MoMLV structure, as purified integrase and recombinant MoMLV DNA formed an intasome-like structure in the absence of BAF protein (Wei et al. 1998). MM-PCR footprinting, however, failed to reveal a similar structure with purified HIV-1 components (H. Chen and A. Engelman, unpublished observations). Because of (a) the relatively high specific activity of BAF, (b) intasome reconstitution by BAF but not HMGA1, and (c) the nearly identical behaviors of bovine RNase A and HMGA1 in some HIV-1 reconstitution assays (Farnet and Bushman 1997; Chen and Engelman 1998), it was proposed that BAF was a specific cofactor for retroviral integration and that HMGA1 acted less specifically (Chen and Engelman 1998; Wei et al. 1998).

Although BAF was significantly more active than HMGA1 at restoring integration to salt-stripped PICs, only HMGA1, and not BAF, has been identified as a bona fide PIC component. Not only was HMGA1 detected in partially-purified HIV-1 PICs by Western blotting, anti-HMGA1 antibodies depleted the functional complementing activity from salt-stripped HIV-1 PIC extracts under conditions in which antibodies against either HIV-1 matrix or nucleocapsid (NC) failed to deplete activity (Farnet and Bushman 1997). These results not only identified HMGA1 as a component of HIV-1 PICs but also implicated HMGA1 as the primary complimenting factor under these assay conditions. Anti-HMGA1 antibodies also immunoprecipitated active MoMLV PICs, and cDNA recovery was prevented by prior salt-stripping (Li et al. 2000). This indicated that HMGA1 was also a component of MoMLV PICs and that salt-stripping destroyed host factor association.

Similar immunoprecipitation experiments have not been reported for BAF because of the lack of sufficient immunochemical reagents. However, the recent identification of an antiserum that can apparently immunoprecipitate BAF protein (R. Craigie, personal communication) should open the door to similar immunoassays. Results of preliminary experiments revealed that this anti-BAF serum immunoprecipitated the majority of endogenous MoMLV cDNA in cytoplasmic extracts of acutely infected cells under conditions in which normal rabbit serum recovered barely detectable cDNA levels, indicating that BAF is also a component of MoMLV PICs (Y. Suzuki and R. Craigie, personal communication).

4.2
Stimulation of Purified Integrase Activity

A variety of host cell proteins have been reported to stimulate the in vitro activity of purified integrase. For example, a mixture of RNase A, RNase T1, histone H1, and bacterial HU increased the strand transfer activity of partially-purified HIV-1 integrase approximately tenfold (Bushman et al. 1990). Because these results were obtained after genetic selection in *E. coli*, it is difficult to assess the mechanism of host cell factor action. It seems likely these nonspecific DNA binding proteins in part protected the mini-HIV substrate from degradation by contaminating cellular nucleases in this early integrase preparation.

Subsequent experiments using radiolabeled mini-RSV revealed that purified HMGB1 (formally HMG-1) stimulated integration three- to fourfold (Aiyar et al. 1996). The physiological relevance of this stimulation is unclear, however, because HMGB1 did not restore activity to salt-stripped HIV-1 (Farnet and Bushman 1997) or MoMLV (Wei et al. 1998) PICs. Results with purified HMGA1, which, as mentioned above, reconstituted salt-stripped HIV-1 (Farnet and Bushman 1997; Chen and Engelman 1998) and MoMLV (Li et al. 1998) PIC activity, have varied. Whereas Hindmarsh et al. (1999) reported an approximate tenfold stimulation with purified HIV-1 integrase and mini-viral DNA, Carteau et al. (1999) failed to detect stimulation with similar assay conditions. These two studies also reported different results for host factor HMGB2 (formally HMG-2). Whereas Carteau et al. (1999) observed similarly weak stimulation by HMGB1 and HMGB2, Hindmarsh et al. (1999) observed significant stimulation by HMGB2 in reactions containing Mg^{2+}. However, HMGB2 failed to reconstitute salt-stripped HIV-1 PIC activity, which was also assayed in Mg^{2+}-containing buffer (Farnet and Bushman 1997). Although the reasons for these different results are unclear, any of a number of parameters, including reaction conditions, protein preparations, and/or mini-viral substrate design, could have contributed. Although HMGB2 can outperform HMGA1 under certain in vitro conditions (Hindmarsh et al. 1999), the current consensus is that HMGA1 may play a physiological role but that neither HMGB1 nor HMGB2 is likely to function as an integration cofactor in vivo.

It is important to note that, although BAF was significantly more active than HMGA1 in PIC reconstitution assays, BAF did not stimulate purified integrase in mini-viral integration assays (Carteau et al. 1999; J. Leis, personal communication; D. Grandgenett, personal communication). Although the reasons for these results are unclear, two possibilities are that (a) BAF is not a physiologically relevant cofactor or (b) the in vivo function of BAF cannot be recapitulated by simply mixing purified components in vitro.

It is also noteworthy that the viral NC protein stimulated HIV-1 integration in vitro, both in PIC reconstitution assays (Farnet and Bushman 1997) and in assays with purified integrase (Lapadat-Tapolsky et al. 1993; Carteau et al. 1997, 1999). Stimulation of concerted integration was quite robust, over 1,000-fold under certain reaction conditions (Carteau et al. 1999). However, the physiological relevance of this stimulation is unclear. Whereas NC protein was identified as a PIC component in some HIV-1 preparations (Gallay et al. 1995, 1997), a separate study failed to detect NC after numerous purification steps, indicating that NC does not play a significant role in HIV-1 PIC activity in vitro (Miller et al. 1997). Consistent with this view, antibodies against NC failed to deplete the functional complementation activity present in high-salt extracts of HIV-1 PICs (Farnet and Bushman 1997).

4.3
Mechanism of Host Factor Function

The mechanisms by which HMGA1 and BAF function in retroviral integration have been investigated. Each is a DNA binding protein; whereas BAF binds DNA nonspecifically (Lee and Craigie 1998; Harris and Engelman 2000; Zheng et al. 2000), HMGA1 preferentially binds A/T-rich regions (reviewed in Bustin and Reeves 1996). Neither protein appears to directly interact with integrase (Farnet and Bushman 1997; Hindmarsh et al. 1999; T. Stoyanova and A. Engelman, unpublished observations). Instead, each protein appears to function via its ability to form higher-order nucleoprotein complexes with DNA (Huth et al. 1997; Li et al. 2000; Zheng et al. 2000; Y. Suzuki and R. Craigie, personal communication).

HMGA1 contains three so-called A·T hook regions or A·T-DNA binding domains (Fig. 3). Deletion mutants containing at least two A·T hooks, either A·T I and A·T II or A·T II and A·T III, restored intermolecular integration activity to salt-stripped MoMLV and HIV-1 PICs and promoted intermolecular ligation of recombinant HIV-1 LTR DNA under dilute conditions (Li et al. 2000). Because single A·T hooks, which bind A/T-rich DNA with significantly less affinity than dual-hooked derivatives (Bustin and Reeves 1996; Huth et al. 1997) failed to (a) restore salt-stripped PIC activity and (b) promote intermolecular ligation under dilute conditions, it was suggested that the role of HMGA1 in retroviral integration was to bridge distant DNA segments together (Li et al. 2000). Consistent with this interpretation, the solution structure of a 50–91 deletion mutant, which contained A·T II and A·T III (Fig. 3), revealed that each A·T hook bound a separate DNA molecule (Huth et al. 1997). The 50–91 derivative also stimulated the mini-viral activity of purified HIV-1

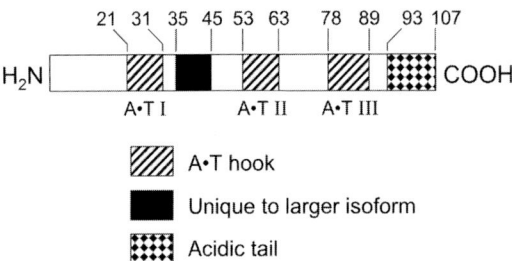

Fig. 3 Domain structure of HMGA1. The 11 amino acids between residues 35 and 45 are unique to a larger isoform (formally HMG-I). The consensus A·T hook binding sequence is TP-KRPRGRPKK (Bustin and Reeves 1996). Although single A·T hooks can weakly bind A/T-rich DNA (Bustin and Reeves 1996; Huth et al. 1997), two such regions were required to stimulate purified HIV-1 integrase in mini-viral integration assays (Hindmarsh et al. 1999) and to reconstitute salt-stripped MoMLV and HIV-1 PIC activity (Li et al. 2000)

integrase under conditions in which a DNA binding-defective mutant failed to function (Hindmarsh et al. 1999).

BAF also binds separate DNA duplexes in forming higher-order nucleoprotein complexes. In this case, the stoichiometry of BAF to DNA is approximately five BAF dimers to five different oligonucleotides (Zheng et al. 2000). Recent results indicate that compaction of retroviral cDNA by BAF is central to its role in protecting MoMLV from autointegration. Salt-stripped MoMLV PICs sedimented more slowly than untreated samples in sucrose gradients, and BAF restored normal sedimentation and intermolecular integration activity in parallel (Y. Suzuki and R. Craigie, personal communication). Neither HMGA1 nor HMGB1 restored normal sedimentation under these conditions, indicating that neither protein plays an important role in compacting preintegrative MoMLV cDNA. These results are consistent with the interpretation that cDNA compaction is central to BAF's role in protecting MoMLV cDNA from autointegration. Additional results suggest that BAF functions during intermolecular strand transfer at the step of target DNA capture. Salt-stripping greatly reduced the ability for MoMLV PICs to bind immobilized target DNA, and BAF in large part restored target DNA binding activity (Y. Suzuki and R. Craigie, personal communication). Thus BAF apparently functions in MoMLV integration (a) by compacting nascent cDNA into a higher-order nucleoprotein structure to prevent autointegration and (b) by capturing a second target DNA molecule for intermolecular DNA recombination. Because analyzing a large number of integration sites did not reveal a preference for A/T-rich sequences, HMGA1 does not appear to function by simply capturing target DNA for intermolecular strand transfer (Carteau et al. 1998; Li et al. 2000).

5
The Roles of Cellular Factors During Gap Repair

As presented in Fig. 1, the final step of retroviral integration requires the repair of the integration intermediate formed by integrase-mediated DNA strand transfer. This entails (a) DNA synthesis across the four- to six-nucleotide gap at each virus-chromosome junction, (b) removing the viral 5' dinucleotide leftover from integrase 3' processing, and (c) sealing the resulting nicks (Fig. 4A). Numerous enzymes, including viral reverse transcriptase, integrase (Chow et al. 1992; Roe et al. 1997), and cellular factors (Daniel et al. 1999; Brin et al. 2000; Yoder and Bushman 2000; Ha et al. 2001) have been implicated in these repair processes.

5.1
Biochemical Assays Using Purified Components

In addition to the physiologically relevant 3' processing and DNA strand transfer activities, purified retroviral integrase catalyzes a third in vitro activity termed disintegration (Chow et al. 1992). During disintegration, integrase uses a 3'-OH to attack a nearby phosphodiester bond, cleaving the acceptor DNA strand and concomitantly joining the attacking strand to the resulting 5'-phosphate (Fig. 4B). It was proposed that integrase's in vitro disintegration or DNA splicing activity might function during gap repair in vivo (Chow et al. 1992). In this scenario the 3'-OH of the filled-in DNA strand would cleave the dinucleotide from the viral 5' end and at the same time join the nascent strand to the cleaved end, essentially accomplishing repair steps b (Fig. 4A, "ii") and c (Fig. 4A, "iii") in a single enzymatic reaction (Fig. 4). Although an attractive model, purified integrase failed to support efficient repair of oligonucleotide substrates that modeled the single-stranded joints of retroviral integration intermediates (Brin et al. 2000; Yoder and Bushman 2000).

Although the results of these experiments cast doubt on the participation of integrase in gap repair, they at the same time highlighted other enzymes that efficiently repaired model substrates. On the basis of these

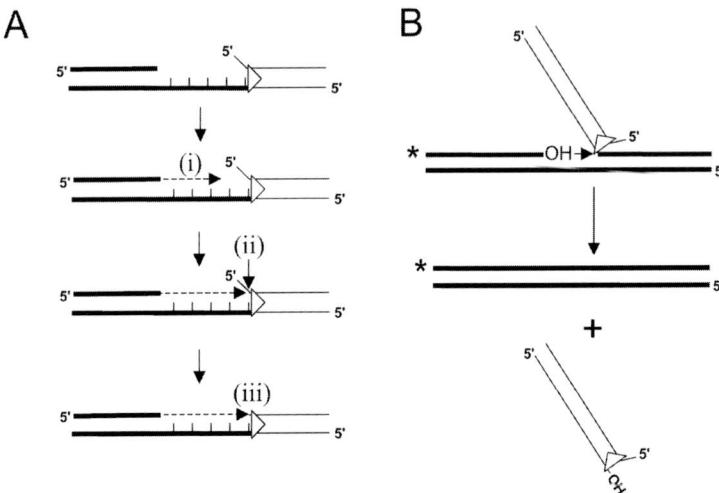

Fig. 4A, B DNA repair of the retroviral integration intermediate. **A** Three theoretical steps of gap repair. (*i*) A DNA polymerase fills in the single-strand gap, (*ii*) an endonuclease activity cleaves the 5′ dinucleotide that remains after integrase 3′ processing, and (*iii*) a DNA ligase seals the nick between the nascent 3′-OH and 5′-phosphate. For simplicity, only one end of the recombination intermediate is shown. **B** Retroviral disintegration. During disintegration, integrase uses a 3′ DNA end to cleave a nearby phosphodiester bond and concomitantly join the attacking oxygen nucleophile to the resulting 5′-phosphate. The substrate represents the product of single-end *att* site integration. In this case disintegration releases the *att* site from the target DNA and at the same time seals the target DNA nick. Placing ^{32}P (*) at the 5′end of the attacking strand is a convenient way to monitor product formation (Chow et al. 1992). *Bold lines*, target DNA; *thin lines*, viral DNA; *triangle*, *att* site

results, it appears that three different enzymatic activities are required to repair retrovirus-induced gaps. DNA polymerase beta, delta, or reverse transcriptase efficiently filled in gaps (step "i" in Fig. 4A). Whereas flap endonuclease I efficiently removed the overhanging 5′ dinucleotide (step b, "ii" in Fig. 4A), DNA ligase I, III, or IV efficiently sealed the nick (step c, "iii" in Fig. 4A). Thus, although these studies indicated that reverse transcriptase may function during gap repair in vivo, they also highlighted that host cell proteins likely participate in the final step of retroviral integration (Brin et al. 2000; Yoder and Bushman 2000).

5.2
Genetic Analyses of Gap Repair

Genetic studies have also implicated the potential involvement of host cell factors in gap repair. Murine *scid* cell lines infected with avian or HIV-1 vectors at a multiplicity of infection (MOI) greater to or equal to 1 died by apoptosis (Daniel et al. 1999). Because *scid* cells are defective for the catalytic subunit of DNA-dependent protein kinase (DNA-PK) and an avian vector carrying an inactivating mutation in the active site of integrase failed to induce apoptosis, it was suggested that (a) the failure to repair integration intermediates induced apoptosis and (b) DNA-PK likely participated in gap repair in vivo (Daniel et al. 1999).

DNA-PK participates in the repair of double-stranded DNA breaks by a process termed nonhomologous end joining (NHEJ) (reviewed in Smith and Jackson 1999). Because integration induces single-stranded gaps in chromosomal DNA as compared to double-stranded breaks (Fig. 1), a potential role for DNA-PK in repairing integration intermediates was somewhat puzzling (reviewed in Coffin and Rosenberg 1999). For example, the retrovirus Abelson murine leukemia virus transformed pre-B cell precursors derived from the bone marrow of *scid* versus normal mice with similar efficiencies (Fulop et al. 1988). Additionally, Baekelandt et al. (2000) failed to detect either an integration defect or apoptosis in DNA-PK-deficient cells infected at MOI <1, indicating that DNA-PK played a protective role against cellular toxicity induced by high MOI compared with a direct role in repairing integration intermediates.

A more recent study indicated that DNA-PK may function before DNA strand transfer. In addition to integrated proviruses, cells infected with retroviruses form two circular species of unintegrated DNA in their nuclei, the so-called 1-LTR and 2-LTR circles (reviewed in Brown 1997). Cells defective for DNA-PK failed to form 2-LTR circles, implicating NHEJ in 2-LTR circle formation (Li et al. 2001). Consistent with this, Ku70 and Ku80, two protein components of DNA-PK, were identified in HIV-1 and MoMLV PIC preparations (Li et al. 2001). In contrast to the report by Daniel et al. (1999), Li et al. (2001) determined that an integrase active site mutant virus efficiently killed DNA-PK-deficient cells by apoptosis. Because integrase active site mutant viruses yield transient increases in unintegrated DNA compared with integration-competent controls (reviewed in Engelman 1999), these results were consistent with the interpretation that unintegrated linear cDNA, which can be thought of as having a double-stranded break, supplied the apoptotic signal and that the role of NHEJ and DNA-PK was to sequester these potentially toxic molecules into benign 2-LTR circles (Li et al. 2001). Thus it seems likely that DNA-PK does play a protective role for the cell during the early phase of retroviral replication. However, it remains unclear whether DNA-PK plays a direct role in repairing retroviral integration intermediates.

Poly(ADP-ribose) polymerase-1 (PARP-1) is a nuclear enzyme implicated in the repair of single-stranded breaks in DNA (reviewed in D'Amours et al. 1999). Antagonizing PARP-1 activity with drugs, antisense oligonucleotides, or dominant-negative PARP-1 mutants reduced integration in vivo, suggesting that PARP-1 may function during the repair of integration intermediates (Gaken et al. 1996). A more recent study reported defective HIV-1 transduction in embryo fibroblasts derived from PARP-1-deficient mice compared with PARP-1-positive controls (Ha et al. 2001). However, other investigators have failed to detect integration defects in cells infected in the presence of PARP-1 inhibitors (Baekelandt et al. 2000) or in PARP-1-minus cells (F. Bushman, personal communication). Thus it is currently unclear whether PARP-1 is important for repair of retroviral integration intermediates.

6
Host Cell Factors Affecting Integration Target Site Selection

As touched on above, retroviruses appear to integrate throughout most of the animal cell genome. Despite this lack of target site specificity, integration is not completely random. Chemical modification of target DNA, for example, can alter the frequency and distribution of in vitro integration (Kitamura et al. 1992). Host cell proteins can likewise alter target site selection. Host proteins prebound to target DNA can either occlude or enhance integration at nearby sites (Pryciak and Varmus 1992; Pryciak et al. 1992; Pruss et al. 1994a,b; Bor et al. 1995). Additionally, host cell factors may direct retroviral PICs to favorable integration sites, as observed for the related Ty1, Ty3 (Chalker and Sandmeyer 1992), and Ty5 (Zou and Voytas 1997) retrotransposons.

6.1
Genetic Analyses of Target Site Selection

Early approaches to the question of target site selection focused on identifying the location of individual proviruses. The results of these studies indicated that retroviruses integrated in the vicinity of actively transcribed genes (Vijaya et al. 1986; Rohdewohld et al. 1987; Scherdin et al. 1990). A subsequent study used PCR to analyze the frequency and distribution of avian virus integration into selected regions of primary fibroblast cell DNA. These results indicated that most of the genome was available for integration (Withers-Ward et al. 1994). Although this study did not rule out a preference for active genes, it indicated that local DNA structure as compared to global regional accessibility was the major determinant behind target site selection (reviewed in Engelman 1994).

To address the relationship between transcription and target site selection more directly, Weidhaas et al. (2000) derived quail cell lines carrying multiple copies of the gene for human growth hormone (hGH) under the control of a chimeric bovine papillomavirus (BPV)/herpes simplex virus promoter. Avian virus integration was examined in parental lines versus subclones expressing the BPV transcriptional activator E2, which yielded five- to sevenfold increases in hGH mRNA. Interestingly, increased transcription suppressed integration in the promoter and hGH coding regions. Although this revealed that increased expression occluded integration into actual transcriptional units, the frequency and distribution of integration into flanking quail cell DNA was not investigated, leaving open the possibility that transcription might direct integration to sites near active genes.

6.2
In Vitro Assays Using Purified Integrase and PICs

In vitro analyses of host factor function in target site selection have focused on integration into naked versus protein-bound target DNA. Purified HIV-1 (Pryciak and Varmus, 1992; Pruss et al. 1994a,b) and MoMLV (Pryciak and Varmus 1992) integrase as well as MoMLV PICs (Pryciak and Varmus 1992; Pryciak et al. 1992) preferentially integrated into nucleosome-induced regions of DNA distortion, indicating that integrase favors distorted DNA over nondistorted target DNA under these assay conditions. A subsequent study expanded on this theme by analyzing the relationship between different types of protein-induced DNA bends and target site preference (Bor et al. 1995). Bacterial integration host factor, which like eukaryotic nucleosomes bends DNA around protein, created integration hot spots. In contrast, lymphoid enhancing factor, which binds to the outside of its induced DNA bend, did not enhance integration. Thus, although protein-induced distortion can create favored sites, the topology of the acceptor nucleoprotein complex apparently influences whether integrase will favor the distortion for integration (Bor et al. 1995).

6.3
Retrotransposons as Model Systems for Retroviral Target Site Selection

Although local influences like CpG methylation (Kitamura et al. 1992) and protein binding (Pryciak and Varmus 1992; Pryciak et al. 1992; Pruss et al. 1994a,b; Bor et al. 1995) can influence the frequency and distribution of retroviral integration, retroviruses for the most part integrate throughout the animal cell genome (Withers-Ward et al. 1994; Carteau et al. 1998). This is in stark contrast to the strong target site preferences of yeast retrotransposons Ty1 (Ji et al. 1993; Devine and Boeke 1996), Ty3 (Chalker and Sandmeyer 1992), and Ty5 (Zou and Voytas 1997; Ke and Voytas 1999), which almost exclusively integrate into benign regions of their host cell genomes. This reflects a basic difference in the lifestyles of viruses versus transposons. Unlike viruses, retrotransposons undergo reverse transcription and integration in the same cell in which they were expressed. Thus, especially considering that the yeast life cycle includes a haploid cell stage, retrotransposons apparently evolved targeted integration to reduce the frequency of integrating into essential genes, which would destroy both their hosts and themselves.

The mechanisms by which yeast retrotransposons select specific target sites have been investigated. Whereas Ty1 and Ty3 preferentially integrate into regions upstream of RNA polymerase III-transcribed genes (Chalker and Sandmeyer 1992; Ji et al. 1993), Ty5 preferentially integrates into silent chromatin at telomeres and mating loci (Zou and Voytas 1997). Ty3 has evolved exquisite target site preference, integrating within one to three nucleotides upstream of the start of transcription (Chalker and Sandmeyer 1992). In this case, targeted integration depends on interactions between integrase and transcription factor (TF) IIIB and TFIIIC components of the RNA polymerase III transcription complex (Kirchner et al. 1995). In the case of Ty5, a direct interaction between integrase and Sir4p, which is a structural component of silent chromatin, mediated preferential integration (Xie et al. 2001).

Do retroviral integrases likewise interact with host cell proteins to guide preferential integration in vivo? The answer to this question is currently unclear. Results of a yeast two-hybrid screen identified a normal human cell protein, Ini1, that tightly bound HIV-1 integrase (Kalpana et al. 1994). Ini1, the human homolog of yeast SNF5, is a component of the large SWI/SNF chromatin-remodeling complex (Wang et al. 1996). Because SWI/SNF contributes to gene expression by altering chromatin structure (reviewed in Sudarsanam and Winston 2000), it seemed possible that a direct interaction between integrase and Ini1 might direct HIV-1 PICs to active regions of chromatin (Kalpana et al. 1994). However, a direct link between Ini1, integrase, and targeted integration in vivo has yet to be established. Although Ini1 is predominantly a nuclear protein, it harbors a nuclear export signal that is apparently unmasked soon after HIV-1 infection (Turelli et al. 2001). Another nuclear protein, the promyelocytic leukemia (PML) protein component of nuclear domain (ND) 10 bodies, was likewise exported from nuclei during HIV-1 infection and, together with Ini1, colocalized with incoming PICs (Turelli et al. 2001). However, the physiological relevance of these interactions is unclear, as a separate study failed to detect unintegrated nuclear HIV-1 DNA in association with ND10 bodies in acutely infected cells (Bell et al. 2001). An additional study revealed that Ini1 was packaged into HIV-1 virions through its interaction with integrase (Yung et al. 2001), suggesting that the major role for an integrase-Ini1 interaction might be during virus egress compared with targeting PICs to integration sites. Additional biochemical analyses, for example, determining the level of Ini1 in purified HIV-1 PICs and possible effects of SWI/SNF on integration frequency and distribution into chromatin templates in vitro, should help decipher the role of Ini1 in the early phase of HIV-1 replication.

7
Future Directions

As alluded to in Sect. 4, the results of numerous experiments have made a strong case for two different cellular factors, BAF and HMGA1, as playing essential roles in PIC structure and function. However, it is currently unclear which factor, if either, predominantly functions in vivo. Because an antiserum that can apparently immunoprecipitate BAF protein was recently described, analyses of PIC activity and BAF and HMGA1 stoichiometries in (a) starting PIC samples, (b) salt-stripped PIC extracts before and after immunodepletion, and (c) reconstituted PICs may help to answer this question. Additionally, the recent discovery that small-interfering (si) RNA can knock down gene expression in transfected mammalian cell lines has opened the door to genetic analyses of host cell factor function (reviewed in Tuschl 2002). At least two different laboratories are currently targeting BAF and HMGA1 with siRNA (M. Owens and A. Engelman, unpublished observations; F. Bushman, personal communication). The results of these experiments may help determine whether BAF and/or HMGA1 are relevant integration cofactors in vivo.

7.1
Inhibiting Retroviral Integration

All retroviruses require the action of three different enzymes, reverse transcriptase, protease, and integrase, to spread from cell to cell. Although antiviral drugs that specifically target reverse transcriptase and protease have been in the clinic for a number of years, anti-integrase drugs have yet to be approved for use with AIDS patients. The identification of a novel class of diketo acids that effectively inhibited purified integrase and PICs in vitro and HIV-1 replication in cell culture, together with the isolation of drug-resistant viral variants containing changes in the integrase region of *pol*, has highlighted integrase as a bona fide target for drug intervention in the fight against HIV/AIDS (Hazuda et al. 2000).

Interestingly, these anti-integrase compounds preferentially inhibited the DNA strand transfer step of HIV-1 integration. Whereas 6 µM of inhibitor L-731,988 was required to inhibit 50% of HIV-1 integrase's 3′ processing activity in an oligonucleotide-based integration assay, 80 nM sufficed to inhibit 50% of the enzyme's DNA strand transfer activity (Hazuda et al. 2000). Similarly, 3′ processing proceeded normally in HIV-1-infected cells treated with 10 µM L-731,988. However, PICs isolated from these drug-treated cells failed to integrate the properly processed viral ends into ΦX174 target DNA in vitro (Hazuda et al. 2000). Additional studies revealed that L-731,988 efficiently interacted with recombinant HIV-1 integrase only after the enzyme was complexed with its viral DNA substrate and that adding target DNA before drug addition abrogated inhibition (Espeseth et al. 2001). Thus

diketo acids like L-731,988 apparently block the ability of properly assembled and processed integrase-viral cDNA complexes from effectively interacting with, and integrating into, target DNA.

Might integration host cofactors also make viable targets for the development of antiviral drugs? The answer to this question is more in its infancy compared with the question of targeting integrase itself. For example, firm evidence for the role of any given host factor in integration is required before that factor could be seriously considered a target for antiviral drug development. Even if an important candidate is identified, cellular toxicity, which is encountered when targeting reverse transcriptase and protease because of the similarities between these viral enzymes and cellular enzymes, will clearly be an issue when targeting a normal cellular protein. For example, inhibiting BAF expression in *Caenorhabditis elegans* arrested embyogenesis at approximately the 100-cell stage, indicating that BAF is most likely essential for normal cellular physiology (Zheng et al. 2000). Despite these caveats, targeting integration host cofactors for antiviral drug development may be feasible in the future. Although the link between BAF function and suppression of autointegration is less clear for HIV-1 than it is for MoMLV, drug-induced autointegration would be an effective way to block HIV-1 replication before integration. First proving that BAF plays a role in protecting HIV-1 from autointegration and then identifying a novel target to disrupt this interaction while at the same time maintaining normal BAF function (Furukawa 1999; Haraguchi et al. 2001) are the types of challenges that await investigators in this area of retrovirology.

Acknowledgements. I thank F. Bushman, R. Craigie, D. Grandgenett, J. Leis, and Y. Suzuki for sharing unpublished information. Work in my laboratory is supported by NIH Grants AI-39394, AI-45313, and AI-28691 (Dana-Farber Cancer Institute Center for AIDS Research).

References

Adzuma K, Mizuuchi K (1989) Interaction of proteins located at a distance along DNA: Mechanism of target immunity in the Mu DNA strand-transfer reaction. Cell 57:41–47

Aiyar A, Hindmarsh P, Skalka AM, Leis J (1996) Concerted integration of linear retroviral DNA by the avian virus integrase in vitro: dependence on both long terminal repeat termini. J Virol 70:3571–3580

Baekelandt V, Claeys A, Cherepanov P, De Clercq E, Strooper BD, Nuttin B, Debyser Z (2000) DNA-dependent protein kinase is not required for efficient lentivirus integration. J Virol 74:11278–11285

Bell P, Montaner LJ, Maul GG (2001) Accumulation and intranuclear distribution of unintegrated human immunodeficiency virus type 1 DNA. J Virol 75:7683–7691

Benkirane M, Corbeau P, Housset V, Devaux C (1993) An antibody that binds the immunoglobulin CDR3-like region of the CD4 molecule inhibits transcription in HIV-infected T cells. EMBO J 12:4909–4921

Bor Y-C, Bushman FD, Orgel LE (1995) In vitro integration of human immunodeficiency virus type 1 cDNA into targets containing protein-induced bends. Proc Natl Acad Sci USA 92:10334–10338

Bowerman B, Brown PO, Bishop JM, Varmus HE (1989) A large nucleoprotein complex mediates the integration of retroviral DNA. Genes Dev 3:469–478

Brin E, Yi J, Skalka AM, Leis J (2000) Modeling the late steps in HIV-1 retroviral integrase catalyzed DNA integration. J Biol Chem 275:39287–39295

Brooun A, Richman DD, Kornbluth RS (2001) HIV-1 preintegration complexes preferentially integrate into longer target DNA molecules in solution as detected by a sensitive, polymerase chain reaction-based integration assay. J Biol Chem 276:46946–46952

Brown PO (1997) Integration. In: Coffin JM, Hughes SH, Varmus HE (eds) Retroviruses, (New York, Cold Spring Harbor Press), pp 161–203

Brown PO, Bowerman B, Varmus HE, Bishop, JM (1987) Correct integration of retroviral DNA in vitro. Cell 49:347–356

Brown PO, Bowerman B, Varmus HE, Bishop, JM (1989) Retroviral integration: structure of the initial covalent product and its precursor, and a role for the viral IN protein. Proc Natl Acad Sci USA 86:2525–2529

Bushman FD (1999) Host proteins in retroviral cDNA integration. Adv Virus Res 52:301–317

Bushman FD, Craigie R (1990) Sequence requirements for integration of Moloney murine leukemia virus DNA in vitro. J Virol 64:5645–5648

Bushman FD, Craigie R (1991) Activities of human immunodeficiency virus (HIV) integration protein in vitro: specific cleavage and integration of HIV DNA. Proc Natl Acad Sci USA 88:1339–1343

Bushman FD, Fujiwara T, Craigie R (1990) Retroviral DNA integration directed by HIV integration protein in vivo. Science 249:1555–1558

Bustin M (2001) Revised nomenclature for high mobility group (HMG) chromosomal proteins. Trends Biochem Sci 26:152–153

Bustin M, Reeves R (1996) High-mobility-group chromosomal proteins: Architectural components that facilitate chromatin function. Prog Nucleic Acid Res Mol Biol 54:35–100

Butler SL, Hansen MS, Bushman FD (2001) A quantitative assay for HIV DNA integration in vivo. Nat Med 7:631–634

Carteau S, Batson SC, Poljak L, Mouscadet J-F, Rocquigny H, Darlix J-L, Roques BP, Kas E, Auclair C (1997) Human immunodeficiency virus type 1 nucleocapsid protein specifically stimulates Mg^{2+}-dependent DNA integration in vitro. J Virol 71:6225–6229

Carteau S, Gorelick RJ, Bushman FD (1999) Coupled integration of human immunodeficiency virus type 1 cDNA ends by purified integrase in vitro: Stimulation by the viral nucleocapsid protein. J Virol 73:6670–6679

Carteau S, Hoffmann C, Bushman F (1998) Chromosome structure and human immunodeficiency virus type 1 cDNA integration: centromeric alphoid repeats are a disfavored target. J Virol 72:4005–4014

Chalker DL, Sandmeyer SB (1992) Ty3 integrates within the region of RNA polymerase III transcription initiation. Genes Dev 6:117–128

Chen H, Engelman A (1998) The barrier-to-autointegration protein is a host factor for HIV type 1 integration. Proc Natl Acad Sci USA 95:15270–15274

Chen H, Engelman A (2000) Characterization of a replication-defective human immunodeficiency virus type 1 *att* site mutant that is blocked after the 3′ processing step of retroviral integration. J Virol 74:8188–8193

Chen H, Engelman A (2001) Asymmetric processing of human immunodeficiency virus type 1 cDNA in vivo: Implications for functional end coupling during the chemical steps of DNA transposition. Mol Cell Biol 21:6758–6767

Chow SA, Vincent KA, Ellison V, Brown PO (1992) Reversal of integration and DNA splicing mediated by integrase of human immunodeficiency virus. Science 255:723–726

Chun T-W, Carruth L, Finzi D, Shen X, DiGiuseppe JA, Taylor H, Hermankova M, Chadwick K, Margolick J, Quinn TC, Kuo Y-H, Brookmeyer R, Zeiger MA, Bartich-Crovo, P Siliciano RF (1997) Quantification of latent tissue reservoirs and total body viral load in HIV-1 infection. Nature 387:183–188

Coffin JM, Rosenberg N (1999) Retroviruses. Closing the joint. Nature 399:413–416

Courcoul M, Patience C, Rey F, Blanc D, Harmache A, Sire J, Vigne R, Spire B (1995) Peripheral blood mononuclear cells produce normal amounts of defective Vif-human immunodeficiency virus type 1 particles which are restricted for the pre-retrotransposition steps. J Virol 69:2068–2074

Craigie R, Fujiwara T, Bushman F (1990) The IN protein of Moloney murine leukemia virus processes the viral DNA ends and accomplishes their integration in vitro. Cell 62:829–837

D'Amours D, Desnoyers S, D'Silva I, Poirier GG (1999) Poly(ADP-ribosyl)ation reactions in the regulation of nuclear functions. Biochem J 342:249–268

Daniel R, Katz RA, Skalka AM (1999) A role for DNA-PK in retroviral DNA integration. Science 284:644–647

Devine SE, Boeke JD (1996) Integration of the yeast retrotransposon Ty1 is targeted to regions upstream of genes transcribed by RNA polymerase III. Genes Dev 10:620–633

Ellison V, Abrams H, Roe T, Lifson J, Brown PO (1990) Human immunodeficiency virus integration in a cell-free system. J Virol 64:2711–2715

Engelman A (1994) Most of the avian genome appears available for retroviral DNA integration. BioEssays 16:797–799

Engelman A (1999) In vivo analysis of retroviral integrase structure and function. Adv Virus Res 52:411–416

Espeseth AS, Felock P, Wolfe A, Witmer M, Grobler J, Anthony N, Egbertson M, Melamed JY, Young S, Hamill T, Cole JL, Hazuda DJ (2000) HIV-1 integrase inhibitors that compete with the target DNA substrate define a unique strand transfer conformation for integrase. Proc Natl Acad Sci USA 97:11244–11249

Farnet CM, Bushman FD (1997) HIV-1 cDNA integration: requirement for HMG I(Y) protein for function of preintegration complexes in vitro. Cell 88:483–492

Farnet CM, Haseltine WA (1990) Integration of human immunodeficiency virus type 1 DNA in vitro. Proc Natl Acad Sci USA 87:4164–4168

Farnet CM, Haseltine WA (1991) Determination of viral proteins present in the human immunodeficiency virus type 1 preintegration complex. J Virol 65:1910–1915

Fitzgerald ML, Vora AC, Zeh WG, Grandgenett DP (1992) Concerted integration of viral DNA by purified avian myeloblastosis virus integrase. J Virol 66:6257–6263

Fujiwara T, Craigie R (1989) Integration of mini-retroviral DNA: A cell-free reaction for biochemical analysis of retroviral integration. Proc Natl Acad Sci USA 86:3065–3069

Fujiwara T, Mizuuchi K (1988) Retroviral DNA integration: structure of an integration intermediate. Cell 54:497–504

Fulop GM, Bosma GC, Bosma MJ, Phillips RA (1988) Early B-cell precursors in *scid* mice: Normal numbers of cells transformable with Abelson murine leukemia virus (A-MuLV). Cell Immunol 113:192–201

Furukawa K (1999) LAP2 binding protein 1 (L2BP1/BAF) is a candidate mediator of LAP2-chromatin interaction. J Cell Sci 112:2485–2492

Gaken JA, Tavassoli M, Gan SU, Vallian S, Giddings I, Darling DC, Galea-Lauri J, Thomas MG, Abedi H, Schreiber V, Menissier-de Murcia J, Collins MK, Shall S, Farzaneh F (1996) Efficient retroviral infection of mammalian cells is blocked by inhibition of poly(ADP-ribose) polymerase activity. J Virol 70:3992–4000

Gallay P, Hope T, Chin D, Trono D (1997) HIV-1 infection of nondividing cells through the recognition of integrase by the importin/karyopherin pathway. Proc Natl Acad Sci USA 94:9825–9830

Gallay P, Swingler S, Song J, Bushman F, Trono D (1995) HIV nuclear import is governed by the phosphotyrosine-mediated binding of matrix to the core domain of integrase. Cell 83:569–576

Goff SP (2001) Intracellular trafficking of retroviral genomes during the early phase of infection: viral exploitation of cellular pathways. J Gene Med 3:517–528

Goodzari G, Im G-J, Brackmann K, Grandgenett DP (1995) Concerted integration of retrovirus-like DNA by human immunodeficiency virus type 1 integrase. J Virol 69:6090–6097

Goodzari G, Pursley M, Felock P, Witmer M, Hazuda D, Brackmann K, Grandgenett D (1999) Efficiency and fidelity of full-site integration reactions using recombinant simian immunodeficiency virus integrase. J Virol 73:8104–8111

Ha HC, Juluri K, Zhou Y, Leung S, Hermankova M, Snyder SH (2001) Poly(ADP-ribose) polymerase-1 is required for efficient HIV-1 integration. Proc Natl Acad Sci USA 98:3364–3368

Hansen MST, Smith GJ, Kafri T, Molteni V, Siegel JS, Bushman FD (1999) Integration complexes derived from HIV vectors for rapid assays in vitro. Nature Biotech 17:578–582

Haraguchi T, Koujin T, Segura-Totten M, Lee KK, Matsuoka Y, Yoneda Y, Wilson KL, Hiraoka Y (2001) BAF is required for emerin assembly into the reforming nuclear envelope. J Cell Sci 114:4575-4585

Harris D, Engelman A (2000) Both the structure and DNA binding function of the barrier-to-autointegration factor contribute to reconstitution of HIV type 1 integration in vitro. J Biol Chem 275:39671-39677

Hazuda DJ, Felock P, Witmer M, Wolfe A, Stillmock K, Grobler JA, Espeseth A, Gabryelski L, Schleif W, Blau C, Miller MD (2000) Inhibitors of strand transfer that prevent integration and inhibit HIV-1 replication in cells. Science 287:646-650

Hindmarsh P, Leis J (1999) Reconstitution of concerted DNA integration with purified components. Adv Virus Res 52:397-410

Hindmarsh P, Ridky T, Reeves R, Andrake M, Skalka AM, Leis J (1999) HMG protein family members stimulate human immunodeficiency virus type 1 and avian sarcoma virus concerted DNA integration in vitro. J Virol 73:2994-3003

Huth JR, Bewley CA, Nissen MS, Evans JNS, Reeves R, Gronenborn AM, Clore GM (1997) The solution structure of an HMG-I(Y)-DNA complex defines a new architectural minor groove binding motif. Nat Struct Biol 4:657-665

Ji H, Moore DP, Blomberg MA, Braiterman LT, Voytas DF, Natsoulis G, Boeke JD (1993) Hotspots for unselected Ty1 transposition events on yeast chromosome III are near tRNA genes and LTR sequences. Cell 73:1-20

Kalpana GV, Marmon S, Wang W, Crabtree GR, Goff SP (1994) Binding and stimulation of HIV-1 integrase by a human homolog of yeast transcription factor SNF5. Science 266:2002-2006

Katz RA, Merkel G, Kulkosky J, Leis J, Skalka AM (1990) The avian retroviral IN protein is both necessary and sufficient for integrative recombination in vitro. Cell 63:87-95

Katzman M, Katz RA (1999) Substrate recognition by retroviral integrases. Adv Vir Res 52:371-395

Katzman M, Katz RA, Skalka AM, Leis J (1989) The avian retroviral integration protein cleaves the terminal sequences of linear viral DNA at the in vivo sites of integration. J Virol 63:5319-5327

Ke N, Voytas DF (1999) cDNA of the yeast retrotransposon Ty5 preferentially recombines with substrates in silent chromatin. Mol Cell Biol 19:484-494

Kirchner J, Connolly CM, Sandmeyer SB (1995) Requirement of RNA polymerase III transcription factors for in vitro position-specific integration of a retroviruslike element. Science 267:1488-1491

Kitamura Y, Lee YMH, Coffin JM (1992) Nonrandom integration of retroviral DNA in vitro: Effect of CpG methylation. Proc Natl Acad Sci USA 89:5532-5536

Lafemina RL, Callahan PL, Cordingley MG (1991) Substrate specificity of recombinant human immunodeficiency virus integrase protein. J Virol 65:5624-5630

Lapadat-Tapolsky M, De Rocquigny H, van Gent D, Roques B, Plasterk R, Darlix, J-L (1993) Interactions between HIV-1 nucleocapsid protein and viral DNA may have important functions in the viral life cycle. Nucleic Acids Res 21:831-839

Lee MS, Craigie R (1994) Protection of retroviral DNA from autointegration: involvement of a cellular factor. Proc Natl Acad Sci USA 91:9823-9827

Lee MS, Craigie R (1998) A previously unidentified host protein protects retroviral DNA from autointegration. Proc Natl Acad Sci USA 95:1528–1533

Lee YMH, Coffin JM (1991) Relationship of avian retrovirus DNA synthesis to integration in vitro. Mol Cell Biol 11:1419–1430

Lewis P, Hensel M, Emerman M (1992) Human immunodeficiency virus infection of cells arrested in the cell cycle. EMBO J 11:3053–3058

Li L, Farnet CM, Anderson WF, Bushman FD (1998) Modulation of activity of Moloney murine leukemia virus preintegration complexes by host factors in vitro. J Virol 72:2125–2131

Li L, Olvera JM, Yoder KE, Mitchell RS, Butler SL, Lieber M, Martin SL, Bushman FD (2001) Role of the non-homologous end joining pathway in the early steps of retroviral infection. EMBO J 20:3272–3281

Li L, Yoder K, Hansen MST, Olvera J, Miller MD, Bushman FD (2000) Retroviral cDNA integration: Stimulation by HMG I family proteins. J Virol 74:10965–10974

McCord M, Stahl SJ, Mueser TC, Hyde CC, Vora AC, Grandgenett DP (1998) Purification of recombinant Rous sarcoma virus integrase possessing physical and catalytic properties similar to virion-derived integrase. Protein Expr Purif 14:167–177

Mighell AJ, Markham AF, Robinson PA (1997) Alu sequences. FEBS Lett 417:1–5

Miller MD, Farnet CM, Bushman FD (1997) Human immunodeficiency preintegration complexes: studies of organization and composition. J Virol 71:5382–5390

Pauza CD (1990) Two bases are deleted from the termini of HIV-1 linear DNA during integrative recombination. Virology 179:886–889

Pruss D, Bushman FD, Wolffe AP (1994a) Human immunodeficiency virus integrase directs integration to sites of severe DNA distortion within the nucleosome core. Proc Natl Acad Sci USA 91:5913–5917

Pruss D, Reeves R, Bushman FD, Wolffe AP (1994b) The influence of DNA and nucleosome structure on integration events directed by HIV integrase. J Biol Chem 269:25031–25041

Pryciak PM, Sil A, Varmus HE (1992) Retroviral integration into minichromosomes in vitro. EMBO J 11:291–303

Pryciak PM, Varmus HE (1992) Nucleosomes, DNA-binding proteins, and DNA sequence modulate retroviral integration target site selection. Cell 69:769–780

Roe T, Chow SA, Brown PO (1997) 3′-End processing and kinetics of 5′-end joining during retroviral integration in vivo. J Virol 71:1334–1340

Rohdewohld H, Weiher H, Reik W, Jaenisch R, Breindl M (1987) Retrovirus integration and chromatin structure: Moloney murine leukemia proviral integration sites map near DNase I-hypersensitive sites. J Virol 61:336–343

Roth MJ, Schwartzberg PL, Goff SP (1989) Structure of the termini of DNA intermediates in the integration of retroviral DNA: dependence on IN function and terminal DNA sequence. Cell 58:47–54

Scherdin U, Rhodes K, Breindl M (1990) Transcriptionally active genome regions are preferred targets for retrovirus integration. J Virol 64:907–912

Sherman PA, Fyfe JA (1990) Human immunodeficiency virus integration protein expressed in *Escherichia coli* possesses selective DNA cleaving activity. Proc Natl Acad Sci USA 87:5119–5123

Sinha S, Pursley MH, Grandgenett DP (2002) Efficient concerted integration by recombinant human immunodeficiency virus type 1 integrase without cellular or viral cofactors. J Virol 76:3105–3113

Smith GCM, Jackson SP (1999) The DNA-dependent protein kinase. Genes Dev 13:916–934

Sonza S, Maerz A, Deacon N, Meanger J, Mills J, Crowe S (1996) Human immunodeficiency virus type 1 replication is blocked prior to reverse transcription and integration in freshly isolated peripheral blood monocytes. J Virol 70:3863–3869

Sudarsanam P, Winston F (2000) The Swi/Snf family nucleosome-remodeling complexes and transcriptional control. Trends Genet 16:345–351

Turelli P, Doucas V, Craig E, Mangeat B, Klages N, Evans R, Kalpana G, Trono D (2001) Cytoplasmic recruitment of Ini1 and PML on incoming HIV preintegration complexes: Interference with early steps of viral replication. Mol Cell 7:1245–1254

Tuschl T (2002) Expanding small RNA interference. Nat Biotech 20:446–448

Vandegraaff N, Kumar R, Burrell CJ, Li P (2001) Kinetics of human immunodeficiency virus type 1 (HIV) DNA integration in acutely infected cells as determined using a novel assay for detection of integrated HIV DNA. J Virol 75:11253–11260

Vijaya S, Steffen DL, Robinson HL (1986) Acceptor sites for retroviral integrations map near DNase I-hypersensitive sites in chromatin. J Virol 60:683–692

Vora AC, Grandgenett DP (1995) Assembly and catalytic properties of retrovirus integrase-DNA complexes capable of efficiently performing concerted integration. J Virol 69:7483–7488

Vora AC, McCord M, Fitzgerald ML, Inman RB, Grandgenett DP (1994) Efficient concerted integration of retrovirus-like DNA by avian myeloblastosis virus integrase. Nucleic Acids Res 22:4454–4461

Wang W, Cote J, Xue Y, Zhou S, Khavari PA, Biggar SR, Muchardt C, Kalpana GV, Goff SP, Yaniv M, Workman JL, Crabtree GR (1996) Purification and biochemical heterogeneity of the mammalian SWI-SNF complex. EMBO J 15:5370–5382

Wei S-Q, Mizuuchi K, Craigie R (1997) A large nucleoprotein assembly at the ends of the viral DNA mediates retroviral DNA integration. EMBO J 16:7511–7520

Wei S-Q, Mizuuchi K, Craigie R (1998) Footprints on the viral DNA ends in Moloney murine leukemia virus preintegration complexes reflect a specific association with integrase. Proc Natl Acad Sci USA 95:10535–10540

Weidhaas JB, Angelichio EL, Fenner S, Coffin JM (2000) Relationship between retroviral DNA integration and gene expression. J Virol 74:8382–8389

Withers-Ward ES, Kitamura Y, Barnes JP, Coffin JM. (1994) Distribution of targets for avian retrovirus DNA integration in vivo. Genes Dev 8:1473–1487

Xie W, Gai X, Zhu Y, Zappulla DC, Sternglanz R, Voytas DF (2001) Targeting of the yeast Ty5 retrotransposon to silent chromatin is mediated by interactions between integrase and Sir4p. Mol Cell Biol 21:6606–6614

Yoder KE, Bushman FD (2000) Repair of gaps in retroviral DNA integration intermediates. J Virol 74:11191–11200

Yung E, Sorin M, Pal A, Craig E, Morozov A, Delattre O, Kappes J, Kalpana GV (2001) Inhibition of HIV-1 virion production by a transdominant mutant of integrase interactor 1. Nat Med 7:920–926

Zheng R, Ghirlando R, Lee MS, Mizuuchi K, Krause M, Craigie R (2000) Barrier-to-autointegration factor (BAF) bridges DNA in a discrete, higher-order nucleoprotein complex. Proc Natl Acad Sci USA 97:8997–9002

Zou S, Voytas DF (1997) Silent chromatin determines target preferences of the *Saccharomyces* retrotransposon Ty5. Proc Natl Acad Sci USA 94:7412–7416

Subject Index

A
A·T hook   221
actin filament   181
AIDS   230–231
AMD3100   11
attachment   3
attachment att site   210
autointegration   216, 218, 222, 231
avian sarcoma and leukosis virus (ASLV)   109

B
barrier-to-autointegration factor (BAF)   217
bio-distribution   160
bridging sheet   5

C
capsid   188
CCR5   2, 8, 10
CD4   5, 10
CD4-independent   8
cDNA compaction   222
chemokine receptor   7
concerted integration   214, 220
cooperativity   16
CXCR4   2, 7, 11
cyclophilin A   189
cytoskeleton   181

D
DC-SIGN   3
dendritic cell   3
diketo acid   230–231
disintegration   223–224
DNA flap   198
DNA recombination   210, 212, 216, 223
DNA-dependent protein kinase (DNA-PK)   225

E
Ebola virus GP2   111
Engineering tropism   143

F
fluorescence in situ hybridization   199
fusion   14, 142, 152–153, 155, 157–158
fusion peptide   110

G
Gag polyprotein   188
gate protein   127
glycoprotein   139, 147
gp41   9
gp120   5

H
haemagglutinin   151, 155
helical region   9
HMGA1   218–222, 229
HMGB1   220, 222
HMGB2   220
HR2 region   12
human immunodeficiency virus type 1 (HIV-1)   211
human immunodeficiency virus type-1   180

I
importin-α 186
importin-β 186
infection of nondividing cell   180
intasome   218
integrase   193, 209–211, 213–216, 218–223, 225, 227, 229–231
integration   193, 209–211, 213–216, 218–231
intermediate filament   181

intravenous administration 138
inverse PCR 215

K
kinetic 14

L
LTR 210, 221, 225

M
matrix 188
membrane 30–33, 38–39, 63, 75, 77–79, 81–82
metastability 142
microbicide 4
microtubule 181
Mini-Viral Substrate 214, 220
MM-PCR footprinting 218
Moloney murine leukemia virus (MoMLV) 211
murine leukemia virus 180

N
Nef 188
nonhomologous end joining (NHEJ) 225
nuclear envelope 183
nuclear import 181
nuclear localization signal 184
nuclear pore complex 181
nucleocapsid 188
nucleocapsid (NC) 219
nucleoporin 184

P
p6 188
pocket 5
Poly(ADP-ribose) polymerase-1 (PARP-1) 226
pre-hairpin 16
preintegration complex 181, 210–211
preintegration complex (PIC) 211
Pro5452 10
promyelocytic leukemia (PML) 229
protease 159, 161–162
pseudotype 145

R
Ran 185
real-time PCR 215
receptor 30–32, 34–45, 47–53, 56–65, 67, 69–82
receptor-primed low-pH entry mechanism 109
retrotransposon 226, 228
γ-retroviral receptor 38, 53, 57–58, 65
retrovirus 30–31, 33–35, 37–39, 41, 45, 49, 56, 63, 69, 71, 74–77, 80–81
γ-retrovirus 30–43, 45, 50, 52–53, 56–58, 63–64, 70, 72, 74–75, 78–82
reverse transcriptase 193, 210, 213, 223–224, 230–231
reverse transcription 210–212, 228
Rous sarcoma virus (RSV) 180, 211

S
SCH-C 11
sequestration 153–154, 156, 160
six-helix bundle 9, 14, 111

T
T20 12–13
T1249 13
TAK-779 11
temperature-arrested state 14
transposon 228
tropism 2, 8, 145, 148
TVA800 114–115
TVA950 114
TVBS1 114, 119
TVBS3 119
Ty1 226, 228
Ty3 226, 228
Ty5 226, 228

U
uncoating 188

V
Vif 188
viral receptor 58, 60, 62, 72
Vpr 187

Current Topics in Microbiology and Immunology

Volumes published since 1989 (and still available)

Vol. 237: **Claesson-Welsh, Lena (Ed.):** Vascular Growth Factors and Angiogenesis. 1999. 36 figs. X, 189 pp. ISBN 3-540-64731-7

Vol. 238: **Coffman, Robert L.; Romagnani, Sergio (Eds.):** Redirection of Th1 and Th2 Responses. 1999. 6 figs. IX, 148 pp. ISBN 3-540-65048-2

Vol. 239: **Vogt, Peter K.; Jackson, Andrew O. (Eds.):** Satellites and Defective Viral RNAs. 1999. 39 figs. XVI, 179 pp. ISBN 3-540-65049-0

Vol. 240: **Hammond, John; McGarvey, Peter; Yusibov, Vidadi (Eds.):** Plant Biotechnology. 1999. 12 figs. XII, 196 pp. ISBN 3-540-65104-7

Vol. 241: **Westblom, Tore U.; Czinn, Steven J.; Nedrud, John G. (Eds.):** Gastroduodenal Disease and Helicobacter pylori. 1999. 35 figs. XI, 313 pp. ISBN 3-540-65084-9

Vol. 242: **Hagedorn, Curt H.; Rice, Charles M. (Eds.):** The Hepatitis C Viruses. 2000. 47 figs. IX, 379 pp. ISBN 3-540-65358-9

Vol. 243: **Famulok, Michael; Winnacker, Ernst-L.; Wong, Chi-Huey (Eds.):** Combinatorial Chemistry in Biology. 1999. 48 figs. IX, 189 pp. ISBN 3-540-65704-5

Vol. 244: **Daëron, Marc; Vivier, Eric (Eds.):** Immunoreceptor Tyrosine-Based Inhibition Motifs. 1999. 20 figs. VIII, 179 pp. ISBN 3-540-65789-4

Vol. 245/I: **Justement, Louis B.; Siminovitch, Katherine A. (Eds.):** Signal Transduction and the Coordination of B Lymphocyte Development and Function I. 2000. 22 figs. XVI, 274 pp. ISBN 3-540-66002-X

Vol. 245/II: **Justement, Louis B.; Siminovitch, Katherine A. (Eds.):** Signal Transduction on the Coordination of B Lymphocyte Development and Function II. 2000. 13 figs. XV, 172 pp. ISBN 3-540-66003-8

Vol. 246: **Melchers, Fritz; Potter, Michael (Eds.):** Mechanisms of B Cell Neoplasia 1998. 1999. 111 figs. XXIX, 415 pp. ISBN 3-540-65759-2

Vol. 247: **Wagner, Hermann (Ed.):** Immunobiology of Bacterial CpG-DNA. 2000. 34 figs. IX, 246 pp. ISBN 3-540-66400-9

Vol. 248: **du Pasquier, Louis; Litman, Gary W. (Eds.):** Origin and Evolution of the Vertebrate Immune System. 2000. 81 figs. IX, 324 pp. ISBN 3-540-66414-9

Vol. 249: **Jones, Peter A.; Vogt, Peter K. (Eds.):** DNA Methylation and Cancer. 2000. 16 figs. IX, 169 pp. ISBN 3-540-66608-7

Vol. 250: **Aktories, Klaus; Wilkins, Tracy, D. (Eds.):** Clostridium difficile. 2000. 20 figs. IX, 143 pp. ISBN 3-540-67291-5

Vol. 251: **Melchers, Fritz (Ed.):** Lymphoid Organogenesis. 2000. 62 figs. XII, 215 pp. ISBN 3-540-67569-8

Vol. 252: **Potter, Michael; Melchers, Fritz (Eds.):** B1 Lymphocytes in B Cell Neoplasia. 2000. XIII, 326 pp. ISBN 3-540-67567-1

Vol. 253: **Gosztonyi, Georg (Ed.):** The Mechanisms of Neuronal Damage in Virus Infections of the Nervous System. 2001. approx. XVI, 270 pp. ISBN 3-540-67617-1

Vol. 254: **Privalsky, Martin L. (Ed.):** Transcriptional Corepressors. 2001. 25 figs. XIV, 190 pp. ISBN 3-540-67569-8

Vol. 255: **Hirai, Kanji (Ed.):** Marek's Disease. 2001. 22 figs. XII, 294 pp. ISBN 3-540-67798-4

Vol. 256: **Schmaljohn, Connie S.; Nichol, Stuart T. (Eds.):** Hantaviruses. 2001, 24 figs. XI, 196 pp. ISBN 3-540-41045-7

Vol. 257: **van der Goot, Gisou (Ed.):** Pore-Forming Toxins, 2001. 19 figs. IX, 166 pp. ISBN 3-540-41386-3

Vol. 258: **Takada, Kenzo (Ed.):** Epstein-Barr Virus and Human Cancer. 2001. 38 figs. IX, 233 pp. ISBN 3-540-41506-8

Vol. 259: **Hauber, Joachim, Vogt, Peter K. (Eds.):** Nuclear Export of Viral RNAs. 2001. 19 figs. IX, 131 pp. ISBN 3-540-41278-6

Vol. 260: **Burton, Didier R. (Ed.):** Antibodies in Viral Infection. 2001. 51 figs. IX, 309 pp. ISBN 3-540-41611-0

Vol. 261: **Trono, Didier (Ed.):** Lentiviral Vectors. 2002. 32 figs. X, 258 pp. ISBN 3-540-42190-4

Vol. 262: **Oldstone, Michael B.A. (Ed.):** Arenaviruses I. 2002, 30 figs. XVIII, 197 pp. ISBN 3-540-42244-7

Vol. 263: **Oldstone, Michael B. A. (Ed.):** Arenaviruses II. 2002, 49 figs. XVIII, 268 pp. ISBN 3-540-42705-8

Vol. 264/I: **Hacker, Jörg; Kaper, James B. (Eds.):** Pathogenicity Islands and the Evolution of Microbes. 2002. 34 figs. XVIII, 232 pp. ISBN 3-540-42681-7

Vol. 264/II: **Hacker, Jörg; Kaper, James B. (Eds.):** Pathogenicity Islands and the Evolution of Microbes. 2002. 24 figs. XVIII, 228 pp. ISBN 3-540-42682-5

Vol. 265: **Dietzschold, Bernhard; Richt, Jürgen A. (Eds.):** Protective and Pathological Immune Responses in the CNS. 2002. 21 figs. X, 278 pp. ISBN 3-540-42668-X

Vol. 266: **Cooper, Koproski (Eds.):** The Interface Between Innate and Acquired Immunity, 2002, 15 figs. XIV, 116 pp. ISBN 3-540-42894-1

Vol. 267: **Mackenzie, John S.; Barrett, Alan D. T.; Deubel, Vincent (Eds.):** Japanese Encephalitis and West Nile Viruses. 2002. 66 figs. X, 418 pp. ISBN 3-540-42783-X

Vol. 268: **Zwickl, Peter; Baumeister, Wolfgang (Eds.):** The Proteasome-Ubiquitin Protein Degradation Pathway. 2002, 17 figs. X, 213 pp. ISBN 3-540-43096-2

Vol. 269: **Koszinowski, Ulrich H.; Hengel, Hartmut (Eds.):** Viral Proteins Counteracting Host Defenses. 2002, 47 figs. XII, 325 pp. ISBN 3-540-43261-2

Vol. 270: **Beutler, Bruce; Wagner, Hermann (Eds.):** Toll-Like Receptor Family Members and Their Ligands. 2002, 31 figs. X, 192 pp. ISBN 3-540-43560-3

Vol. 271: **Koehler, Theresa M. (Ed.):** Anthrax. 2002, 14 figs. X, 169 pp. ISBN 3-540-43497-6

Vol. 272: **Doerfler, Walter; Böhm, Petra (Eds.):** Adenoviruses: Model and Vectors in Virus Host Interactions. Virion and Structure, Viral Replication, Host Cell Interactions. 2003, 63 figs., approx. 280 pp. ISBN 3-540-00154-9

Vol. 273: **Doerfler, Walter; Böhm, Petra (Eds.):** Adenoviruses: Model and Vectors in Virus Host Interactions. Immune System, Oncogenesis, Gene Therapy. 2003, 33 figs., approx. 280 pp. ISBN 3-540-06851-1

Vol. 274: **Workman, J. L. (Ed.):** Protein Complexes that Modify Chromatin. 2003, 38 figs., XII, 296 pp. ISBN 3-540-44208-1

Vol. 275: **Fan, Hung (Ed.):** Jaagsiekte Sheep Retrovirus and Lung Cancer. 2003, 63 figs., XII, 252 pp. ISBN 3-540-44096-3

Vol. 276: **Steinkasserer, A. (Ed.):** Dendritic Cells and Virus Infection. 2003, 24 figs., X, 296 pp. ISBN 3-540-44290-1

Vol. 277: **Rethwilm, A. (Ed.):** Foamy Viraces. 2003, 40 figs., X, 214 pp. ISBN 3-540-44388-6

Vol. 278: **Salomon, Daniel R.; Wilson, Carolyn (Eds.):** Xenotransplantation. 2003, 22 figs., IX, 254 pp. ISBN 3-540-00210-3

Vol. 279: **Thomas, George; Sabatini, David; Hall, Michael N. (Eds.):** 1OR. 2004, 49 figs., approx. 270 pp. ISBN 3-540-00534-X

Vol. 280: **Heber-Katz, Ellen (Ed.):** Regeneration Beyond the Stem Cells. 2004, 42 figs., approx. 160 pp. ISBN 3-540-02238-4

Printing: Saladruck Berlin
Binding: Stürtz AG, Würzburg